Nutrition in Early Life

Edited by

Jane B. Morgan
and
John W. T. Dickerson

School of Biomedical and Life Sciences
University of Surrey, Guildford, UK

WILEY

Other Wiley Editorial Offices

John Wiley & Sons Inc., 111 River Street,
Hoboken, NJ 07030, USA

Jossey-Bass, 989 Market Street,
San Francisco, CA 94103-1741, USA

Wiley-VCH Verlag GmbH, Boschstr. 12,
D-69469 Weinheim, Germany

John Wiley & Sons Australia Ltd, 33 Park Road,
Milton, Queensland 4064, Australia

John Wiley & Sons (Asia) Pte Ltd, 2 Clementi Loop #02-01,
Jin Xing Distripark, Singapore 129809

John Wiley & Sons Canada Ltd, 22 Worcester Road,
Etobicoke, Ontario, Canada M9W 1L1

Library of Congress Cataloging-in-Publication Data

Nutrition in early life : concepts and practice / edited by Jane Morgan & J.W.T. Dickerson.
    p. ; cm.
  Includes bibliographical references and index.
  ISBN 0-471-88064-7 (alk. cased)
  ISBN 0-471-49624-3 (alk. paper)
    1. Infants — Nutrition. 2. Children — Nutrition. I. Morgan, Jane. II. Dickerson, John W.T.
  [DNLM: 1. Infant Nutrition. 2. Child Nutrition. WS 115 N9838 2002]
RJ216.N8585 2002
612.3'083 — dc21   2002033050

British Library Cataloguing in Publication Data

A catalogue record for this book is available from the British Library

ISBN 0471 49624 3 (paperback)
ISBN 0470 88064 7 (cased)

Typeset by Dobbie Typesetting Ltd, Tavistock, Devon
Printed and bound in Great Britain by Antony Rowe, Chippenham, Wilts
This book is printed on acid-free paper responsibly manufactured from sustainable forestry

Nutrition in Early Life

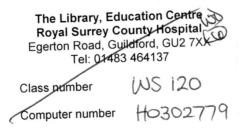

CONTENTS

3: Maternal physiology and nutrition during reproduction   73
Elisabet Forsum

4: Physiological and nutritional aspects of the placenta   91
Michael E. Symonds, Helen Budge and Terence Stephenson

5: Lifestyle and maternal health interactions between mother and fetus   123
Mohammed Ibrahim and J. Stewart Forsyth

6: The fetus at birth: maternal and fetal preparations for postnatal development

145

Mary McNabb

9: Complementary feeding for the full-term infant 233
Nilani Sritharan and Jane B. Morgan

10: Nutrition of the low-birth-weight and very-low-birth-weight infant 257
Caroline King and Michael Harrison

12: Practical advice on food and nutrition for the mother, infant and child   325
Margaret Lawson

PREFACE

The developing bodies of multicellular organisms are in a condition of 'plasticity', for changes in structure and function are continually taking place. There is a harmony in these processes as the multitude of changes associated with growth and development are interdependent and time-related. Moreover, the various processes are subject to moderation and control by genetic, nutritional, hormonal and other influences.

Each of us, the Editors, of the present book, has had an extensive interest over a long period of time in aspects of growth and development in both teaching and research. In these activities we drew considerable inspiration and help from a book, *Developmental Nutrition* by Lucille Hurley published in 1980. This book is now out of print and out of date. Moreover, increase in knowledge and the recognition of the importance of developmental aspects of nutrition in the training of health professionals pointed to the need for an up-to-date and extended text incorporating scientific aspects of the subject and their practical application. The recognition that disturbances in biochemical programming during development, resulting in aberrations of the normal harmony of growth, can influence the development of disease later in life provided a further incentive. The seeds of much that is in the book can be traced back to the work of R. A. McCance FRS and E. Widdowson FRS in the 1950s and 1960s. To them we would like to dedicate the book.

We have tried to trace the development of the human organism from the time when this can be investigated in the fetus through to maturity. We have approached the subject from structural, physiological and nutritional standpoints through to the application of these scientific principles in the feeding of babies and children. Also, we have recognized that the nutrition of the mother is central to the adequate provision of care and nutrition for infants at particular times in their lives. In developing these themes we have had to recognize that certain aspects of the subject are not amenable to direct observation or measurement in mothers and babies and alternative sources of information have had to be used.

We are grateful to our colleagues who have shared our enthusiasm for the theme of the book and have generously contributed to it in their particular field of interest. With two exceptions the authors are currently located in the UK, and this has led inevitably to the text having a UK focus. If the focus had been extended this would have resulted in a larger book with the danger of taking it beyond our prime aim, the provision of a student textbook.

We are deeply grateful to our publishers, John Wiley and Sons, for their unstinting support of this venture and we are particularly grateful to Nicky McGirr for her help in so many ways.

Jane B. Morgan and **John W.T. Dickerson**
Brook, Surrey
April 2002

FOREWORD

The effects of nutrition and nutritional stress depend on a triad of influences, the genes of an individual, the stage of development he or she has reached and the circumstances in which they live. This book describes the middle factor of the triad. If we take folic acid as an example then, depending on the stage of development, the effects of its presence or absence in the diet will vary from a neural tube defect during organogensis, to megaloblastic anaemia in pregnancy or malabsorption, cardiovascular disease due to homocystinaemia in middle age, and precipitation of spinal cord disease by masking the haematological clues to vitamin B_{12} deficiency in older people.

Conventional textbooks of nutrition describe in great detail the situation for healthy adults. They then dispose of the developmental aspects with a few added chapters on so called 'vulnerable groups' such as children, pregnant women and older people. This book therefore comes as a breath of fresh air with its developmental approach acknowledging that all individuals are either going through or have previously experienced various stages of development – hardly special vulnerable groups but rather the whole population.

The editors are well versed in the developmental approach – Morgan from her studies of dietary intake, in particular energy, and their effects on growth, initially in London and Southampton, and Dickerson from his studies of normal and retarded growth on body composition, initially in Cambridge and London. They came together at the University of Surrey and began a fruitful collaboration, including the concept and organization of this book. The authors are committed to the view that nutrition plays a vital role in growth and development throughout the entire life cycle. The contents of this book are an interpretation of this view. They, and their distinguished panel of contributors, describe the crucial role of biological age and developmental clocks in the nutritional health of people.

Professor Brian Wharton
Honorary Professor of
University College London
MRC Childhood Nutrition Research Centre
Institute of Child Health
Guilford Street
London, UK

LIST OF CONTRIBUTORS

David J.P. Barker, MRC Environmental Epidemiology Unit, Southampton General Hospital, Southampton, UK

Helen Budge, Academic Division of Child Health, School of Human Development, University Hospital, Nottingham, UK

Jane Coad, European Institute for Health and Medical Sciences, University of Surrey, Guildford, UK.
Current address: Institute of Food, Nutrition and Human Health, Massey University, Palmerston North, New Zealand

John W.T. Dickerson, School of Biomedical and Life Sciences, University of Surrey, Guildford, UK

Elisabet Forsum, Division of Nutrition, Department of Biomedicine and Surgery, University of Linköping, Linköping, Sweden

J. Stewart Forsyth, Tayside Institute of Child Health, University of Dundee, Dundee, UK

Keith M. Godfrey, MRC Environmental Epidemiology Unit, Southampton General Hospital, Southampton, UK

Michael Harrison, Department of Paediatrics and Neonatal Medicine, Hammersmith Hospital, London, UK

Mohammed Ibrahim, Tayside Institute of Child Health, University of Dundee, Dundee, UK

Caroline King, Department of Nutrition and Dietetics, Hammersmith Hospital, London, UK

Margaret Lawson, MRC Childhood Nutrition Research Centre, Institute of Child Health, London, UK

Mary McNabb, Division of Midwifery, South Bank University, London, UK

Jane B. Morgan, School of Biomedical and Life Sciences, University of Surrey, Guildford, UK

Elizabeth Poskitt, Public Health Nutrition Unit, London School of Hygiene and Tropical Medicine, London, UK

Ann Prentice, MRC Human Nutrition Research, Elsie Widdowson Laboratory, Cambridge, UK

Nilani Sritharan, School of Biomedical and Life Sciences, University of Surrey, Guildford, UK. *Current address*: The Dairy Council, 5–7 John Princes Street, London, UK

Terence Stephenson, Academic Division of Child Health, School of Human Development, University Hospital, Nottingham, UK

Michael E. Symonds, Academic Division of Child Health, School of Human Development, University Hospital, Nottingham, UK

Lawrence T. Weaver, Department of Child Health, Royal Hospital for Sick Children, University of Glasgow, UK

1

GROWTH, DEVELOPMENT AND THE CHEMICAL COMPOSITION OF THE BODY

John W. T. Dickerson

LEARNING OUTCOMES

- Knowledge of the mechanisms of growth, and how it can be measured and recorded.

- How to assess developmental age and the factors that affect it.

- How the chemical composition of the body changes before and after birth.

- How the composition of organs and tissues changes during growth and development.

- What effects protein-energy malnutrition has on growth and development.

Introduction

Growth and development are the processes by which the fertilized ovum is transformed into a mature individual. Growth occurs by cell multiplication (hyperplasia), by cell enlargement (hypertrophy) and by the synthesis of extracellular tissue. This latter process includes an expansion of the volume of extracellular fluid and an increase in the amounts of specific, but diverse proteins such as those in the plasma and the organic matrix of the skeleton. In most organs, cell multiplication ceases at a tissue-specific age and further growth is by enlargement of existing cells (Winick and Noble, 1965). We can measure the number of cells in an organ which has only mononuclear diploid cells by measuring the amount of DNA in the organ and dividing this by the amount of DNA in a diploid nucleus, which is about 6.2 pg. Changes in the size of cells can be estimated from the ratio of the amount of protein associated with a diploid nucleus or, to put it simply, by the protein/DNA ratio. Cell multiplication continues throughout life in the hair follicles, the epidermis and the mucosa of the alimentary tract. Increase in body fat does not constitute growth, although it may greatly increase body weight. The synthesis of new tissue uses energy and the energy cost of weight gain has been calculated to be 4.6 kJ/g after deducting the energy stored (Passmore and Eastwood, 1986).

Development constitutes those changes in structure, function and composition which are an essential part of the maturation process. Growth and development are complex, integrated processes that are closely related to time and are dependant on appropriate nutrition (McCance, 1962). If the food supply is reduced at an early age, including early postnatal life, growth and development are separated from time and are retarded in ways that are organ- and tissue-specific. Following such a period of growth retardation due to malnutrition or severe illness, nutritional rehabilitation is accompanied by a period of 'catch-up' growth during which the growth velocity is greater than normal for the age of the child. The magnitude of the increase in growth velocity depends on the age of the child and the severity and duration of the growth retardation. It may be as much as twice the normal velocity in young children with prolonged retardation. The ability of a malnourished animal or child then to return to its normal growth trajectory

depends on the magnitude of the catch-up growth. The biological basis for failure of 'catch-up' growth to return the individual to the normal trajectory for the individual is at present not clear. An early hypothesis that it is due to a reduction in the period of hyperplastic growth has not been confirmed in the rat (Sands *et al.*, 1979).

The growth curve of the whole body and of its constituent parts has a sigmoid shape, but different organs and tissues grow at different rates and at different times. The four main types of growth curve are shown in Figure 1.1 (Tanner, 1962; from Scammon, 1930). The period of rapid increase in the 'General' curve

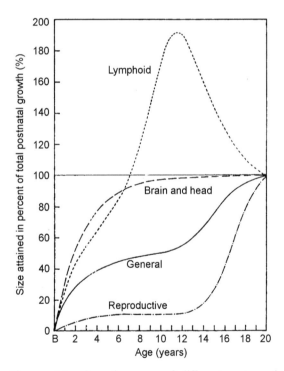

Figure 1.1 Growth curves of different parts and tissues of the body. All the curves are of size attained and plotted as percentages of total gain from birth to 20 years so that size at age 20 is 100 on the vertical scale. Data from Scammon [reproduced by permission of Blackwell Science from Tanner (1962) *Growth at Adolescence*, 2nd edn].

Table 1.1 Relative lengths (percentage) of parts of the human body during growth; values calculated from Medawar (1944) (from Tanner, 1962)

Age (years)[a]	Head	Trunk	Upper limbs	Lower limbs
0.42	33	43	26	24
2.75	21	41	34	37
6.75	16	41	34	41
25.75	12	43	37	43

[a]Age from 5 months postconception.

from about 12 to 15 years is called the 'adolescent spurt' and involves every muscular and skeletal dimension in the body. Maturity is not achieved until this has been completed, and again this is related to time and is separated from time by nutritional deprivation. The early rapid growth of the head and brain shown in Figure 1.1 is an example of a 'growth gradient', and this particular one is called the 'cephalocaudal' gradient. The head of a young child may be almost the same size as that of its mother. The changes in the relative size of different parts of the body with growth and development are also shown in Table 1.1, in which the sizes of different parts of the body are expressed as a percentage of the total body length. The proportion accounted for by the head and neck decreases from approximately 30 per cent in the 5-month-old fetus to approximately 12 per cent in the adult. In contrast, the percentage of length accounted for by the lower limbs increases from approximately 24 per cent in the fetus to 43 per cent in the adult. The percentage of the body length contributed by the trunk (about 40 per cent) hardly changes during growth. In the leg, another gradient may be distinguished, as growth in foot length ceases before that of the calf, and that of the calf before that of the thigh. Material in Chapters 2 and 7 should be read in relation to this chapter.

Growth curves

Each individual has his or her own growth curve, or 'trajectory', as it is called, if measured longitudinally. The oldest such curve is that of a boy measured every 6 months for 18 years by Count de Montbeillard (Figure 1.2; from Tanner, 1962). The longitudinal construction

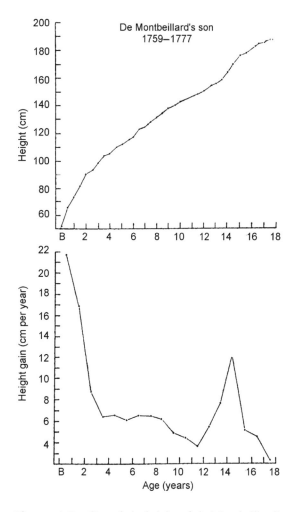

Figure 1.2 Growth in height of de Montbeillard's son from birth to 18 years, 1759–1777. Top, distance curve, height attained at each age; bottom, velocity curve, increments in height from year to year. Data from Scammon [reproduced by permission of Blackwell Science from Tanner (1962) *Growth at Adolescence*, 2nd edn]

of such growth curves for individual children is of considerable value in clinical paediatrics. There are many causes of growth failure, or 'failure to thrive', one of which is malnutrition; the construction of an individual child's growth curve permits the degree of growth failure to be assessed and the progress of rehabilitation to be followed. To help in this process, standard growth curves, and particularly percentile charts, have been constructed from measurements of large numbers of children of different ages, that is from cross-sectional measurements. In percentile charts (Figs 10.2a–d, the height or weight, or whatever other measurement is being considered, follows the 50th percentile for 50 per cent of the children measured at a particular age. Similar percentiles are drawn in such a way that a greater or a smaller number of children have values below the line. Ideally, growth charts should be available nationally in different countries. Perhaps the best known are those for the USA (Hamill *et al.*, 1977), and in the UK the curves produced by Tanner *et al.* (1966) have been replaced by those published by Freeman *et al.* (1995). It is often some time after the measurements were made before the charts become available. Thus, the US charts are based on data collected between 1929 and 1975 and Tanner *et al.*'s UK charts were based on data collected between 1952 and 1954. This poses a problem if infant feeding practices change as this might result in changes in infant and children's growth rates. Differences in infant feeding practices, for instance, in developing countries, suggest that growth charts should be kept under review (Whitehead and Paul, 2000). Prentice (1998) has suggested using body mass index (BMI; defined as weight/height^2, kg/m^2) charts available from the Child Growth Foundation (London W4 1PW, UK) for the assessment of nutritional status in children. Cole (2001) has discussed the use and abuse of centile curves for the BMI. The application of BMI charts to children was first suggested by Cole (1979).

Developmental age and physiological maturity

The age of a child can be expressed in two ways. It is usually quoted simply as the number of years, months or weeks since it was born. This is its 'chronological' age. Then we can also determine its 'developmental' age, which is a measure of how far the child has progressed towards maturity. This can be assessed in a number of different ways (Table 1.2). Each method has its own limitations and it is necessary to consider each method in some detail.

Skeletal age is the most commonly used indicator of physiological maturity (Tanner, 1962). It is a measure of the degree of development of the skeleton as measured by the appearance and size of the epiphyses of certain bones. Each bone begins with a primary centre of ossification. It then enlarges, changes shape and secondary centres of ossification develop in the cartilaginous epiphyses. Eventually, the epiphyses fuse and the epiphysial plate disappears. This sequence of changes is the same for all indivduals, whatever the rate of development. Skeletal maturity is judged both on the number of centres present and on the stage of development of each. The appearance of the epiphyses at birth may differ from one child to another with different numbers of primary centres developed and larger areas ossified. Areas of ossification are not of themselves considered good indicators of bone development as they differ according to the size of the individual.

Assessment of skeletal maturity is accomplished by comparing an X-ray with a set of

Table 1.2 Assessment of developmental age – systems in use (Tanner, 1962)

Skeletal age
Dental age
Morphological or shape age
Secondary sex characteristics age

standards. There are two ways of doing this. An older, atlas method involved matching an X-ray with standards representing the 'norm' for different ages, with a skeletal age being assigned to a test X-ray according to the age of the nearest match in the atlas. Tanner *et al.* (1961) refined this method by assigning a score to different changes in bone maturity. In this method, a test X-ray scored a number of development points. The bones for which there are standard atlases are the wrist and the knee, with separate standards for the two sexes. This is because girls are more mature at birth, before it and throughout the whole period of growth up to adolescence. It is to be noted that skeletal age can be assessed throughout the period of growth of the bones.

Dental age can be obtained using the same principle as skeletal age, with eruption and noneruption of teeth as the index corresponding to the appearance and non-appearance of an ossification centre. A refinement of this method involves more detailed observation and scoring of degrees of tooth eruption and root development. The use of dental age is clearly limited to the period when the deciduous and permanent teeth are erupting. For deciduous dentition this is from about 6 months to 2 years. The corresponding period for permanent dentition is from 6 to 13 years. There is a marked sex difference in the eruption of teeth, with all teeth appearing earlier in girls than in boys by an amount varying from 2 months for the first molars to 11 months for the canines (Tanner, 1962). It may be considered that the times of the eruption of teeth are just as crude a method of assessing developmental age as the timing of the presence of ossification centres. It has been suggested that in the absence of a birth certificate the state of teeth eruption can be used to estimate chronological age. To this end, published data from 42 studies of children's dentition transformed into chronological age have been examined (Towsend and Hammel, 1990). Lack of significant differences

between the estimates of age seemed to justify the use of a single set of data. However, results of a longitudinal study of 129 Finnish children based on deciduous teeth (Nystrom *et al.*, 2000) led to the conclusion that estimates of age should not be based on teeth eruption alone because of marked variation in their homogeneous group of children.

Morphological or shape age has been considered as a means of assessing development. The idea that changes in shape of the body might be quantified and used in this way was probably first suggested by Godin in France in 1903 (quoted by Tanner, 1962) and was later developed by Medawar (1944) with reference to the shape change in vertical proportions (see Table 1.1). Tanner (1962) quotes Richards and Kavanagh (1945) as having outlined the mathematical procedures by which this might be achieved. The concept seems not to have been pursued further.

Sexual age is derived from observations of the development of secondary sex characteristics. The adolescent growth spurt, and the development of these characteristics, occurs later in boys than in girls. The age ranges over which the changes begin and end are shown in Table 1.3. A scoring system of 2–5 is used to

Table 1.3 The sequence of events at adolescence in boys and girls used to assess developmental age (adapted from Tanner, 1962)

	Beginning (years)	End (years)
Boys		
Height spurt	10.5–13	16–17.5
Penis growth	11–13.5	14.5–17
Testis growth	10–14.5	13.5–18
Pubic hair (grades 2–5)	10–14	15–18
Girls		
Height spurt	9.5–14.5	
Menarche	10–16.5	
Breast (grades 2–5)	8–13	
Pubic hair (grades 2–5)	8–14	

assess breast development in girls and pubic hair in both sexes (Tanner, 1962). Sexual development, and particularly the age of menarche, is occurring earlier now than it was, say, 100 years ago due to what is called the 'secular trend' (Wyshak and Frisch, 1982). Obviously, the ages over which these assessments of development can be used are limited to those ages over which the changes occur. Key factors which influence their development are sex hormones and nutrition. In the disease anorexia nervosa, which occurs most commonly in adolescent girls, who are often severely emaciated although secondary sex characteristics are usually well developed, amenorrhoea is a common feature. This feature of the disease is closely linked with body weight (Frisch, 1994).

Factors which influence growth and development

The rate of development can be assessed, as we have seen, by the age at which certain milestones of development occur. This age can be affected by genetic constitution, nutritional status (often associated with poverty), severe illness, psychological disturbance and the secular trend.

Early observations about the influence of genetics pertained to the age of menarche in mothers and daughters (quoted by Tanner, 1962). Pairs of identical twins were closest in age of menarche, with an average difference of 2.8 months; non-identical twins, with a difference of 12 months, were not very different from sisters (12.8 months), with unrelated women showing a difference of 18.6 months. According to Tanner, evidence of genetic control has also been noted for the reaching of peak growth velocity, skeletal maturity and in the growth of specific muscles. Undernutrition and, often with it, poverty or famine can have a profound effect on growth, separating it from time. The effects may manifest themselves in the fetus, with the result that the baby is born 'small-for-dates', or after birth, when the child's growth is stunted. In rats, which are born at an earlier stage of development than humans, it is easy to show a permanent stunting when the animals are nutritionally deprived at an early age. In human babies, in which there is, by comparison, an extended period of growth and development, it is much more difficult to show permanent stunting. The greater a mother's size before pregnancy, the more likely she is to have a normal birth-weight baby (Naeye, 1981). For women who are underweight when they conceive, the amount of food they consume during pregnancy affects the birth-weight (Papoz et al., 1981). In mothers with protein-energy malnutrition (PEM), or who have a preconception daily energy intake of 7.5 MJ (1800 kcal) or less, appropriate food supplementation during pregnancy, depending on the size of the deficiency, increases fetal growth and decreases the number of low-birth-weight babies (Lechtig and Klein, 1981). As to the effect of supplementation after birth, the following examples will suffice. During the post-war famine in Europe in 1947–1948, children in a German orphanage whose diets averaged about 80 per cent of their desirable nutrient intake were supplemented for a year with bread and other foods (see Widdowson, 1951). During the period of the supplement their heights and weights increased at a greater than normal rate (that is they showed 'catch-up' growth) and their skeletal maturity changed in parallel with their growth. In a second example, a group of 141 Korean girls were admitted to the USA and adopted into American families (Winick et al., 1975). The girls were divided into three groups of whom 42 were severely malnourished and below the 3rd percentile for both height and weight by Korean standards. Another 52 were marginally malnourished, between the 3rd and 25th percentile for height and weight, and 47 were well-nourished and above the 50th percentile for height and weight. The families who adopted them before their second birthday had no idea of the children's previous nutritional history. By the time they were 7 years of age there were no differences in the average weight of the three groups of children although the average height of the previously malnourished Korean children remained statistically below those of the well-nourished children. All the Korean children remained shorter and lighter than the American standards.

Illness only has a transient effect on children's growth unless it is severe; then its effects mimic those of malnutrition. That the psychological state of children affects the effects of food on body growth was a serendipitus observation during the supplementation study in the German orphanages mentioned above (Widdowson, 1951). During the supplementation it was found that it was the presence of a Sister (called 'B', in the write-up) in the orphanage, rather than the food available, that determined the children's growth, as the mealtimes were chosen by her as an opportunity to severely reprimand the majority of the children, other than those who were 'B's favourites; it was these favourites who gave the expected response to the rations. There was no doubt that the children who did not respond consumed the supplements.

The 'secular trend' is the term used to describe the striking tendency for the age of adolescence, for example menarche, and the growth spurt to take place earlier than they did 100 years ago. Similar trends have been reported in all Western countries. These trends are greater than the differences between social classes (Tanner, 1978). In countries with large populations such as India, trends in growth and development may be induced by racial, ethnic and genetic factors as well as those caused by socioeconomic status and nutrition. This may make it necessary to construct local/regional growth standards (Singh, 1995). The secular trend has had sociological and medical effects; the latter are shown by the occurrence of myopia in children at the earlier age of puberty (Tanner, 1962).

Body Composition

The composition of the mammalian body can be considered from three different viewpoints – anatomical, physiological and chemical – each of which has importance for the nutritionist and implications for public health and clinical medicine. Anatomically, our bodies consist of a number of organs and tissues which contribute varying proportions to the total body weight. Physiologically, our bodies contain 60–70 per cent water, which is distributed between the cellular and extracellular compartments, with the different composition of the intracellular fluid (ICF) and the extracellular fluid (ECF) being maintained by energy-dependent mechanisms in the cell membranes. Also, physiologically, our bodies can be divided into energy-expending tissues, collectively called the 'lean body mass' (LBM) and energy-storing adipose tissue, collectively called the 'fat mass' (FM). Chemically, the body consists of various organic and inorganic substances that are functionally integrated, with the mineral composition of the body necessarily depending on its organic structure. There are nevertheless three factors which predominantly affect the proportion of inorganic elements in the body and its tissues. The first is the amount of fat, as fatty tissue contains comparatively little inorganic material, so that it acts mainly as a diluent. The second is the amount of ECF in the body or tissue at the moment of analysis. Structurally and functionally this is important in the process of development, in which there is a decrease in the volume of ECF consequent upon the increase in the cell mass (CM), and in disease, in which malnutrition produces the opposite changes – an increase in the volume of ECF consequent upon a decrease in the CM. The magnitude of the changes in the proportion of ECF far outweigh the changes in its composition or in that of the cells. The third factor is the amount of bone and its degree of calcification, as the adult skeleton contains 99 per cent of the body's calcium. Changes in the concentration of calcium in the body fluids have important physiological consequences, but they have no appreciable effect on the composition of the body.

It is important to remember, as we discuss the chemical composition of the body, that we are considering a static picture of a dynamic scene, for the molecules of which our bodies are composed are in a state of individual and collective activity, and what we are considering is like a snapshot of a busy street full of pedestrians and automobiles (Widdowson and Dickerson, 1964).

Methods for determining whole body composition

Chemical analysis

Detailed discussion of the methods available for the analysis of the human body is outside the scope of this chapter. However, it should be noted that chemical analysis is essentially a destructive process and can be carried out only after death or on tissue obtained by biopsy. Quantitative analysis of whole bodies presents considerable difficulties. In the first place, it is necessary for the investigator to obtain permission from the relatives or guardians of the body to deal with it in this way. This is not easy. It is even more difficult to obtain the body of a healthy person. This problem, together with that of handling such a large amount of material in a quantitative fashion, has limited the number of adult human bodies that have been analysed. In fact, up to 1945, our knowledge about the chemical composition of the adult human body was derived from

work carried out in Europe about 100 years ago; since that time the composition of five more human bodies (four men and one woman) has been determined (see Widdowson and Dickerson, 1964). It is likely that this will remain the total information that we have of the elemental composition of the adult human body. The bodies of human fetuses and stillborn babies are much easier to deal with and the results of the analysis of these will be considered here. Again, though, trends in public opinion and ethical considerations make it unlikely that there will be any further analyses of this nature. This adds value to the work of Fomon *et al.* (1982) in producing calculated data for the composition of 'reference' children up to 10 years of age, and these will be considered later.

Other methods

There has been, and is continuing to be, research into other methods for the determination of aspects of the composition of the living human body. Much of this development has stemmed from a concept of the body as consisting of two components, fat and lean tissue (Behnke *et al.*, 1942). This is now referred to as the 'two-compartment model' of body composition. A four-compartment model for the assessment of body composition of humans has been devised which involves the determination of body fat by underwater weighing, total body water (TBW) by deuterium, total body mineral by dual-energy X-ray absorptiometry (DXA) and fat-free body mass as body weight minus fat (Fuller *et al.*, 1992). Coward *et al.* (1988) reviewed the established techniques available at that time: measurement of body fat from measurements body density, TBW, total body potassium and determination of body fatness by anthropometry. They also reviewed the newer technique of electrical conductivity and impedence. In a study in which body fat was measured in lean and obese individuals (McNeill *et al.*, 1989) by six different methods [skinfold thickness, underwater weighing, whole body ^{40}K counting, deuterium dilution of body water, tetrapolar bioelectrical impedence and magnetic resonance imaging (MRI)], it was found that, despite high correlations between any two different methods over a wide range of fatness, there was substantial disagreement between the results by the different methods in the same individual. Measurements of gross body fat in rats by DXA, compared with absolute values determined by carcase analysis (Jebb *et al.*, 1994), showed that this method overestimated body fat in the rats by 30–39 per cent. Bioelectrical impedance analysis has been shown to be of greater value in assessing lower limb muscle area in groups of subjects rather than in individuals (Fuller *et al.*, 1999). The need for simple (and preferably inexpensive) methods for the determination of aspects of body composition at the bedside has led to research into methods that could be used to calibrate such instruments (Elia and Ward, 1999). The BOD POD body composition system developed in the US (Life Measurement Systems, Concord, CA, USA) can be used to measure body volume by air, rather than by water, displacement, as in the method described by Behnke *et al.* (1942) for the determination of body density. This method of determining body fat then becomes possible in children. Alternatively, deuterium dilution can be measured by infrared spectroscopy rather more cheaply than by mass spectroscopy. Bioelectrical impedance can be used to accurately measure skinfold thickness. Again, both these methods can be used in children.

The main conclusion that can be drawn from the literature on this subject is that a variety of expensive research tools are available which are essentially difficult to calibrate against absolute values. Reproducibility of results, availability, cost and expertise all need to be considered in the use of any of them. The reason for making the measurement also needs to be considered, whether it is for research or to follow the progress of treatment in a single individual. If it is simply a matter of assessing a change in nutritional status, repeated careful measurement of body weight under standard conditions together with triceps skinfold thickness may suffice.

The composition of the whole body

The effect of development

Table 1.4 shows the changes in the chemical composition, determined by chemical analysis, of human fetuses and stillborn babies varying in weight from 0.75 to 4373 g. The smallest of the foetuses contained 924 g of water per kg of body tissue, which is about the same amount that exists in serum after birth. The heaviest stillborn baby (4373 g) contained only 585 g of water per kg of tissue. Part of the difference in the amount of water was due to the difference in fat content, 5 g compared with 282 g per kg, and on a fat-free basis the proportion of water in the body fell from 930 to 820 g per kg of body tissue. It is important to note that the amount of fat in the body did not rise above 100 g per kg until a fetus weighed more than 2600 g and reference will be made to this again later. When information from other workers is included (Figure 1.3), we find that the water content of the body falls rapidly during early growth, reaching 880 g per kg fat-free tissue when the fetus weighs 50–100 g and then declining more gradually to 820 g per kg when the fetus reaches full term. This fall in water content is due to a reduction in the amount of ECF consequent on an increase in the CM and is reflected in a fall in the concentrations of the EC ions, sodium and chloride, and a rise in the concentration of the predominantly intracellular ion, potassium. However, not all the sodium in the body is located in the ECF and it has been calculated

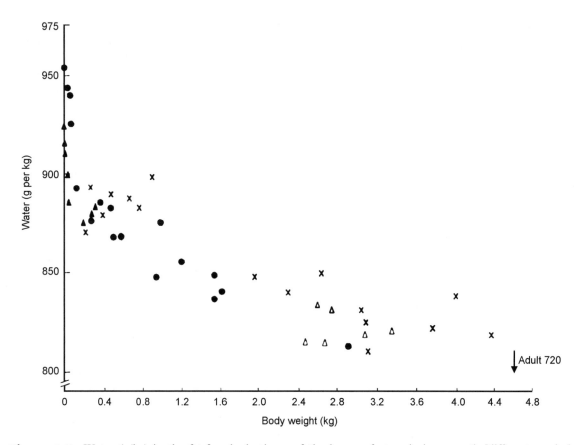

Figure 1.3 Water (g/kg) in the fat-free body tissue of the human foetus during growth [different symbols signify different sources of data; reproduced from Widdowson and Dickerson (1964). *Mineral Metabolism*, Vol. 2A, pp. 1–217, by permission of Academic Press]

that at term about 13 per cent of the body's sodium is found in the bones and that from about the seventh month of prenatal life the fall in the proportion of extracellular sodium is approximately counter-balanced by increases in sodium in the skeleton. The skin also contains much sodium and chloride at all ages and the concentration of chloride in adult skin is at least as high as that in the skin of a full-term baby. The changes in the amount of calcium in the body are a reflection of the ossification of the skeleton and this begins to occur when the fetus weighs between 700 and 900 g and rises to term. The increase in the mineralization of the skeleton also contributes

to the rise in the amount of phosphorus in the body; the soft tissues also contain phosphorus and thus the increase in the CM also contributes to the increase in the body's content of this mineral. The concentrations of iron, copper and zinc in Table 1.4 show little evidence of regular trends with the progress of gestation.

Using information obtained by 'dilution' methods, it is possible to extend the developmental curve for some body constituents to find what Moulton (1923) described as the age of 'chemical maturity'. Using this information (Widdowson and Dickerson, 1964) it is possible to conclude that total water, 'exchangeable'

Table 1.4 Chemical composition of human fetuses and newborn babies [reproduced from Widdowson and Dickerson (1964) *Mineral Metabolism*, Vol. 2A, pp. 1–217; reproduced by permission of Academic Press]

Body weight (g)	Per kg whole body			Per kg fat-free body tissue										
	Water (g)	Nitrogen (g)	Fat (g)	Water (g)	Nitrogen (g)	Sodium (mmol)	Potassium (mmol)	Chloride (mmol)	Calcium (mmol)	Phosphorus (mmol)	Magnesium (mmol)	Iron (mmol)	Copper (mmol)	Zinc (mmol)
0.75	924	8.1	5	930	8.1	—	—	—	—	—	—	—	—	—
7.6	915	8.6	5	920	8.6	—	38	—	—	—	—	—	—	—
11.1	910	9.4	5	915	9.4	108	49	84	41	56	3.3	—	—	—
29.5	885	11.5	5	890	11.6	125	49	80	—	—	—	—	—	—
32.5	898	12.3	5	900	12.4	111	48	77	64	80	4.9	—	—	—
198	875	17.7	5	880	17.8	106	44	80	114	103	9.0	—	—	—
225	870	16.3	6	875	16.4	—	44	71	106	100	8.0	0.92	0.06	0.39
271	880	13.3	5	885	13.4	96	46	76	76	75	6.2	—	—	—
286	893	12.9	5	895	13.0	—	38	—	118	112	8.2	1.18	0.05	0.26
314	882	13.1	5	885	13.2	99	39	78	114	104	7.4	—	—	—
400	879	14.9	6	880	15.0	—	47	—	106	100	6.2	1.33	0.03	0.39
478	889	13.5	5	890	13.6	—	45	—	110	97	7.0	0.85	0.06	0.25
673	876	13.6	15	890	13.8	—	42	—	142	114	6.7	0.88	0.06	0.25
787	875	14.5	9	880	14.6	—	41	—	153	120	8.6	0.98	0.05	0.32
911	887	12.3	12	900	12.5	—	45	—	142	112	8.6	1.16	0.05	0.27
1966	813	18.6	42	850	19.4	—	41	—	197	143	9.2	1.51	0.07	0.17
2295	778	18.9	75	840	20.4	—	47	—	194	154	9.5	1.59	0.04	0.30
2652	797	17.6	67	850	18.8	—	41	—	202	132	8.6	1.40	0.06	0.23
3050	726	19.1	125	830	21.8	—	53	—	219	170	9.5	2.03	0.07	0.17
3090	699	18.8	155	825	22.2	—	55	—	242	168	10.7	2.20	0.08	0.31
3105	721	22.1	110	810	24.9	—	53	—	234	187	11.1	1.48	0.06	0.22
3767	697	19.7	152	820	23.2	—	50	—	220	177	10.7	2.09	0.09	0.47
3994	722	17.4	139	840	20.3	—	48	—	257	182	11.4	1.04	0.07	0.29
4373	585	16.9	283	820	23.5	—	55	—	257	194	11.1	1.24	0.09	0.30

Table 1.5   Body composition of reference boys from birth to age 10 years (from Fomon *et al.*, 1982)

	Fat percentage body weight	Components of fat-free body mass (% body weight)					
		Protein	Total body water	Extracellular body water	Intracellular body water	Osseous minerals	Non-osseous minerals
Birth	13.7	12.9	69.6	42.5	27.0	2.6	0.6
1 month	15.1	12.9	68.4	41.1	27.3	2.6	0.6
2 months	19.9	12.3	64.3	38.0	26.3	2.4	0.6
3 months	23.2	12.0	61.4	35.7	25.8	2.3	0.6
6 months	25.4	12.0	59.4	33.4	26.0	2.3	0.5
12 months	22.5	12.9	61.2	32.9	28.3	2.3	0.6
5 years	14.6	15.8	65.4	30.0	35.4	3.1	0.6
8 years	13.0	16.6	65.8	28.3	37.5	3.4	0.6
9 years	13.2	16.8	65.4	27.6	37.8	3.5	0.6
10 years	13.7	16.8	64.8	26.7	38.0	3.5	0.6

chloride, and 'exchangeable' sodium have reached adult proportions in terms of body weight by the time a child is 3 years old. This is approximately 4.5 per cent of the total expected life-span, which is the proportion suggested by Moulton to be that required by mammals to reach chemical maturity. However, it is known that certain aspects of body composition do not reach mature values by 3 years of age. For example, the proportion of ECF may continue to fall until puberty, ossification of some of the long bones is not complete until 20–30 years of age, and the amounts of calcium and phosphorus must continue to increase throughout the period of growth.

Using the values for the calculated body composition of reference boys (Fomon *et al.*, 1982) shown in Table 1.5, it can be seen that the composition of boys is approaching maturity by the age of 9 or 10 years. The composition of girls follows a similar pattern. However, all these values for gross body composition ignore the differences in the rate of chemical development of individual organs and tissues (see later). There is also considerable variability in the composition of the fat-free mass in children

of the same age (Wells *et al.*, 1999). In the study of the body composition of 30 children, Wells and colleagues concluded that half the variability in the values for the water, mineral and protein content of the FFM was methodological and the other half was biological. From the values for the amounts of Ca in the newborn baby and the results of balance experiments and known gains in weight, it has been calculated that the concentration of Ca in the bodies of breast-fed babies in the suckling period is probably lower at 6 months than at birth. The concentration of calcium in the long bones certainly falls during the suckling period and then rises again (see the section 'The Skeleton' below).

The premature baby

The outstanding difference in the body composition of a premature baby compared with that of a full-term baby is the amount of fat in the body (Table 1.6). At a weight of 1.5 kg the premature baby probably contains less than one-tenth as much fat as the one born full-term and this has important implications for the

Table 1.6 Total amounts of fat, nitrogen (g) and minerals (mmol) in the bodies of premature babies compared with those in a full-term baby [adapted from Widdowson and Dickerson (1964) *Mineral Metabolism*, Vol. 2A, pp. 1–217; reproduced by permission of Academic Press]

	More premature	Less premature	Full-term (FT)	More premature as percentage (FT)	Less premature as percentage (FT)
Body weight (kg)	1.5	2.5	3.5	43	72
Fat (kg)	0.03	0.17	0.53	6	32
Fat-free body weight (kg)	1.47	2.33	2.97	49	79
Total nitrogen	25.5	46.6	66.0	39	71
Sodium	134	200	243	55	82
Potassium	64	108	150	43	72
Chloride	95	139	160	60	87
Calcium	255	475	705	36	68
Phosphorus	210	384	523	40	74
Magnesium	13.3	24.2	31.7	42	76
Iron	1.89	3.57	5.71	33	63
Copper	0.08	0.14	0.22	35	64
Zinc	0.40	0.61	0.81	49	75

baby's care, since it represents a difference in subcutaneous insulation and energy store. A premature baby has considerably less calcium in its body than one born full-term, as the skeleton grows relatively faster than the body as a whole and the bones become more highly calcified during the last 3 months of gestation. The premature baby is also very short of iron and is therefore likely to suffer from a more severe degree of 'suckling' anaemia than the full-term baby unless dietary supplementary iron is supplied.

Postnatal changes in body fat

We have seen that fat accounts for about 13 per cent of a baby's weight at full term. The proportion of fat continues to increase for approximately 6 months until it reaches approximately 25 per cent. By this age, babies are becoming more active and some are walking by 12 months. This increase in activity, combined with the ingestion of solid food, results in a gradual proportional decrease in body fat content. The 'fatness' of the human body can be assessed by the calculation of the BMI. During the first 6 months or so of postnatal life the BMI rises rapidly, then gradually falls to about 4 years of age, subsequently rising again. These changes are a normal occurrence and need to be interpreted with care. As commented earlier, the BMI ranges used for the assessment of obesity in adults are not appropriate for children (Prentice, 1998). The BMI charts for British children from birth to 20 years of age published by the Child Growth Foundation have been recommended (see p. 4).

Composition of the newborn of different species

In the context of this book it is not intended to discuss in any detail the body composition of species other than man. However, it is of interest to draw attention to the fact that the

Table 1.7 Chemical composition of newborn mammals. Values expressed per kg of fat-free body tissue [adapted from Widdowson and Dickerson (1964) *Mineral Metabolism*, Vol. 2A, pp. 1–217; reproduced by permission of Academic Press]

	Man	Pig	Dog	Cat	Guinea-pig	Rabbit	Rat	Mouse
Body weight (g)	3560	1260	328	118	80	54	5.9	1.6
Fat (g/kg body tissue)	150	<10	<10	<10	70	<10	<10	<10
Water (g)	823	820	845	822	775	865	862	850
Total nitrogen (g)	22.6	18.0	20.9	24.4	29.2	18.1	15.6	20.5
Sodium (mmol)	82	93	81	92	71	78	84	–
Potassium (mmol)	53	50	58	60	69	53	65	70
Chloride (mmol)	55	52	60	66	–	56	67	–
Calcium (mmol)	240	250	122	165	307	120	77	85
Phosphorus (mmol)	181	187	130	140	240	116	116	110
Magnesium (mmol)	11	11	7	11	20	10	10	10
Iron (mmol)	1.68	0.52	–	0.98	1.20	2.41	1.05	1.20
Copper (mmol)	0.07	0.05	–	0.05	0.11	0.06	0.07	0.11
Zinc (mmol)	0.29	0.15	–	0.44	0.54	0.35	0.37	0.71

stage of chemical development reached at the same milestone of growth, birth, is related to a mammal's physiological development. The newborn human baby is different from newborn pigs, dogs, cats rabbits, rats and mice in containing much more fat in its body (Table 1.7). Newborn guinea-pigs also contain a substantial amount of fat, but they contain rather more calcium and phosphorus, indicating that their skeletons are more highly calcified. Whilst the concentrations of these minerals is similar in the newborn piglet to those in the human baby, they are rather higher than in the less mature rabbit, rat and mouse. The newborn piglet has the lowest concentration of iron in its body and suckling anaemia used to be a considerable cause of mortality in young piglets.

Effect of Dietary Deficiency and Excess

Protein-energy deficiency

In man at all ages a dietary deficiency of energy leads to a loss of fat, a loss of cellular material and an increase in the proportion of the LBM occupied by ECF. This inevitably causes a change in the mineral composition of the body, so that as far as sodium and chloride and potassium are concerned it comes to resemble one that is chemically immature. The only infant bodies that have been analysed any time after birth are five that died of gastrointestinal disorders – a premature baby aged 13 days, three aged 3–4 months and one aged 4 months who weighed only 3.7 kg when she died (quoted by Widdowson and Dickerson, 1964). These were all undernourished. Interest in children with PEM in Jamaica led to measurements of TBW with tritium oxide in such infants under 2 years of age with oedema, and showed a mean value of 85 per cent of the body weight (Smith, 1960). After losing the oedema, the TBW was 73 per cent of the body weight and decreased to 63 per cent on recovery, when the body weight was increasing rapidly. Exchangeable potassium has been found to be greatly reduced in babies suffering from PEM and it has been suggested that the tissue cells in such bodies may be overhydrated.

Dehydration

A baby has a much larger turnover of water than an adult in proportion to its body weight. More water is lost via the lungs because it breathes a greater volume of air per kg of body weight each minute; more is also lost through the skin because it has a relatively larger surface area than an adult in relation to its weight. The baby also requires a greater volume of water to excrete the same amount of urea and salts because it cannot concentrate its urine to the same extent. A newborn baby may not be supplied with any food or water during the first 2 days after birth and minerals/electrolytes and water are lost from its body. A premature baby has a bigger surface area relative to its weight; it also has a lower metabolic rate than the full-term baby, so it loses relatively more water by insensible perspiration and it catabolizes less solid matter as a source of energy. In a hot environment more water and fewer solids would probably be lost; on the other hand, anything that increases the metabolic rate is likely to increase the loss of solids, and particularly cell solids (Widdowson, 1959).

Sodium chloride excess

The newborn baby, like the adult, can excrete an excess of sodium chloride if given sufficient water, but since at this time of life the concentrating power of the kidney is low, more water has to be given in proportion to the salt. If a newborn baby is given a solution of sodium chloride as dilute as 0.7 per cent, it retains relatively more salt than water, and the extracellular fluids become not only expanded in volume but hypertonic as well (McCance and Widdowson, 1957). This may well have implications in relation to the amount of salt in weaning diets, particularly if babies are weaned early, before renal function has fully developed.

Iron deficiency

Iron forms an essential part of the body's structure, but the amount in the body, in health, can vary much more widely than that of the electrolytes or calcium. The average amount found in the bodies of full-term babies at birth is 320 mg. The liver is the main organ where iron is stored and at birth it contains no more than 30–50 mg of iron that can be used for growth. This is only some 15 per cent of the total body iron and cannot constitute an important reserve. The blood of a newborn baby acts to a certain extent as a reserve, if the clamping of the cord is delayed, as up to 100 ml of blood may be gained containing 40 mg iron. By following the fate of red cells tagged with ^{55}Fe in the mother during pregnancy it has been found that at birth the infant had 170 mg of iron as haemoglobin in the body which had reached it through the placenta (Smith et al., 1955). At one year there were 200 mg of haemoglobin iron which had been obtained through the placenta, and this was about 70 per cent of the total haemoglobin iron. Thus, at birth about 30 mg of transplacental iron must have been deposited in some part of the body other than the blood and used for haemoglobin formation during the first year. Possibly little or none of the dietary iron is utilized for haemoglobin until 3–4 months after birth. Human milk contains about 0.1 mg iron per 100 ml (Macy et al., 1953). If the breast-fed baby is assumed to take an average of 800 ml of milk per day throughout the first 6 months of life and to have no other source of iron, its iron intake might amount to about 150 mg by 6 months. This is less than the amount in the body at birth and less, therefore, than the amount required to maintain the concentration of iron in the body while the birth-weight is being doubled. Since no baby can absorb and utilize 100 per cent of the iron in its food, the proportion of iron stored in the breast-fed baby will fall (resulting in anaemia) unless the baby is given a supplementary dietary source of iron.

Changes in Organ and Tissue Proportions During Growth

As the human body grows and develops, its form changes due to differential growth of its component parts. The chemical development of the body is also a differential process, with organs and tissues changing in composition at different rates and at different times. For some organs these changes are closely age-specific and we are now learning that this phenomenon, which has been called 'biochemical programming', may hold the key to the development of diseases such as coronary heart disease and diabetes mellitus later in life (Barker, 1994) (see Chapter 7). The chemical composition of the body at any age is the result of the contribution of the different organs and tissues and of their composition at that age. Both these parameters change during development. Skeletal muscle is the most abundant single soft tissue in the fetus at 20–24 weeks, when it accounts for 25 per cent of the body weight (Table 1.8). This proportion does not change during fetal life, but greatly increases after birth when it contains the bulk of the body's protein. In contrast, the skin and brain account for more of the body weight before birth than in the adult. The skeleton, on the other hand contributes rather more to the weight of the fetus than it does at birth. Organs such as the heart and kidneys contribute little to the body weight and hence only a small amount to the the body's composition. Because of their composition some organs contribute greater amounts of a particular constituent than their weight would signify. Thus, as mentioned above, the skeleton contains 99 per cent of the body's calcium and a considerable proportion of its phosphorus. The skeleton and skin account for a considerable

Table 1.8 Contribution of organs and tissues to the body weight of man during growth; values expressed as a percentage of the body weight (Widdowson and Dickerson (1964) *Mineral Metabolism*, Vol. 2A, pp. 1–217; reproduced by permission of Academic Press]

	Fetus (20–24 weeks)	Newborn baby	Adult
Skeletal muscle	25	25	40
Skin	13	15	7
Skeleton	22	18	18
Heart	0.6	0.5	0.4
Liver	4	5	2
Kidneys	0.7	1	0.5
Brain	13	13	2

proportion of the body's connective tissue and hence of the protein collagen, and because of this of a specific amino acid, hydroxyproline.

Adipose tissue with its content of fat may be considered to be an 'organ' since one form of it, brown adipose tissue (BAT), can quickly generate heat, whilst its other form, white adipose tissue, acts as an energy store and stores and produces hormones. Fat cells, or adipocytes, multiply in early life from stem cell precursors. They occur not only in depots such as under the skin and in the abdomen, but also as discrete masses in other tissues and organs such as skeletal muscle and the liver. The size of adipocytes depends on the amount of fat they contain and this varies at any one time in different parts of the body. The chemical composition of the fat depends on the kinds of fatty acids in the diet and this also affects the physical nature of the fat. The higher the amount of polyunsaturated fatty acids in the diet, the 'softer' will be the fat. There have been attempts to determine the number of fat cells in infants from determinations of total body fat and of the number and the fat content of fat cells in biopsies of subcutaneous fat. However, this is not possible because, as stated above, the size of adipocytes varies in different parts of the body. For further information about adipose tissue, readers are referred to Chapters 2 and 4 of this book.

The Composition of Organs and Tissues

Limitations of space preclude a consideration of the chemical composition of all the individual organs and tissues of the body. From an anatomical viewpoint the body's organs and tissues can be divided into muscle, connective tissue, glandular organs and nervous tissue. Skeletal muscle has been chosen because it is the largest soft tissue and changes most in composition and bulk during postnatal life. Bone and skin have been chosen as rather different examples of connective tissue, whilst the liver has been chosen as the largest glandular organ. For nervous tissue, discussion has concentrated on the brain.

Skeletal muscle

Effect of growth and development

Skeletal muscle cells, more accurately called fibres, originate as myotubes, which are formed by differentiation of myoblasts and these in turn are formed by the differentiation of mesenchymal cells (Figure 4.10). As discussed in Chapter 4, three kinds of muscle fibres, primary, secondary and tertiary, may be distinguished during growth and development. The number of primary muscle fibres is genetically determined. The major fibre population in mature muscle is composed of secondary fibres. Tertiary muscle fibres, produced in late gestation, are found only in large animals. The factors that regulate the differentiation and early development of muscle are discussed by Symonds and his colleagues

(Chapter 4). The total muscle mass is distributed between individual muscles of different shapes and sizes. In the mature individual, the fibres in the different muscles differ considerably in size, in their growth potential in response to hormones and exercise and in their susceptibility to nutritional deprivation. As far as the effects of growth and development on their chemical composition are concerned, attention has mostly been given to easily dissected discrete muscles that constitute a relatively substantial proportion of the total muscle mass. Most investigators have worked on the quadriceps muscle in the leg. When considering the effects of growth on the number of fibres it is essential to restrict attention to a muscle, the sartorius (one of the quadriceps group), in which the fibres are arranged longitudinally and mostly occupy the length of the muscle.

Skeletal muscle cells are multinucleate and therefore their number cannot be determined from the amount of DNA in the tissue, and the size of the cells cannot be determined from the protein/DNA ratio. In spite of these limitations, DNA has been used as an index of human postnatal muscle growth (Widdowson, 1970). Measurements of DNA in biopsy samples of gluteal muscles were assumed to be representative of all the muscles in the body and from determinations of the total muscle mass, derived from creatinine excretion, the total number of muscle nuclei was calculated. Samples obtained from 33 boys and 19 girls showed that there was an increase in the number of nuclei throughout childhood and that in boys there was a spurt in the rate of multiplication of nuclei at the time of puberty (DB Cheek; quoted by Widdowson, 1970). The number doubled between 10 and 16 years of age. Overall, there was a 14-fold increase in the number of nuclei in the muscle of boys after birth. The increase was smaller in girls. The changes in the chemical composition of human quadriceps muscle during growth are shown in Table 1.9.

Table 1.9 Effect of development on the composition of skeletal muscle; values expressed per kg of muscle (Dickerson and Widdowson, 1960)

	Fetus		Baby		
	13–14 weeks	20–22 weeks	Newborn	4–7 months	Adult
Water (g)	907	887	804	785	792
Total nitrogen (g)	11.2	14.8	20.7	29.1	30.8
Intracellular protein N (ICPN), percentage total nitrogen	86.0	81.4	70.7	74.6	87.6
Extracellular protein N (ECPN), percentage total nitrogen	5.5	11.8	18.2	15.6	4.6
Sodium (mmol)	101	90.6	60.1	50.1	36.3
Potassium (mmol)	56.3	57.6	57.7	89.5	92.2
Chloride (mmol)	76.4	65.6	42.6	35.5	22.1
Phosphorus (mmol)	36.5	40.0	47.0	64.9	58.8
Magnesium (mmol)	5.8	5.3	7.4	10.0	8.3
Calcium (mmol)	2.8	3.5	2.1	1.5	1.3
Derived data					
Extracellular water (g/kg)[a]	672	577	350	293	183
Intracellular water (g/kg)	235	310	454	492	609
Intracellular protein N (g/kg)	10.5	12.0	14.6	21.8	27.0
Total cations/ICPN (mmol/g ICPN)	6.7	6.2	5.0	4.9	4.1

[a]Calculated as the 'chloride space', assuming that all the chloride is outside the cells at the same concentration as that in plasma water.

The amount of water per kg of muscle falls as the amount of nitrogen ($\times 6.25 =$ protein) rises. The rise in the amount of nitrogen during fetal life is partly due to a rise in the amount of extracellular protein (ECPN – collagen, elastin and reticulin) found in connective tissue. After birth, the concentration of ECPN falls. The fall in water content is accounted for by the expansion of the cell mass and the consequent fall in the amount of ECF calculated as the 'chloride' space, that is the amount of fluid containing chloride ions at the concentration at which they are present in plasma water at that age. The 'space' occupied by sodium ions, calculated in the same way as the chloride space, also falls but the sodium space is always greater than the chloride space because some sodium is always present in muscle cells. The composition of muscle cells with respect to their content of cations and protein, expressed as the 'total cation/intracellular protein nitrogen (ICPN) ratio' gives a measure of the composition of the cells. This ratio falls from 6.7 to 5.0 in fetal life with a continued fall to 4.1 in adult tissue. Similar evidence for a change in composition of muscle cells during growth and development has been found in both pig (Dickerson and Widdowson, 1960) and fowl (Dickerson, 1960) muscle. The changes in the chemical composition of muscle described above are accompanied by changes in histological structure (Figure 1.4). In the photomicrograph of transverse sections of quadriceps muscle samples it is seen that in the fetus of 20 weeks gestation the fibres are small, relatively few in number and widely

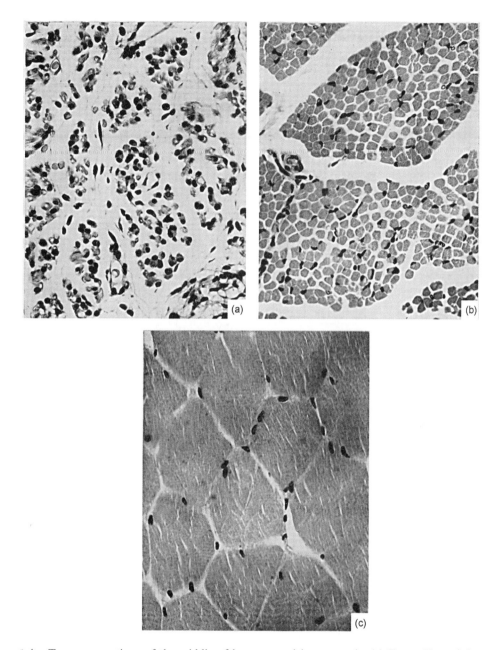

Figure 1.4 Tranverse sections of the middle of human quadriceps muscle: (a) Fetus, 28 weeks' gestation; (b) newborn baby at term; (c) adult [reproduced from Dickerson and Widdowson (1960) *Biochem. J.* **74**, 247–257, by permission of the *Biochemical Journal*]

separated by extacellular material. The nuclei occupy a larger proportion of the cells than they do at later stages. At term, the fibres are still small, but there are many more of them and they are more closely packed together. In adult muscle the fibres are much larger in diameter, the nuclei are relatively small and on the edge of the fibres, and there is little space between the fibres for extracellular material. Thus the decrease in the proportion of ECF in muscle during growth and development is accounted for firstly by increase in the number of fibres and later by the increase in the size of fibres. These changes also account for the fact that the connective tissue proteins increase in concentration during fetal life and decrease in concentration during postnatal life. From a study of the human sartorius muscle (Montgomery, 1962) it seems likely that the baby at birth, or soon afterwards, has got its adult number of muscle fibres and that muscle growth postnatally is entirely due to hypertrophy of existing fibres. The growth and integrity of skeletal muscles depend on their activity: inactive muscles atrophy.

Maternal muscle during pregnancy

The protein available to the fetus during gestation seems not to be derived directly from the mother's diet at that time but to come from the breakdown of maternal muscle proteins. The amino acid, 3-methylhistidine, is located mainly in skeletal muscle. When skeletal muscle proteins are catabolized during pregnancy this amino acid cannot be re-utilized and is excreted quantitatively in the urine. Naismith (1981) and his colleagues have shown that the excretion of 3-methylhistidine during human pregnancy rises sharply during the last trimester of pregnancy when the baby is growing at its most rapid rate and have interpreted this as evidence that maternal muscles are the source of fetal nitrogen. It appears not to be known if a similar breakdown of maternal protein occurs in mothers who are undernourished.

Effects of protein-energy malnutrition

Normal growth depends on an adequate supply of energy and nutrients. When the supply is inadequate, either before or after birth, the growth of animals, including human babies, is retarded. Undernourished infants and children lose lean body tissue and gain fluid. The effect on the composition of skeletal depends on the severity of the undernutrition and its timing. Studies in experimental animals, including chickens and pigs (Dickerson and McCance, 1960), have shown that, when growing animals are maintained at almost constant body weight for periods of up to a year, the growth of muscle cells almost ceases, whereas that of the connective tissue proceeds, albeit slowly. The result is that the composition of the tissue reverts to that characteristic of younger animals, with an increase in the concentration of ECF and extracellular protein and a relative decrease in the concentration of cellular fluid and protein. When experimental animals (Dickerson and McCance, 1960) and children (Mendes and Waterlow, 1958; Montgomery, 1962) lose weight as a result of undernutrition, there is a similar effect on the composition of skeletal muscle, but the mechanism by which it is brought about is rather different, as in this condition more protein is lost from the muscle cells than from the surrounding connective tissue in which the proteins are relatively metabolically 'inert' (Neuberger and Slack, 1953). It is important to recognize that the muscles do not contain a 'store' of protein corresponding to the store of fat found in adipose tissue. Thus, when protein is lost from muscle, it is the cellular fibrillar and sarcoplasmic proteins that are catabolized and their loss affects the strength of muscles and their ability to do 'work' decreases. This loss also happens after injury, whether the result of accidental trauma or elective surgery (Cuthbertson, 1932). In these conditions, the breakdown of muscle proteins results from the effects of cytokines produced by leucocytes (Grimble, 1990) and the magnitude of protein catabolism depends on the severity of the injury. In some patients, undernutrition also contributes to the protein breakdown and minimizing the nitrogen loss is one of the challenges in the care of seriously ill patients.

Not all muscles are affected to the same extent by malnutrition. In experimental animals it has been shown that those muscles that mature late tend to be affected more than those that mature early (Dickerson and McCance, 1960) and to be associated with differences in the rates of DNA and intracellular protein accretion (Dickerson and McAnulty, 1975).

The skeleton

We speak of 'bone' and 'bones'. The word 'bone' is used to describe a specialized form of connective tissue. 'Bones' are organs which are largely composed of this tissue. The individual bones together make up the skeleton which holds and protects the soft tissues. The hollow cavities of the long bones and ribs are also the sites where many of the blood corpuscles are made in the bone marrow. A long bone is, therefore, a composite structure consisting of bone tissue, bone marrow and cartilage. In the long bones of adult animals the amount of cartilage is small and restricted to the articular surface of the epiphyses, but in young animals the whole of the epiphyses may be composed of cartilage. During development the proportion of cartilage in the epiphyses falls, due to the enlargement of the secondary centres of ossification.

'Bone' contains cells and a matrix. The cells (osteoblasts, osteocytes and osteoclasts) are derived during fetal and post-fetal life from mesenchymal cells. The matrix consists of the same kind of substances – collagen, mucopolysaccharides and extracellular water – which constitute the connective tissue of other tissues such as skeletal muscle and skin, but it differs from the connective tissue of these organs in its characteristic 'hardness' which is due to the deposition of 'bone mineral' within the collagen fibres. The crystals of bone mineral are very small, of the order of 200–300 Å in length and breadth, with a thickness of 20–50 Å. Owing to their small size the crystals have an enormous total surface area. One gramme of bone mineral is reported to have a surface area in excess of 100 square metres and the mineral in the bone of a 70 kg man to have a surface area exceeding 100 acres (McLean and Urist, 1961).

Chemically, bone mineral has long been thought to be similar to the terrestrial mineral hydroxyapatite $[Ca_3(PO_4)_2.2Ca(OH)_2]$. The composition of bone mineral is, however, not pure hydroxyapatite because it also contains carbonate, citrate, sodium, magnesium and traces of fluoride. It is likely that the minor constituents of bone mineral arise as a passive consequence of the solution from which the mineral was formed (Neuman and Neuman, 1958). The proportion of the total nitrogen in bone tissue accounted for by collagen increases at certain stages in the development of bone (Dickerson, 1962a), but the stage of development at which the increase occurs varies from one species to another. Thus in human bone the main increase occurs before 22 weeks' gestation, in the pig it occurs before 65 days gestation, and in the rat not until after 65 days after birth (Dickerson, 1962b). In the cortex of the human femur collagen accounts for 89–96 per cent of the total nitrogen after 9 months of age (Rogers et al., 1952; Dickerson, 1962a).

The effect of growth on the calcification of bone

The degree of calcification of the different parts of a long bone can be conveniently assessed from measurements of total nitrogen and calcium in dry bone tissue and calculation of the calcium/nitrogen ratio. This ratio was found by Rogers et al. (1952; Figure 1.5) to increase from about 4.4 at 8 months of age to about 5.7 at about 20–30 years of age and then to increase much more slowly up to about 5.8 at about 60 years of age. Bone begins to be laid

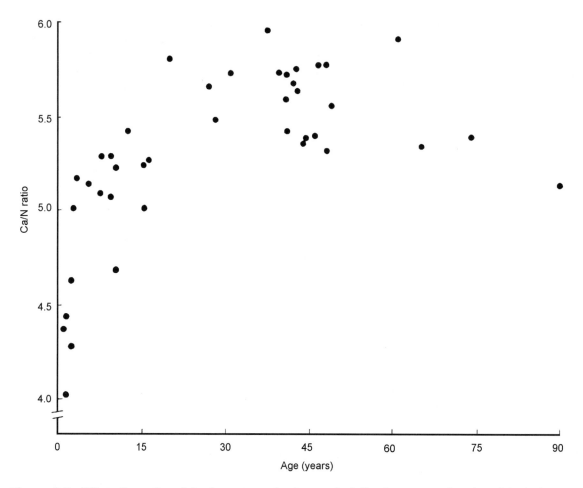

Figure 1.5   Effect of growth and development on the degree of calcification measured as the calcium–nitrogen (Ca/N) ratio of bone tissue from the cortex of the human femur [reproduced from Rogers *et al.* (1952) *Biochem. J.* **50**, 537–542, by permission of the *Biochemical Journal*]

down in the cartilage model of the human femur at about 8 weeks' gestation (Hamilton *et al.*, 1945) and before this the calcium/nitrogen ratio may be assumed to be practically zero. In the 12–14 week fetal human bones analysed by Dickerson (1962a) the calcium/nitrogen ratio was 3.2. The ratio at 25–28 weeks had risen to 5.05, but no further increase occurred until after a postnatal age of 12–24 months. Of course the bones greatly increased in size during this time, but the calcium/nitrogen ratio in the epiphyses showed that there was very little increase in the development of the secondary centres of ossification, as the calcium/nitrogen ratio in this part of the femur did not rise between the 15–16 week fetal bones and those in the infants of 2–4.5 months (0.14 and 0.13, respectively). The values for the calcium/nitrogen ratio in the whole femur suggest that no increase in the degree of calcification occurred until after the infants were 24 months of age. This period from the beginning of the last third of gestation to the end of the second year of postnatal life is one of rapid growth and change of nutrition, first from parenteral to enteral feeding and

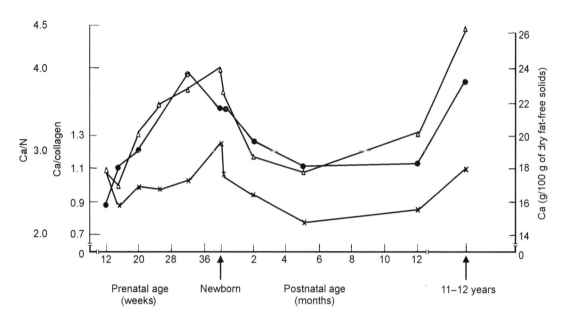

Figure 1.6 Effect of growth and development on the calcification of the non-epiphysial parts of the human femur [reproduced from Dickerson (1962a) *Biochem. J.* **82**, 56–61, by permission of the *Biochemical Journal*]

then the enteral feed changing from milk to solids. Studies in other species, particularly the kitten, showed that the biggest fall in the degree of calcification occurred in the meta-physis rather than in the diaphysis (the shaft) from which the cortical bone samples were taken. Exclusion of the epiphyses with their low degree of calcification showed clear evidence of a fall in the degree of calcification of the human femur during the first 6 months or so of postnatal life with a later rise (Figure 1.6; Dickerson, 1962a).

Using the kitten as an experimental model, Slater and Widdowson (1962) found that administration of calcium phosphate (CaHPO$_4$) during the first week of life to some extent prevented the normal fall in the degree of calcification in the femur and in the humerus. The normal fall in the calcification of the parietal bone of the kitten's skull was also partially prevented. It is interesting to note that narrow borders of uncalcified osteoid have been described in the shaft of bones of rapidly growing premature infants. From their studies

in the kitten, Slater and Widdowson (1962) concluded that phosphorus was probably the limiting nutrient since at this time the animal's soft tissues were competing for the dietary phosphorus. King and Harrison (Chapter 10) have discussed the question of phosphorus being the first limiting nutrient for bone growth in preterm infants and its role in the reduction of bone disease of prematurity (Holland *et al.*, 1990). There is also the possibility that relative deficiency of phosphorus is not the only problem, since a shortage of calcium in premature babies may be linked to poorer growth of the skeleton (Fewtrell *et al.*, 2000a,b).

Effects of undernutrition

In conditions of prolonged undernutrition more bone is resorbed than is deposited, and this results in the so-called 'starvation osteoporosis'; malnutrition, whether marasmus or kwashiorkor, also results in a decreased rate of growth and of skeletal maturation. Chemically, femoral epiphyses of malnourished children contain less calcium than controls (Dickerson and John, 1969), and this is in keeping with their smaller degree of development. Information about the differential effect of undernutrition on the different bones of the skeleton cannot be acquired in man for ethical reasons. This matter has been studied longitudinally by whole body radiography in rats that were undernourished before and after birth (Dickerson and Hughes, 1972). The results showed that skeletal development was retarded less than bone size. After rehabilitation for 119 days the fore and hind limbs and the skull were restored to their normal size, but the length of the spine and the dimensions of the pelvis were not. The findings in this study could be explained from a knowledge of the different timing of the peak velocity of growth of the individual bones (Hughes and Tanner, 1970). A smaller than normal size pelvis is often seen in previously malnourished women (Birch, personal communication).

Effects of senescence and inactivity

The degree of calcfication of the cortex of the human femur does not fall during old age, but the bones may have thin cortices and there may be resorption of cancellous bone due to osteoporosis. This disease is now defined as a metabolic bone disease 'characterized by low bone mass and microarchitectural deterioration of bone tissue, leading to enhanced bone fragility and a consequent increase in fracture risk' (Consensus Development Conference, 1991, 1993). The bones are also more brittle, and this together with osteoporosis accounts for the high incidence of femoral fractures and collapsed vertebrae seen in older people, especially women (Cooke 1955). These conditions are exacerbated by inactivity. Indeed, inactivity can cause the atrophy of bones (loss of bone tissue) at any age. This was clearly shown by

Whedon and his colleagues (Whedon, 1960), who found a prompt and increasing excretion of calcium in young men immobilized in plaster casts. Bone loss was a problem in the early astronauts as a result of weightlessness and has been studied in Russian cosmonauts (Vico et al., 2000). There is no doubt that weight-bearing physical activity is important in maintaining the structural integrity of the skeleton, but the interaction of this with nutritional and genetic factors requires further study (New, 2001).

The skin

The importance of the skin to body composition is often overlooked. In adult man it may account for 7 per cent of the fat-free body weight and contain about 10 per cent of the total body nitrogen. At maturity, human skin consists of three layers – the epidermis, the dermis or corium and a variable layer of subcutaneous fat. Downgrowths of the epidermis into the corium constitute the hair follicles and their associated sebaceous glands, whilst also embedded in the corium are the sweat glands, whose secretion plays an important role in controlling body temperature. The corium makes a vital contribution to the function of the skin in protecting and supporting the underlying soft tissues.

The composition of skin varies considerably between different species and within species, according to the site from which the samples are taken (Dickerson and John, 1964). Table 1.10 shows the composition of human skin from the abdomen or thigh at different ages (Widdowson and Dickerson, 1960). As with skeletal muscle, there is a considerable fall in the proportion of water in the tissue between the 13–14 week fetus and the adult, and overall this is due to the increase in the amount of nitrogen as protein. In mature skin the bulk of the protein is collagen present in the corium. However, it is important to note that by 20–22

Table 1.10 Effect of development on the composition of skin; values expressed per kg of fat-free skin (Widdowson and Dickerson, 1960)

	Fetus		Baby		
	13–14 weeks	20–22 weeks	Newborn	4–7 months	Adult
Water (g)	917	901	828	675	694
Total nitrogen (g)	11.6	11.9	26.5	54.5	53.0
Collagen nitrogen (g)	–	2.4	16.8	39.2	45.7
Sodium (mmol)	–	120	87.1	65.4	79.3
Potasium (mmol)	23.8	36.0	45.0	43.7	23.7
Chloride (mmol)	90.6	96.0	66.9	72.3	71.4
Phosphorus (mmol)	41.8	28.2	31.7	34.9	14.0
Magnesium (mmol)	–	1.9	2.3	3.7	1.5
Calcium (mmol)	2.2	3.0	5.0	5.7	4.7
Distribution of skin water (values expressed as a percentage of total water)					
Cell water	–	6.9	33.3	10.3	13.2
Interstitial water	–	90.6	47.3	34.0	23.1
Connective tissue water	–	2.5	19.4	55.7	63.7
Total extracellular water	–	93.1	66.7	89.7	86.8

weeks the skin still consists of 90 per cent water and only 20 per cent of its small amount of nitrogen is estimated as collagen. At birth the skin still contains 83 per cent water, although 63 per cent of its increased amount of nitrogen is now present as collagen. Comparative values for adult skin are 69 and 86 per cent, respectively. From the values at birth, it is quite easy to appreciate how easily the skin of newborn babies, and particularly that of premature babies, can be damaged and how easily they may become dehydrated. Histological examination of fetal skin has, in fact, shown no mature collagen fibres but that what was determined as 'collagen' was, in fact, 'reticulin'.

Collagen and reticulin, together with elastin, constitute the extracellular protein of all tissues, but connective tissue also contains non-fibrous material, e.g. mucopolysaccharides and plasma proteins. It will be appreciated that the disposition of ECF in the skin is more complex than that in most other tissues. The extracellular water of skin, calculated as in skeletal muscle, as the 'chloride space' is partitioned between the 'fibres' (called 'fibre'

water) and the non-fibrous (called 'non-fibre' water) phases. The values given in Table 1.10 show that, before birth, 'fibre' water rises from 2.5 to 19.4 per cent of the ECF, whereas 'non-fibre' water falls from 91 to 47 per cent. After birth, 'fibre' water rises from 19 to 64 per cent of the extracellular water, whereas 'non-fibre' water falls from 47 to 23 per cent.

The skin of the newborn baby contains fewer cells scattered in the corium than that of the fetus, but glands of mature appearance are present and the epidermis is also more mature than in the fetus. It is probable that the glands and epidermis contribute to the increase in the amount of potassium (Table 1.10) that occurs in the latter part of gestation. The skin increases in thickness during postnatal growth, and the combination of this, with a decrease in cell density in the corium, is largely responsible for the fall in the level of potassium after a postnatal age of 7 months.

The collagen of skin is less inert metabolically than that of other tissues. Evidence for this has come from studies of the effects of undernutrition in rats (Cabak et al., 1963) and mice (Harkness et al., 1958). In the former study, 60 per cent of the total collagen lost from the bodies of the undernourished animals came from the skin. If the collagen of the skin of malnourished babies and children behaves in the same way, it will result in the thinning of the skin with breakdown and the risk of infection, which may be life-threatening. Bed sores in the chronically sick and elderly may have a similar origin, particularly as many such individuals are poorly nourished.

Hair

The apparent nakedness of human skin, except in certain areas, is illusory, for most of the apparently 'naked' areas are covered with very fine and inconspicuous hair. The organic constituent of hair shafts is mainly keratin and this is characterized by little or no metabolic turnover. The sulphydryl groups of the follicular proteins have a high affinity for heavy metals and poisons, such as arsenic, which are not reabsorbed. The composition of hair is therefore important from a medicolegal standpoint.

Changes in scalp hair shaft coloration, thickness and appearance have long been recognized in children with kwashiorkor. The cells of hair matrix normally multiply at a rate which probably exceeds that of any other tissue, with the possible exception of bone marrow (Bradfield *et al.*, 1967). Hair root diameter is reduced significantly in children with mild to moderate malnutrition and the changes occur early enough and regularly enough to be used to differentiate between normal and moderately malnourished children (Bradfield and Jelliffe, 1970). The ease with which hair samples can be obtained from the scalp seems to justify further assessment of hair follicles as a means of diagnosing malnutrition in individuals of any age.

The liver

The form and structure of the adult organism is reached by a process of differential growth.

This is true also of its chemical development and the liver matures more rapidly than skeletal muscle. Associated with this is the fact that during gestation and throughout postnatal life the liver acts as a storage organ, for example for iron and vitamin A. Moreover, variations in dietary intake bring about bigger changes in chemical structure in this organ than in most other tissues. During fetal life it also participates in blood formation (Hamilton *et al.*, 1945). Besides being the largest glandular organ, the liver has attracted most attention as far as the composition of its cells is concerned because of analyses based on the constancy of the amount of DNA in a diploid nucleus (Harrison, 1953), although in the liver this is complicated by polyploidy.

Effects of growth and development

The contribution of the liver to the total body weight in man changes little between a fetus of 13–14 weeks and a baby of 4–7 months (4 per cent; Table 1.11) but is smaller in adults (2.4 per cent). As with all other organs, growth is associated with a fall in the proportion of water and a rise in that of nitrogen. The livers of the fetuses that have been analysed contained quite a high concentration of potassium for which there is no obvious explanation unless they are associated with the haemopoietic activity of the organ. The concentration of sodium is not correspondingly lower and the sum of the sodium and potassium is higher than at any other age. Immature livers contain more sodium and chloride than the adult organ, suggesting that they contain more extracellular fluid, but the possibility that the cells contain varying amounts of both these ions suggests that it is unwise to use either as a basis for the calculation of the proportion of extracellular fluid.

The liver of the newborn baby, like that of the newborn of other species, contains glycogen (Shelley, 1961), which decreases rapidly

Table 1.11 Changes in the chemical structure of human liver with development; values expressed per kg of fresh liver (Widdowson and Dickerson, 1960)

	Fetus		Baby		
	13–14 weeks	20–22 weeks	Newborn	3–5 months	Adult
Water (g)	849	812	786	764	711
Total nitrogen (g)	20.2	22.1	22.6	24.4	28.2
Sodium (mmol)	–	54.8	59.8	51.0	42.5
Potassium (mmol)	81.8	92.9	58.7	66.2	75.0
Chloride (mmol)	62.2	57.1	55.8	42.8	38.3
Phosphorus (mmol)	82.5	88.0	56.5	82.5	86.0
Magnesium (mmol)	–	7.3	5.2	5.9	7.6
Calcium (mmol)	–	1.1	1.5	2.2	1.4
Zinc (mmol)	–	–	1.1	–	0.8
Copper (mmol)	–	–	3.6	–	0.6

after birth. Concentrations differ in different species. Thus, half-way through gestation, human fetal liver contains about 50 mg/g, whereas that of the pig fetus at the same stage contains only about 4 mg/g. The factors that control the deposition of glycogen in the fetus are complex, although it seems clear that the enzymes concerned with its synthesis occur before those concerned with its degradation (Dawkins, 1963).

Effects of malnutrition

Studies in experimental animals have shown that the effects of undernutrition on the liver depend on the timing of the deprivation and its length. If the deprivation occurs at a time when the liver is normally growing at a faster rate than the remainder of the body, in the rat at 3–7 weeks, the weight of the liver continues to increase, but if it occurs after the liver has passed the peak of its growth curve, 6–10 weeks, it will decrease (Jackson, 1915). The livers of children suffering from kwashiorkor accumulate fat and microscopically there may be only a thin rim of cytoplasm surrounding a large fat globule. Serial biopsies of the livers of children suffering from kwashiorkor and undergoing treatment (Waterlow and Weisz, 1956) showed that after 3–8 weeks the proportion of fat had fallen from 338 to 83 g/kg fresh weight. The ratio of protein nitrogen/DNA-P rose from 49 to 69 over the same period.

The liver as a storage organ

Iron exists in the liver in several forms. There is some iron that forms part of the cellular structure and the iron-containing enzymes. Iron is also part of the haemoglobin molecule and therefore is present because of the blood contained in the organ. Haemosiderin, a colloidal ferric hydroxide-phosphate, occurs as a brownish yellow granular pigment. Ferritin consists of a globulin, apoferritin, to which iron in the form of ferric hydroxide–phosphate micelles is bound on the surface of the protein. Haemosiderin and ferritin are the forms in which iron is stored in the liver. Up to 35 per cent of the haemosiderin molecule may consist of iron, and 23 per cent of the molecule of ferritin.

More iron crosses the placenta than the fetus requires for growth, and a human fetus weighing less than 300 g may have as high a concentration of iron in its liver as a full-term baby (Widdowson and Spray, 1951). The concentration of iron in human liver both before and after birth is very variable. However, in spite of this variability there is a characteristic life curve, the value being high at birth, falling to a minimum at 2 years and then rising again. The values for adults are very variable, and one reason for this is that the subjects may have taken medicinal iron preparations at some time in their lives or have received blood transfusions. Iron which is absorbed and deposited in the liver cannot be removed unless the individual suffers from severe repeated haemorrhages. Iron-deficiency anaemia leads to a reduction in the storage of iron in the liver. This form of anaemia occurs during suckling because of a diet poor in iron during a period of rapid growth.

Copper is mainly stored in the liver but the concentration varies enormously from species to species and from one age to another within each species. In man, and some other species (calf and pig) the concentration is very much higher at birth than in the adult. In man, and some other species (rat, rabbit, cat and pig) the 'adult' concentration is reached soon after the end of the weaning period.

The brain

The growth and development of the brain is influenced by a complex interplay of factors. It is generally recognized that intelligence, a manifestation of brain function, is in part genetically determined and that there is for each individual a genetically determined potential. The attainment of this potential is then influenced by both the external environment and the internal milieu. These factors include nutrition, endocrine status, infections, sensory stimulation, parental care and many others. Any attempt at a detailed discussion of the effects of these factors is beyond the scope of

this chapter. However, the effects of nutrition on brain growth are clearly of importance in children with PEM, and these are primarily found in developing countries. The discussion is also relevent to two groups of children in Western societies – the 'small-for-dates' baby and the infant with disease which impairs the absorption or the metabolism of nutrients. The latter group includes children with cystic fibrosis, coeliac disease and phenylketonuria. Deficiencies or excesses of single nutrients may have profound effects on brain organogenesis. Excesses which can cause problems include that of vitamin A, which can cause anencephaly.

Brain growth

The period of maximum growth of the brain with reference to birth and when expressed as a rate curve is species-specific (Figure 1.7; (Davison and Dobbing, 1966). For the human brain, this 'growth spurt' occurs perinatally, in contrast to that of the guinea-pig, which occurs prenatally, and that of the rat, which occurs postnatally. Davison and Dobbing suggested that the growth spurt of the brain constituted a 'vulnerable' or 'critical' period, when adverse influences would have their greatest effect on brain growth. It should be remembered, however, that anatomical, physiological, biochemical and psychological functions of the brain all have a critical period of development when they are maturing at their most rapid rates. Moreover, within each aspect of growth there are also different critical periods. Thus, the period of most rapid cellular division is not the same as that for myelination or that when the growth of dendrites, dendritic arborization, is at its maximum. Also, the brain consists of a number of discrete parts such as the cerebrum, cerebellum and brain stem and the critical periods of different aspects of growth and function will differ from one part to another. What we are

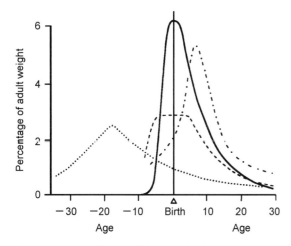

Figure 1.7 Velocity of human brain growth (wet weight) compared with that of other species. Prenatal and postnatal age is expressed as follows: human (——) in months; guinea-pig (·····) in days; pig (- - - - -) in weeks; rat (- · - · -) in days [reproduced from Davison and Dobbing (1966) *Br. Med. Bull.* **22**, 40–44, by permission of Oxford University Press]

considering in this chapter is an overview of brain composition.

Cellular growth

We have seen that tissue growth can occur by hyperplasia and by hypertrophy and that these processes can be assessed by measuring the DNA content and the protein/DNA ratio, respectively. Although the DNA content gives an accurate assessment of the number of cells, it does not differentiate between different cell types. The brain contains many kinds of cells which can be broadly categorized into glial cells and neurones. The ratio of the numbers of these cell types differs in different species. Within the glial cells, astrocytes differ from oligodendroglia in size and shape and, within the neurones, large cerebral neurones differ from small cerebellar neurones.

In man, the wet weight of the brain increases until about 6 years of age (Dobbing and Sands, 1973). Before birth, DNA synthesis is fairly linear but soon after birth there is a decline in the rate; synthesis continues until at least 6 years of age. If the data are plotted in a semi-logarithmic fashion it is possible to identify a sharp decline in the rate of DNA accretion at about 18 weeks gestation, which is considered to be due to the end of maximal neuronal multiplication (Figure 1.8). Continued DNA accretion is probably largely due to glial cell multiplication. The forebrain and brain stem DNA levels reach 70 per cent of mature values by 2 years of age and thereafter gradually increase to reach a maximum at 6 years of age. In the cerebellum, DNA replication proceeds more rapidly and achieves adult levels by 2 years. Although the cerebellum accounts for only 10 per cent of the brain weight it contains 30 per cent of the total brain DNA.

The effect of development on the composition of the human brain

We have seen that the brain weight increases rapidly early in life. Although it contributes a falling percentage of the body weight before birth, at birth it still accounts for more than 10 per cent of the body weight compared with about 2 per cent in the adult. The changes in its gross composition (Table 1.12) follow the pattern that we have seen in the other organs and tissues. Although the fall in water content and rise in nitrogen content are small during fetal life compared with those that occur after birth, they are accompanied by changes in sodium, potassium and chloride similar to those that occur in other tissues. It is to be noted, however, that the biggest changes in composition occur after birth, with large decreases in water, sodium and chloride and large increases in the concentrations of potassium and particularly of phosphorus. More detailed analysis of different parts of the human brain (MacArthur and Doisy, 1919) showed that the brain stem had the lowest percentage of water in the adult brain, but this

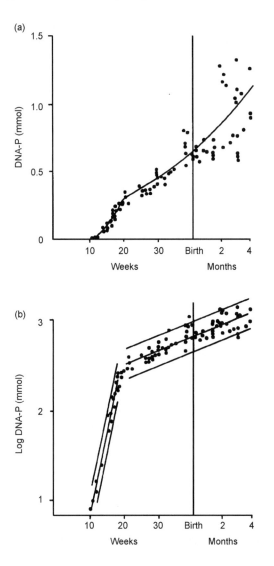

Figure 1.8 Total amounts of DNA phosphate, equivalent to cell number, in the forebrain of human foetuses and infants, (a) amounts per forebrain and (b) a semi-logarithmic plot of the same data with regression lines with 95% confidence limits added [reproduced from Dobbing and Sands (1973) *Arch. Dis. Child.* **48**, 757–767]

was only a little lower than in the forebrain. In both the brain stem and forebrain, the main decrease in water content took place between 8 months and 21 years and was due to a large increase in lipid content. Analysis of white and grey matter (Johnson *et al.*, 1949) has shown no difference in the percentage of water during intrauterine life. After birth the proportion of water in grey matter falls to an adult level of about 84 per cent between 5 and 10 years of age. In white matter, there is a much larger fall in the percentage of water due to the accumulation of myelin. This appears from crude analysis to be completed between 5 and 10 years of age. The distribution of water in the brain is difficult to assess since there is controversy about the size and nature of the extracellular space. Some scientists, mainly electron microscopists, seem to favour a small space, whilst physiologists favour one of conventional size. A consideration of the development of the blood–brain barrier and its nature is also involved (Dobbing, 1968). Detailed microscopic study of the process of myelination (Yakovlev and Lecours, 1967) has shown that this process may not be completed in some parts of the brain until about 30 years of age.

The brain contains practically no neutral fat, that is triglyceride. The bulk of its lipid content is in the form of cholesterol and complex lipids – phospholipids, glycolipids and other esters which contain various fatty acids. Esterified cholesterol is not present in the mature brain. The proportion of the total cholesterol which is esterified falls from about 5 per cent in early foetal life in the forebrain and cerebellum to about 1 per cent at about 30 weeks gestation, with a small rise and subsequent fall during early postnatal life (Yusuf *et al.*, 1981). The changes in the proportion of cholesterol esters in the brain stem are rather smaller.

In the central nervous system (CNS), the bulk of the complex lipids is present in myelin, which is formed from the membranes of oligodendroglial cells, and myelination begins when these cells have ceased dividing (Altman, 1969). These glial cells then surround the nerve axons in a spiral fashion and a progressive

Table 1.12 Effects of development on the composition of the human brain; values expressed per kg of fresh whole brain (Widdowson and Dickerson, 1960)

	Fetus		Newborn baby	Adult
	13–14 weeks	20–22 weeks		
Weight of brain (g)	4.65	34	365	1438
Weight of brain as percentage body weight	15.0	13.4	13.4	2.3
Water (g)	914	922	897	774
Total nitrogen (g)	9.6	8.4	9.3	17.1
Sodium (mmol)	97.5	91.7	80.9	55.2
Potassium (mmol)	49.6	52.0	58.2	84.6
Chloride (mmol)	72.1	72.6	66.1	40.5
Phosphorus (mmol)	57.0	52.2	54.0	109
Magnesium (mmol)	–	4.2	3.9	5.7
Calcium (mmol)	–	2.4	2.4	2.0

deposition of lipids occurs within the developing myelin sheath, resulting in the transformation of the glial cell membranes into the specialized mature myelin with its lamellated structure. Myelin accounts for about 50 per cent of the total lipid in the adult brain and over 25 per cent of its weight (Chase, 1976). Evidence from the rate of accumulation of cerebroside sulphate (a glycolipid selectively located in myelin) shows that myelin rises rapidly between 12 and 24 weeks, and between 34 weeks' gestation and term the content rises by some 300–400 per cent. The adult amount is probably formed before 4 years of age. The replication of the oligodendroglial cells whose membranes form myelin is a key factor in the formation of new myelin.

Phospholipids are important constituents of all cell membranes, including myelin. Before birth, the phospholipid pattern of the human forebrain, cerebellum and brain stem is similar, with choline phosphoglycerides as the major phospholipids (Yusuf and Dickerson, 1977). After birth the brain stem shows the greatest change in pattern with ethanolamine phosphoglyceride becoming dominant. This change is probably due to the large amount of white matter accumulating in this part of the brain.

Besides cerebrosides, the other principal glycolipids in the brain are the gangliosides. These substances contain N-acetylneurominic acid, sphingosine and three molecules of either glucose or galactose. A number of different species of ganglioside are found in the human brain but four of them contribute about 95 per cent of the total ganglioside content. While small amounts of gangliosides are present in glial cells, the bulk is found in the neurones (Dekirmenjian et al., 1969). In the rat, the microsomal disialoganglioside, GD1a (according to the Svennerholm classification, Dickerson, 1981) has been found to be concentrated in synaptic membranes (Yusuf and Dickerson, 1978) and can be used as a marker for dendritic arborization with the accompanying synaptogenesis. The changes in the ganglioside pattern with growth and development in different parts of the human brain are complex (Yusuf et al., 1977). However, since the ganglioside GD1a has been found to be specifically located in synaptic membranes in the rat, it is tempting to suggest that the sharp increase in the amount of this substance in the human forebrain between about 30 weeks' gestation and about 9 months after birth is due to an increase in dendritic arborization during this time consequent upon increases in brain stimulation and function.

Effects of PEM on brain composition

It was for some time considered that the brain was 'spared' the effects of undernutrition, but recognition that the 'growth spurt' constitutes a 'critical' period for its growth and development has led to a re-assessment of the matter. Studies in experimental animals, principally the rat, have shown that if the animal's growth is retarded at the time of the growth spurt the brain will never achieve its appropriate number of cells and degree of myelination on rehabilitation (Dobbing, 1974). The smaller brains of undernourished children contain smaller amounts of DNA than the larger brains of

controls of the same age (Winick, 1976), but probably the appropriate amount for their weight (Figure 1.9; Dickerson et al., 1982). The same is also true of the amount of cholesterol in the brain and it may be concluded that malnutrition does not have a specific effect on either cell multiplication or on myelination. In contrast, the absolute amounts of the disialoganglioside, GD1a, are specifically reduced, being too small for the weight of the brain (Figure 1.10). It would seem that PEM reduces dendritic arborization and possibly brain function. However, care is necessary in making this interpretation as, in undernourished rats, Morgan and Winick (1980) have shown that

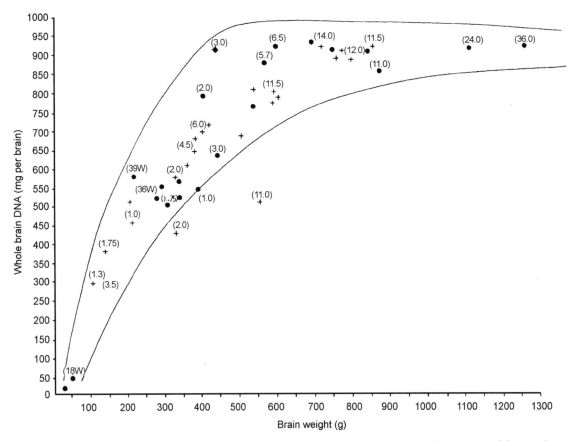

Figure 1.9   The DNA content of brains from 'normal' (●) and malnourished (+) children. Age of fetuses shown in weeks and that of children shown in months [reproduced from Dickerson (1981) *Maturation and Development*, pp. 110–130, by permission of Heinemann]

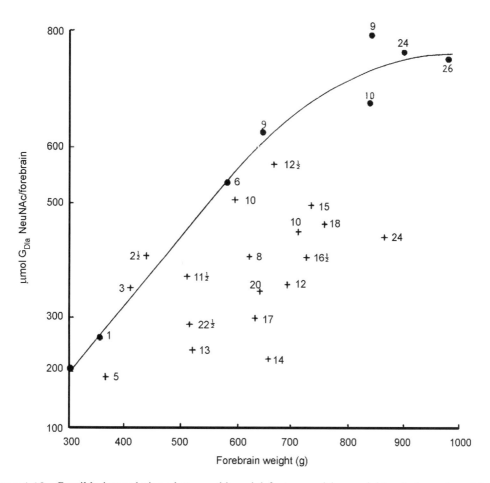

Figure 1.10 Possible interrelations between biosocial factors and low weight gain in malnourished children. (After Cravioto *et al* (1967), reproduced with permission.)

positive environmental stimulation, such as handling and stroking, causes changes in behaviour and increases the ganglioside content of the brain. This leads to the possibility that the abnormally low values for GD1a in the brains of malnourished children are not due primarily to the nutritional deprivation, but to lack of environmental stimulation. Cravioto *et al.* (1966) have emphasized the complexity of the conditions (Figure 1.11) to which the malnourished child may be subject and the difficulty of identifying cause and effect relationships.

Contribution of Major Soft Tissues to Total Amounts of Body Constituents During Growth

Table 1.13 shows that the major soft tissues considered in this chapter together contribute a greater proportion of water, nitrogen, sodium, potassium and chloride to the total body content at birth than in the 20–22 week fetus. Whilst the proportion of water and nitrogen which they contribute in the adult shows practically no change, the proportions of

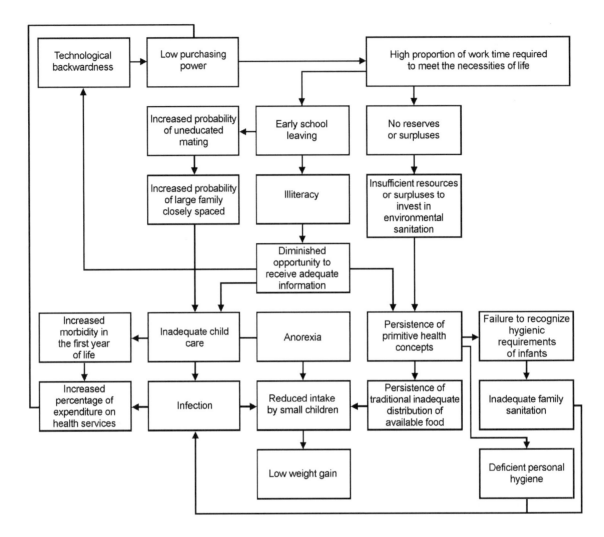

Figure 1.11 Interrelation between biosocial factors and low weight gain [reproduced from Cravioto *et al.* (1966) *Pediatrics* **38**, 319–372, by permission]

sodium and chloride fall. In the case of chloride, the fall is likely to be accounted for by the decrease in the volume of ECF. Whilst this also contributes to the fall in the proportion of sodium, there is also an accumulation of sodium in the skeleton during postnatal development. The major soft tissues account for only about 10 per cent of the body's phosphorus and probably less than 1 per cent of the body's calcium. The bulk of the body's content of these two minerals is located in the skeleton and if the dietary intake of either is deficient the main effect will be on the bones.

Conclusion

The growth, development and consequent changes in chemical composition of our bodies and organs are differential processes whose timing is subject to nature, nurture and

Table 1.13 Contribution (percentage) of the constituents of skeletal muscle, skin, liver and brain to the total amounts of water, nitrogen and minerals in the human body during growth (Widdowson and Dickerson (1964) *Mineral Metabolism*, Vol. 2A, pp.1–217; reproduced by permission of Academic Press)

	Fetus	Newborn	Adult
Water	56	68	65
Total nitrogen	52	62	62
Sodium	53	61	39
Potassium	69	74	74
Chloride	53	70	56
Phosphorus	25	18	9
Magnesium	35	33	23
Calcium	1.6	1.1	0.4

nutrition. The interaction of these factors may have both short-term and long-term effects. With reference to the latter, the results of careful observations and studies in man, and of experiments in animals, on the effects of timing of nutritional deprivation laid an early basis for the current interest in the effects of biochemical programming on the development of disease in later life. In the words of the Psalmist, 'I am fearfully and wonderfully made' (Psalm 139 v. 14).

References

Altman J (1969) DNA metabolism and cell proliferation. In: *Handbook of Neurochemistry*. Vol. 2, ed. Lajtha A. Plenum Press, London.

Barker DJP (1994) *Mothers, Babies, and Disease in later Life*. BMJ Publishing Group, London.

Behnke AR, Feen BG and Welham WC (1942) The specific gravity of healthy men, body weight/volume as an index of obesity. *JAMA* **118**, 495–498.

Bradfield RB and Jelliffe EFP (1970) Early assessment of malnutrition. *Nature* **225**, 283–284.

Bradfield RB, Bailey MA and Margen S (1967) Morphological changes in human scalp hair roots during deprivation of protein. *Science* **157**, 438–439.

Cabak V, Dickerson JWT and Widdowson EM (1963) Response of young rats to deprivation of protein or of calories. *Br. J. Nutr.* **17**, 601–606.

Chase HP (1976) Undernutrition and growth and development of the human brain. In: *Malnutrition and Intellectual Development*, ed. Lloyd-Still JD, pp. 13–38. MTP, Lancaster.

Cole TJ (1979) A method for assessing age-standardized weight-for-height in children seen cross-sectionally. *Ann. Hum. Biol.* **6**, 249–268.

Cole TJ (2001) Use and abuse of centile curves for BMI. In: *Nutrition in the Infant*, ed. Preedy V, Grimble G and Watson R, pp. 39–43. Greenwich Medical Media, London.

Consensus Development Conference (1991) Diagnosis, prophylaxis and treatment of osteoporosis. *Am. J. Med.* **90**, 107–110.

Consensus Development Conference (1993) Diagnosis, prophylaxis and treatment of osteoporosis. *Am. J. Med.* **94**, 646–650.

Cooke AM (1955) Osteoporosis. *Lancet* **i**, 877–937.

Coward WA, Parkinson SA and Murgatroyd PR (1988) Body composition measurements for nutrition research. *Nutr. Res. Rev.* **1**, 115–124.

Cravioto J, Delicardie ER and Birch HG (1966) Nutrition, growth and neurointegrative development: an experimental ecological study. *Pediatrics* **38**, 319–372.

Cravioto J, Birch HG, de Licardia ER, Rosales L (1967) The ecology of infant weight gain in a pre-industrial society. *Acta Paediatr. Scan.* **56**, 71–84.

Cuthbertson DP (1932) Observations on the disturbance of metabolism produced by injury to the limbs. *Q. J. Med.* **25**, 233–246.

Davison AN and Dobbing J (1966) Myelination as a vulnerable period in brain development. *Br. Med. Bull.* **22**, 40–44.

Dawkins MJR (1963) Glycogen synthesis and breakdown in rat liver at birth. *Q. J. Exp. Physiol.* **48**, 265–272.

Dekirmenjian H, Brunngraber EG, Lemkey-Johnston N and Larramendi LMH (1969) Distribution of gangliosides glycoprotein-NANA and acetylcholinesterase in axonal and synaptosomal fractions of cat cerebellum. *Exp. Brain Res.* **8**, 97–104.

Dickerson JWT (1960) The effect of growth on the composition of avian muscle. *Biochem. J.* **75**, 33–37.

Dickerson JWT (1962a) Changes in the composition of the human femur during growth. *Biochem. J.* **82**, 56–61.

Dickerson JWT (1962b) The effect of development on the composition of a long bone of the pig, rat and fowl. *Biochem. J.* **82**, 47–55.

Dickerson JWT (1981) Nutrition, brain growth and development. In: *Maturation and Development*, ed. Conolly KJ and Prechtl HFR, pp. 110–130. Spastics International Medical Publications, Heinemann, London.

Dickerson JWT and Hughes PCR (1972) Growth of the rat skeleton after severe nutritional intra-uterine and post-natal retardation. *Resuscitation* **1**, 163–170.

Dickerson JWT and John PMV (1964) The effect of sex and site on the composition of skin in the rat and mouse. *Biochem. J.* **92**, 364–368.

Dickerson JWT and John PMV (1969) The effect of protein-calorie malnutrition on the composition of the human femur. *Br. J. Nutr* **23**, 917–924.

Dickerson JWT and McAnulty PA (1975) The response of hind-limb muscles in the weanling rat to undernutrition and subsequent rehabilitation. *Br. J. Nutr.* **33**, 171–180.

Dickerson JWT and McCance RA (1960) Severe undernutrition in growing and adult animals 3. Avian sleletal muscle. *Br. J. Nutr.* **14**, 331–338.

Dickerson JWT and Widdowson EM (1960) Chemical changes in skeletal muscle during development. *Biochem. J.* **74**, 247–257.

Dickerson JWT, Merat A and Yusuf HKM (1982) Effects of malnutrition on brain growth and development. In: *Brain and Behavioural Development*, ed. Dickerson JWT and McGurk H, pp. 73–108. Surrey University Press Blackie, Glasgow.

Dobbing J (1968) The development of the blood–brain barrier. *Prog. Brain Res.* **29**, 417–427.

Dobbing J (1974) The later development of the brain and its vulnerability. In: *Scientific Foundations in Paediatrics*, ed. Davis JA and Dobbing J, pp. 565–577. Heinemann, London.

Dobbing J and Sands J (1973) Quantitative growth and development of human brain. *Arch. Dis. Child.* **48**, 757–767.

Elia M and Ward LC (1999) New techniques in nutritional assessment: body composition methods. *Proc. Nutr. Soc.* **58**, 33–38.

Fewtrell MS, Cole TJ, Bishop NJ and Lucas A (2000a) Neonatal factors predicting childhood in preterm infants: evidence for a persisting effect of early metabolic bone disease? *J. Paediatr.* **137**, 668–673.

Fewtrell MS, Prentice A, Cole TJ and Lucas A (2000b) Effects of growth during infancy and childhood on bone mineralization and turnover in preterm children aged 8–12 years. *Acta Paediatr.* **89**, 148–153.

Fomon SJ, Haschke F, Zeigler EE and Nelson SE (1982) Body composition of reference children from birth to age 10 years. *Am. J. Clin. Nutr.* **35**, 1169–1175.

Freeman JV, Cole TJ, Chin S, Jones PRM, White EM and Preece MA (1995) Cross sectional stature and weight reference curves for the UK. *Arch. Dis. Child.* **73**, 17–24.

Frisch RE (1994) The right weight: body fat, menarche and fertility. *Proc. Nutr. Soc.* **53**, 113–129.

Fuller NJ, Jebb SA, Laskey MA, Coward WA and Elia M (1992) Four component model for the assessment of body composition in humans: comparison with alternative methods, and evaluation of the density and hydration of fat-free mass. *Clin. Sci.* **82**, 687–693.

Fuller NJ, Hardingham CR, Groves M, Screaton N, Dixon AK, Ward LC and Elia M (1999) Comparison of fundamental bio-electrical impedence analysis and anthropometric methods for predicting magnetic imaging estimates of lower limb muscle cross-sectional area. *Proc. Nutr. Soc.* **58**, 134A.

Grimble RF (1990) Nutrition and cytokine action. Nutrition and cytokine action. *Nutr. Res. Rev.* **3**, 193–210.

Hamill PVV, Drizd TA, Johnson CL, Reed RB and Roche AF (1977) *NCHS Growth Curves for Children, Birth to 18 years.* US Department of Health, Education and Welfare Publications no. PHD 78-1650. National Center for Health Statistics, Hyattsville, MD.

Hamilton WJ, Boyd JD and Mossman HW (1945) *Human Embryology*, ed. Heffer W. Cambridge University Press, Cambridge.

Harkness MLR, Harkness RD and James DW (1958) The effect of a protein-free diet on the collagen content of mice. *J. Physiol.* (*Lond.*) **144**, 307–313.

Harrison MF (1953) Composition of the liver cell. *Proc. R. Soc. Lond. B* **141**, 203.

Holland P, Wilkinson A, Diez J and Lindsell D (1990) Prenatal deficiency of phosphate, phosphate supplementation and rickets in very low birth weight infants. *Lancet* **335**, 697–701.

Hughes PCR and Tanner JM (1970) A longitudinal study of the growth of the black hooded rat; methods of measurement and rates of growth for skull, limbs, pelvis, nose–rump and tail lengths. *J. Anat.* **106**, 349–371.

Jackson CM (1915) Changes in the relative weight of the various organs of young albino rats held at constant weight by underfeeding for various peroids. *J. Exp. Zool.* **19**, 99.

Jebb SA, Garland SW, Jennings G and Elia M (1994) Measurement of gross body fat using dual energy X-ray absorpsiometry. *Proc. Nutr. Soc.* **53**, 222A.

Johnson AC, McNabb AR and Rossiter RJ (1949) Concentration of lipids in the brain of infants and adults. *Biochem. J.* **44**, 494–498.

Lechtig A and Klein RE (1981) Prenatal nutrition and birth weight: is there a causal association? In: *Maternal Nutrition in Pregnancy – Eating for Two?*, ed. Dobbing J, pp. 131–174. Academic Press, London.

MacArthur CG and Doisy EA (1919) Quantitative chemical changes in the human brain during growth. *J. Comp. Neurol.* **30**, 445–486.

Macy IG, Kelly HS and Sloan RE (1953) *The Composition of Milks*. National Academy of Sciences National Research Council Publication no. 254 (revision of Publication no. 119).

McCance RA (1962) Food, growth and time. *Lancet* **ii**, 621–626.

McCance RA and Widdowson EM (1957) Hypertonic expansion of the extracellular fluids. *Acta Paediatr.* **46**, 337–353.

McLean FC and Urist MR (1961) *Bone – an Introduction to the Physiology of Skeletal Tissue*, 2nd edn, p. 51. University of Chicago Press, Chicago, IL.

McNeill G, Fowler PA, Maughan RJ, McGaw BA, Gvozdanovic S, Gvozdanovic D and Fuller MF (1989) Body fat in lean and obese women by six methods. *Proc. Nutr. Soc.* **48**, 23A.

Medawar PB (1944) The shape of the human being as a function of time. *Proc. R. Soc. Lond. B* **132**, 133–141.

Mendes CB and Waterlow JC (1958) The effect of a low-protein diet, and of refeeding, on the composition of liver and muscle in the weanling rat. *Br. J. Nutr.* **12**, 74–88.

Montgomery RD (1962) Growth of human striated muscle. *Nature* **195**, 194–195.

Morgan BLC and Winick M (1980) Effects of environmental stimulation on brain *N*-acetyl-neuraminic acid content and behaviour. *J. Nutr.* **110**, 425–432.

Moulton CR (1923) Age and chemical development in mammals. *J. Biol. Chem.* **57**, 79.

Naeye RL (1981) Maternal nutrition and pregnancy outcome. In: *Maternal Nutrition in Pregnancy –*
Eating for Two, ed. Dobbing J, pp. 81–111. Academic Press, London.

Naismith DJ (1981) Diet during pregnancy – a rationale for prescription. In: *Maternal Nutrition in Pregnancy – Eating for Two?*, ed. Dobbing J, pp. 21–40. Academic Press, London.

Neuberger A and Slack HGB (1953) The metabolism of collagen from liver, bone, skin and tendon in the normal rat. *Biochem. J.* **53**, 47–52.

Neuman WF and Neuman MW (1958) *The Chemical Dynamics of Bone Mineral*. University of Chicago Press, Chicago, IL.

New SA (2001) Exercise, bone and nutrition. *Proc. Nutr. Soc.* **60**, 265–274.

Nystrom M, Peck L, Kleemola-Kujula E, Evalahti M and Kataja M (2000) Age estimation in small children: reference values based on counts of deciduous teeth in Finns. *For. Sci. Int.* **110**, 179–188.

Papoz L, Eschwege E. Pequignot G and Barrat J (1981) Dietary behaviour during pregnancy. In: *Maternal Nutrition in Pregnancy – Eating for Two?*, ed. Dobbing J, pp. 41–69. Academic Press, London.

Passmore R and Eastwood MA (1986) *Human Nutrition and Dietetics*, 8th edn. Churchill Livingstone, Edinburgh.

Prentice AM (1998) Body mass index standards for children. *Br. Med. J.* **317**, 1401–1413.

Richards OW and Kavanagh AJ (1945) The analysis of growing form. In: *Essays on Growth and Form, Presented to D'Arcy Wentworth Thompson*, ed. Le Gros Clark WE and Medawar PB, pp. 188–230. Clarendon Press, Oxford (quoted by Tanner, 1962).

Rogers HJ, Weidmann SM and Parkinson A (1952) Studies on the skeletal tissues 2. The collagen content of bone from rabbits, oxen and humans. *Biochem. J.* **50**, 537–542.

Sands J, Dobbing J and Gratrix CA (1979) Cell number and cell size: organ growth and development and the control of catch-up growth in rats. *Lancet* **ii**, 503–505.

Scammon RE (1930) *The Measurement of Man*. University of Minnesota Press, Minneapolis, MN (quoted by Tanner, 1962).

Shelley HJ (1961) Glycogen reserves and their changes at birth and in anoxia. *Br. Med. Bull.* **17**, 137–143.

Singh R (1995) Secular increase in body size and nutritional anthropometric measurements of Indian children. In: *Essays on Auxology*, ed. Hauspie R, Lindgren G and Falkner F, pp. 322–333. Castlemead Publications, Welwyn Garden City.

Slater JE and Widdowson EM (1962) Skeletal development of suckling kittens with and without supplementary calcium phosphate. *Br. J. Nutr.* **16**, 39–48.

Smith CA, Cherry RB, Maletskos CJ, Gibson JG, Roby CC, Cation WL and Reid DE (1955) Persistence and utilization of maternal iron for blood formation during infancy. *J. Clin. Invest.* **34**, 1391–1402.

Smith R (1960) Total body water in malnourished infants. *Clin. Sci.* **19**, 275–285.

Tanner JM (1962) *Growth at Adolescence*, 2nd edn. Blackwell Scientific, Oxford.

Tanner JM (1978) *Foetus into Man*, pp. 150–153. Open Books, London.

Tanner JM, Whitehouse RH and Healy MJR (1961) Standards for skeletal maturity based on a study of 3000 British children. 2. The scoring system for all 28 bones of the hand and wrist. Thesis. Institute of Child Health, University of London.

Tanner JM, Whitehouse RH and Takaishi M (1966) Standards from birth to maturity for height, weight, height velocity and weight velocity: British children, 1965. *Arch. Dis. Child.* **41**, 454–471; 613–635.

Townsend N and Hammel EA (1990) Age estimation from the number of teeth erupted in young children an aid to demographic surveys. *Demography* **27**, 165–174.

Vico L, Collet P, Guignandon A, Lafage-Proust MH, Thomas T, Rehaillia M and Alexandre C (2000) Effects of long-term micro-gravity exposure on cancellous and cortical weight-bearing bones of cosmonauts. *Lancet* **355**, 1607–1611.

Waterlow JC and Weisz T (1956) The fat, protein and nucleic acid content of the liver in malnourished human infants. *J. Clin. Invest.* **35**, 346–354.

Wells JCK, Fuller NJ, Dewit O, Fewtrell MS, Elia M and Cole TJ (1999) Variability in the composition of the fat-free mass in children aged 8–12 years. *Proc. Nutr. Soc.* **58**, 17–23.

Whedon GD (1960) Osteoporosis: atrophy of disuse. In: *Bone as a Tissue*, ed. Rodahl K, Nicholson JT and Brown EM, p. 67. McGraw–Hill, New York.

Whitehead RG and Paul AA (2000) Long-term adequacy of exclusive breast feeding: how scientific research has led to revised opinions. *Proc. Nutr. Soc.* **59**, 17–23.

Widdowson EM (1951) Mental contentment and physical growth. *Lancet* **i**, 1316–1318.

Widdowson EM (1959) Chemical structure, functional integration and renal regulation as factors in the physiology of the newborn. In: *Physiology of Prematurity*, p. 97. Transactions of the 4th Conference, Josiah Macy Jr Foundation, New York.

Widdowson EM (1970) Harmony of growth. *Lancet* **i**, 901–905.

Widdowson EM and Dickerson JWT (1960) The effect of growth and function on the chemical composition of soft tissues. *Biochem. J.* **77**, 30–43.

Widdowson EM and Dickerson JWT (1964) Chemical composition of the body. In: *Mineral Metabolism*, vol. 2A, ed. Comar CL and Bronner F, pp. 1–217. Academic Press, New York.

Widdowson EM and Spray CM (1951) Chemical development *in utero*. *Arch. Dis. Child.* **26**, 205–214.

Winick M (1976) Nutrition and cellular growth of the brain. In: *Malnutrition and Brain Development*, pp. 63–97. Oxford University Press, London.

Winick M and Noble A (1965) Quantitative changes in DNA, RNA and protein during prenatal and postnatal growth in rats. *Devl. Biol.* **12**, 451–466.

Winick M, Meyer KK and Harris RC (1975) Malnutrition and environmental enrichment by adoption. *Science* **190**, 1173–1175.

Wyshak G and Frisch RE (1982) Evidence for a secular trend in age of menarche. *New Engl. J. Med.* **306**, 1033–1035.

Yakovlev PI and Lecours A-R (1967) The myelogenetic cycles of regional maturation of the brain. In: *Regional Development of the Brain in Early Life*, ed. Minkowski A, pp. 3–65. Blackwell Science, Oxford.

Yusuf HKM and Dickerson JWT (1977) The effect of growth and development on the phospholipids of the human brain. *J. Neurochem.* **28**, 783–788.

Yusuf HKM and Dickerson JWT (1978) Disialoganglioside GD1a of rat brain subcellular particles during development. *Biochem. J.* **174**, 655–657.

Yusuf HKM, Dickerson JWT, Hey EN and Waterlow JC (1981) Cholesterol esters of the human brain during fetal and early postnatal development: content and fatty acid composition. *J. Neurochem.* **36**, 707–714.

Yusuf HKM, Merat A and Dickerson JWT (1977) Effect of development on the gangliosides of human brain. *J. Neurochem.* **28**, 1299–1304.

2

PRE- AND PERICONCEPTUAL NUTRITION

Jane Coad

LEARNING OUTCOMES

- Discuss the association between body size and puberty, describing possible mechanisms of control.

- Describe the effects of undernutrition, obesity and weight fluctuations on fertility and outcomes of pregnancy.

- Describe the evidence and implications of recommendations to consume folic acid supplements during the periconceptual period.

- Critically discuss the role and effects of deficiency of other specific nutrients on reproductive potential.

- Discuss the effects of lifestyle choices on fertility.

Introduction

Nutritional status in women is linked to reproductive outcome. Unfavourable conditions result in the suspension of reproductive function, but adaptation to poor nutrition can occur. Nutrition before pregnancy can affect fertility, early development and nutritional status throughout pregnancy and this might affect a woman's ability to withstand nutritional insults during pregnancy. Recently, it has become evident that there are also a

number of potential links between nutrition
and male reproductive performance.

Because nutrition and growth appear to be
crucial in determining the onset of puberty, as
well as affecting the success of fertilization,
implantation and subsequent development and
growth, nutrition is also closely associated with
reproductive potential throughout the life-
span. Historically, the sensitivity of the hypothalamus to environmental influences, such as
nutrient availability, was probably of immense
importance in promoting pregnancy in seasons
when the fetus and infant had optimal chances
of survival. Although the greatest nutritional
vulnerability is probably before a woman
realizes she is pregnant, preconceptual nutrition has a broader remit than considering how
nutrition affects fertility alone. It is the 'take-
home' baby rate rather than fertility *per se* that
is important. Practically, the question is whether there is an advantageous diet or an
advantageous body weight which favours conception and early development and maximizes
the chances of the baby being born healthy and
of optimum birth-weight. Material in Chapters
1, 4 and 10 should be read in relation to this
chapter.

The Relationship Between Body Size and Reproductive Potential

The onset of puberty and body size

The age of menarche has been getting progressively earlier over the last century, although it
now seems to have reached a plateau (Cole,
2000). Menarche requires sufficient oestrogen
production from the ovarian follicles to permit
endometrial build-up and breakdown. The
cascade of events, from increased gonadotrophin secretion from the anterior pituitary
gland to increased gonadal production of
sex steroids resulting in changes in the

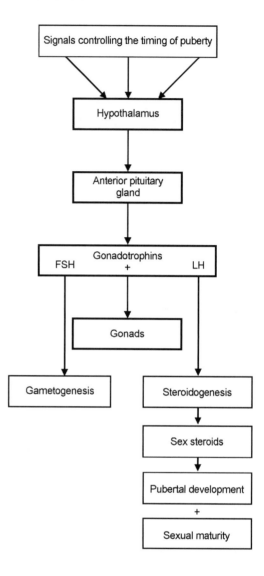

Figure 2.1 Signals controlling puberty. The physical
changes of puberty are controlled by gonadal, adrenal and
pituitary hormones. Hypothalamic pulsatile secretion of
gonadotrophin-releasing hormone (GnRH) controls
pituitary secretion of the gonadotrophins, follicular-
stimulating hormone (FSH) and luteinizing hormone
(LH). Immediately after birth, levels of gonadotrophins
are in the adult range, but they decline over the first year of
life and remain at a low level throughout childhood until
the onset of puberty. Early puberty is marked by a
dramatic change in LH secretion which increases in
magnitude and exhibits a circadian pattern

reproductive systems, leading to puberty and sexual maturity, is driven by increased secretion of gonadotrophin-releasing hormone (GnRH) from the hypothalamus (Figure 2.1). Whereas the age of menarche in Western countries is decreasing, a woman's body size at menarche has remained constant. It was first suggested in the 1960s that body weight and food intake initiated puberty in rats (Kennedy and Mitra, 1963). Frische and Arthur (1974) hypothesized that the maintenance of weight above a threshold level and body fat above a threshold mass are critical in permitting the onset and regularity of menstrual cycles and hence reproductive function. The critical fat hypothesis proposed that, to be reproductively mature, girls require a fat-to-lean ratio of about 24 per cent fat, a proportion of fat approximately equivalent to the energy demands of pregnancy and lactation (Frische, 1990). The association between body size and menarche was supported by the findings that undernourished women, such as ballet dancers and those with anorexia nervosa, had delayed puberty.

As the rate of sexual maturity is clearly more dependent on growth and body size than on chronological age, the regulating factor appears to be nutrition. However, the data linking body weight to age at menarche show a broad individual range. The critical fat hypothesis can be criticized because both the rate of growth and age at the onset of menarche can be considered to be end-points of a genetic body plan established much earlier, before the changes in puberty. This is supported by observations that children entering puberty earlier than their peers tend to be taller and heavier throughout early life. The recent rise in childhood obesity has led to an appreciable weight increase prior to puberty in many children without any effect on menarche (Cole, 2000). The hormonal changes heralding puberty occur before the peak height velocity, fat deposition and menarche. Late maturers may simply gain fat more slowly than early maturers. This is supported by the finding that height rather than weight seems to be the better predictor of timing of menarche (Ellison, 1982).

Although Frische identified the association between fatness and reproductive function, the putative mechanism remained more elusive. Adipose tissue is an important site of steroid hormone production and metabolism (Pasquali et al., 1997). Indeed, in postmenopausal women, adipose tissue is a significant source of extra-ovarian oestrogen and, therefore, important in bone and cardiovascular health. The amount and also the position of body fat affect the production of different oestrogens. Frische suggested several possible mechanisms centring on steroid hormone metabolism by the endocrinologically active adipose cells (Frische, 1990). Metabolic pathways in adipose tissue can convert androgens to oestrogens, oestradiol to oestrone and dihydroepiandrosterone to androstenediol (Pasquali et al., 1997). Although oestrone is less metabolically active than oestradiol, it adds to the level of circulating oestrogens, which have a negative feedback effect at the pituitary. As adrenarche precedes menarche, peripheral precursors of adipose-derived oestrogen would be available for metabolism by fat tissue. Steroid hormone metabolism by adipose tissue could also modify oestrogen production, producing more or less potent forms (see Table 2.1).

Adipose tissue also acts as a store of steroid hormones and so might influence levels of steroid hormone binding globulin (SHBG), although how these factors could affect the timing of puberty is not clear. The major criticism of fat cell metabolism triggering the onset of puberty is that a gradually increasing

Table 2.1 Biological activity of oestrogens

Oestradiol 17β E_2 (100%)
Oestriol E_3 (10%)
Oestrone E_1 (1%)

level of oestrogen from adipose tissue is more likely to inhibit GnRH, and therefore pre-ovulatory follicular development, via negative feedback, rather than stimulate it.

Despite the lack of demonstrated mechanisms, the association between better nutrition and growth and the timing of reproductive function has received much attention. Although critical levels of body weight and fat mass are associated with normal reproductive function, other factors are clearly involved (Bringer *et al.*, 1997). Low body fat is not invariably associated with reduced fecundity (Sinning and Little, 1987). On the other hand, a substantial proportion of anorexic young women do not resume normal menstrual function within a year of their weight being restored to the normal range (Schweiger *et al.*, 1987). Most species in the wild reproduce when they are in positive energy balance rather than when a threshold level of fat is deposited, and fertility can be suspended by disrupted energy intake in mammals before body fat content diminishes (Bronson, 2000). These observations led to the emphasis changing from a critical weight or level of fatness to a critical level of a metabolic signal (Foster and Nagatani, 1999). The metabolic fuel hypothesis proposed that the availability and oxidation of 'metabolic fuels' could link nutrition and reproduction, possibly by metabolites being sensed by the brain and liver (Wade *et al.*, 1996). The altered level of circulating metabolic intermediates would then be signalled centrally, thus tying nutritional status mechanistically to control of the reproductive axis. The essential concept is that the neuro-endocrine mechanisms controlling reproduction respond to acute changes in energy balance rather than energy reserves so the intracellular sensory signals generated by changes in energy balance have a greater role than those signals arising from changes in body fat content. The two theories as described above, critical body fat mass vs a metabolic signal, rather than being mutually exclusive, seemed to be integrated with the discovery of leptin (Zhang *et al.*, 1994). Leptin has now become a subject of major interest and research and, because of this, a detailed account of its importance in reproductive function is given below.

The role of leptin in reproductive function

Leptin, the 16 kDa (167 amino acid) protein product of the *ob* gene, is produced predominantly by adipocytes. Concentrations of leptin in plasma directly reflect the amount of body fat (Dagogo-Jack *et al.*, 1996). Leptin binds to specific receptors in the hypothalamus (Pelleymounter *et al.*, 1995) and plays a significant role in the control of adiposity and energy balance by suppressing food intake and stimulating energy expenditure. It thus acts as a satiety signal regulating appetite and energy balance (Saladin *et al.*, 1995). Leptin is secreted in a pulsatile pattern and has a circadian rhythm with a nocturnal rise, peaking between 01:00 and 02:00 h (Licinio *et al.*, 1998). This pattern of secretion synchronizes with the secretory pattern of luteinizing hormone (LH).

The model of action is that leptin is released from adipose tissue and binds to receptors in the arcuate region of the hypothalamus. Many of the peptides and neurotransmitters implicated in appetite and food intake are also known to influence secretion of GnRH. Cells from the arcuate nucleus project to a number of regions including the lateral hypothalamic nuclei, such as the ventromedial area, which is involved in appetite regulation, the paraventricular nucleus, which can be considered to be the stress centre, and the preoptic area, which has GnRH-containing cells and is important in reproduction. In the hypothalamus, leptin stimulates two classes of neuron which independently regulate adipose tissue mass and control reproduction (Figure 2.2). Regulation of adipose mass occurs via the

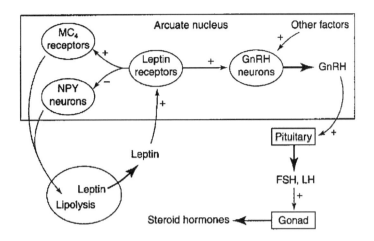

Figure 2.2 Leptin regulation of lipolysis and reproduction. Adipocytes secrete leptin which activates the leptin receptor expressing neurons in the arcuate nucleus of the hypothalamus. Projections from these neurons stimulate the melanocortin MC_4 receptors and the neuropeptide Y (NPY)-containing neurons to activate the sympathetic nervous system which regulates lipolysis in the adipose tissue. Leptin receptors also interact with the GnRH-containing neurons affecting the reproductive axis. [Reprinted from Chehab FF (2000) *Trends Pharmac. Sci.* **21**, 309–314, with permission from Elsevier Science]

melanocortin MC_4-receptor-expressing neurons. The neuropeptide Y (NPY) neurons activate the sympathetic nervous system controlling lipolysis. Occupation of the leptin receptors of the hypothalamus stimulates the GnRH neurons and triggers secretion of GnRH. Other factors affecting the reproductive axis, such as NPY, growth hormone and insulin, also mediate activation of the GnRH neurons (Chehab, 2000).

Leptin is thought to exert its metabolic effects by suppressing NPY expression and secretion. NPY is a potent orexigenic (appetite-stimulating) agonist which stimulates food intake. Leptin also has endocrine effects on the gonadotrophin axis mediated by NPY. Increased NPY activity is inhibitory to the gonadotrophin axis, which is a mechanism for inhibiting sexual maturation and reproductive function if food is restricted or energy expenditure is high (Schubring *et al.*, 2000). Under optimum nutritional conditions, the levels of leptin would increase, thus suppressing NPY activity and lifting inhibition on the gonadotrophin axis (Kiess *et al.*, 1997), so

secretion of gonadotrophins and sex steroids would increase. Leptin also has direct effects on the pituitary gland and gonads. It is suggested that it affects the growth and development of the pituitary cells and increases sensitivity of the pituitary by amplifying signals from the hypothalamus (Caprio *et al.*, 2001).

Genetically obese (*ob/ob*) mice have a homozygous mutation of the *ob* gene and are leptin-deficient (Figure 2.3). They have reduced GnRH levels and low circulating gonadotrophin levels. The female *ob/ob* mice are infertile and male *ob/ob* mice have impaired spermatogenesis. Leptin treatment, but not energy restriction, can promote maturation of the hypothalamic–pituitary–gonadal axis of *ob/ob* mice and allow them to reproduce successfully (Chehab *et al.*, 1996). This suggests that leptin deficiency rather than obesity is the cause of the infertility. Genetically obese mice with a mutation of the *db* gene, which encodes for the leptin receptor, are leptin-insensitive and have chronically high levels of leptin. Administration of leptin to *db/db* mice has no effect on

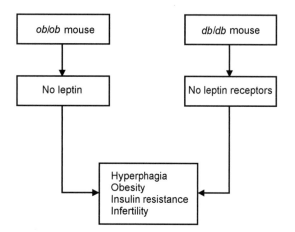

Figure 2.3 Mouse models of leptin deficiency and insensitivity. The genetically obese mouse (*ob/ob*) is leptin deficient. It has reduced levels of GnRH and gonadotrophins and is infertile. It is hyperphagic, insulin resistant and obese. Leptin treatment, but not energy restriction, restores fertility. The *db/db* mouse, which has a mutation of the leptin receptor, has a similar phenotype. However because the defect is at the receptor level, the mouse is leptin-insensitive so exogenous leptin does not affect appetite or restore fertility

food intake, body weight and fertility (Campfield *et al.*, 1995). Although reproductive function in both *db/db* and *ob/ob* mice is similarly disrupted, leptin does not either affect appetite or restore fertility in *db/db* mice, because the defect is at the receptor level (Caprio *et al.*, 2001).

As well as its effects on weight regulation in *ob/ob* mice, the administration of leptin also restores fertility (Chehab *et al.*, 1996). This critical discovery suggested that leptin might be the pivotal signal from fat to the brain, indicating that the fat stores are adequate to support reproduction. Underweight women and those with eating disorders produce low levels of leptin, presumably below the critical threshold to permit reproduction (Köpp *et al.*, 1997).

As fat stores increase during growth, production of leptin gradually rises in proportion. When body mass index (BMI) is adjusted for,

leptin levels at puberty in both girls and boys are elevated (Blum *et al.*, 1997). At menarche, leptin levels can be correlated with increased adipose tissue mass (Ahmed, 1999) and the rise in serum leptin concentration precedes the changes in gonadotrophin and oestrogen production (Garcia-Mayor *et al.*, 1997). After puberty, there is a sexual dimorphism; in males, leptin levels reach a peak in early puberty and then decline, whereas in females leptin levels continue to rise, so females have three to four times as much circulating leptin. Although it has been demonstrated that there is a prepubertal nocturnal leptin surge in monkeys (Suter *et al.*, 2000), a similar surge has not been identified in humans, possibly because of the difficulty in the continuous blood sampling protocols necessary to demonstrate the leptin surge in other species (Chehab, 2000).

Dieting, self-induced weight loss and low body weight are all associated with delayed menarche. Effectively, the initiation of puberty can be delayed by undernutrition or excess energy expenditure relative to intake. Prepubertal women have a lower proportion of body fat and a greater strength-to-weight ratio (Cumming *et al.*, 1994). Strenuous athletic training is associated with a pubertal delay which correlates to the level of competition (Cumming *et al.*, 1994). In athletic amenorrhoea, the ovarian events of puberty (breast development and menarche) are affected but not those of adrenarche (pubic hair growth). During periods of inactivity, there is advancement of the pubertal stages.

The link between puberty and leptin is supported by findings that treatment of prepubertal mice with recombinant leptin accelerates their onset of puberty (Chehab *et al.*, 1997) and allows onset of puberty in severely food-restricted rats (Gruaz *et al.*, 1998). Transgenic mice with elevated leptin levels exhibit precocious puberty (Yura *et al.*, 2000). It seems that leptin alters the pulse frequency of GnRH secretion (Nagatani *et al.*, 1998); fasting reduces leptin release, which suppresses LH secretion, by affecting the pulsatile release of GnRH (Foster and Nagatani, 1999).

Despite the identification of a metabolic signal apparently associated with reproduction, the definitive mechanism underlying the link between nutrition and fertility has not yet been elucidated. The critical fat hypothesis lacked a link between fat mass and the hypothalamus. Although leptin appears to fulfil a number of the criteria identified for a blood-borne signal between adipose tissue and brain, there are a number of reservations in accepting that leptin induces puberty rather than acting in concert with a number of other factors. Leptin levels and body fat content can be dissociated; the extent of leptin fluctuations does not correlate with the proportion of body fat. Leptin concentrations fall during fasting without discernible changes in body weight or fat mass. Leptin levels are labile, fluctuating with short-term energy intake rather than with levels of energy reserves (Schneider and Wade, 2000). Although there are diurnal changes in leptin concentration, mean levels are maintained over a longer period. Also, paradoxically, in the medical literature there are case studies of women who are leptin-deficient having normal reproductive progression and being fertile (Chehab, 2000).

A number of different models have been proposed to explain how leptin regulates GnRH release and reproduction. Firstly, leptin could regulate GnRH independently of other nutritional factors. Although there are leptin receptors in the hypothalamus and supporting evidence that leptin can stimulate GnRH release, this model does not explain why short-term fluctuations in dietary intake can affect reproduction and how other metabolic fuels could act as signals. Inhibitors of metabolic oxidation suppress reproductive function long before fat stores and leptin production change (Wade and Scheneider, 1996). Thus it is debatable whether leptin acts as a primary stimulus of the reproductive axis or acts as a permissive factor in the onset of puberty (Clarke and Henry, 1999). Instead of being the primary trigger which determines the pubertal spurt, leptin may play a permissive role in the onset of puberty rather than acting to regulate reproductive function in the short term. As a tonic mediator, leptin might be required to be present above a certain threshold, acting permissively as a metabolic gate before other factors can trigger puberty (Cheung et al., 1997).

There is evidence from a number of sources that the effect of leptin on GnRH secretion, LH release and the onset of puberty can be modified by glucose availability and insulin (Foster and Nagatani, 1999), suggesting that leptin works in collaboration with other metabolic signals. This led to a second model being proposed whereby signals about reserve energy (fatness signalled by leptin) determine the threshold for current energy (glucose availability) and are integrated to regulate GnRH neuronal activity (Figure 2.4). Alternatively, there could be a cascade of GnRH regulation steps whereby leptin-induced changes in glucose availability, possibly mediated by leptin-induced recruitment of insulin-dependent glucose transporters such as GLUT4, relayed information to the GnRH neuro-secretory system. Leptin might also interact with other signals such as GH and insulin-like growth factor-I (IGF-I; Caprio et al., 2001).

There is still an on-going debate about the mechanisms underlying nutritional infertility. Most of the factors that increase hunger and affect food intake also decrease reproductive function. A number of signals have been proposed, such as hormones, neurotransmitters and metabolic substrates, but levels of these probably change secondary to the true primary sensory signal, the metabolic events that occur on the transition to negative energy balance and metabolic adaptations to conserve energy during seasonal changes in food availability and climatic conditions (Schneider and Wade, 2000). In humans and primates, sexual

Possible models:

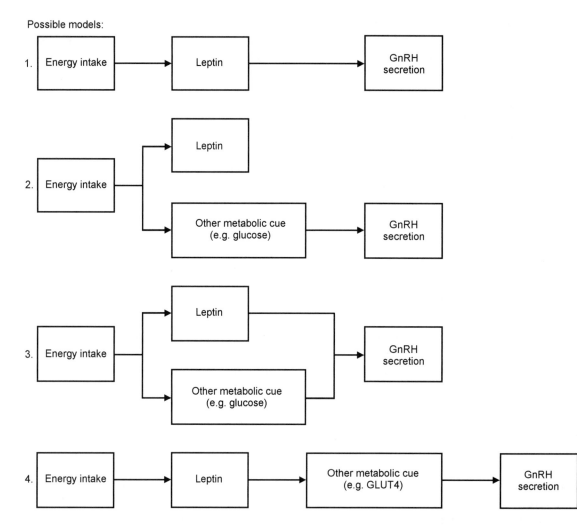

Figure 2.4 Possible models of leptin regulation of reproduction. (1) Energy intake affects leptin secretion which regulates GnRH secretion and regulates reproduction. (2) Reproduction is controlled by another metabolic cue which, like leptin, increases in response to feeding. (3) Both leptin and another metabolic cue interact to affect GnRH secretion and regulate reproduction. (4) The effect of leptin is mediated by the metabolic cue

behaviour and fertility may be dissociated, but sexual desire and activity, as well as reproductive function, are adversely affected by metabolic challenges (Juiter *et al.*, 1993).

In conclusion, there are three types of hypotheses about the control of nutritional infertility: (1) adipostatic theories where the critical signal is a long-term energy reserve in the form of fat; (2) hormone theories where the level of hormone(s) signal the state of short-term energy balance; and (3) metabolic theories where availability or oxidation of metabolic substrates generates the primary signal. Currently, the support for reproduction being controlled by availability and oxidation of intracellular levels of metabolic fuels is growing. Leptin continues to have a role, but the emphasis is on its effects on fuel availability and oxidation in cells of specific tissues and consequent responsiveness to energetic challenges. The suggestion that reproduction might be controlled, not directly by an alteration in hormone concentration, but by a metabolic event is analogous to the control of insulin secretion from pancreatic β cells being dictated by the metabolic flux (Malaisse, 1998).

Effect of Body Weight on Reproductive Success

In developing children, it is obviously difficult to dissociate growth-induced signals affecting reproductive potential from those induced by nutrition alone. However, in adults, who are somatically mature, growth is complete so the effects of nutrition and associated metabolism can be resolved by studying the effect of extremes of body weight on reproductive success.

Undernutrition

The relationship between reproductive success and seasonal fluctuations in nutrient supply has been extensively studied in animals (Stein and Susser, 1991; Short, 1994). Evolutionary aspects of human feeding patterns with periods of feast and famine led to the suggestion that humans only had adequate nutrition to allow a fairly short period of fertility each year. Van der Walt *et al.* (1978) reported that fluctuations in availability of food and physical exercise associated with food-seeking resulted in a seasonal cycle of fertility in women of the South African *!Kung San* (Bushman) tribes. Both long-term undernutrition and short-term periods of nutritional imbalance have been associated with adverse effects on reproductive outcome. Examples include the effect of undernutrition on fertility seen in whole populations, such as the effects of famine and war, and chronic undernutrition associated with poverty

and eating disorders. Women who were exposed to nutrient deficiency during the early stages of pregnancy had an increased likelihood of having a baby with a developmental problem (Stein *et al.*, 1975).

Normal reproductive function appears to be suspended when nutritional intake is significantly compromised. During the famines of World War II, which produced useful results about the effect of undernutrition in pregnancy, the severe food deprivation resulted in a significant increase in amenorrhoea. This suspension of reproductive function can be viewed as protective to the mother as she can conserve energy for her own needs. Also poor nutrition appears to act as a signal to prevent investment in a pregnancy that might result in an infant with poor potential for survival. However, some women did conceive during the war (Figure 2.5); the rates of spontaneous abortions, congenital abnormalities, perinatal mortality and low birth-weight were increased in these poorly nourished women (Stein *et al.*, 1975). At the end of the periods of food deprivation, fertility and reproductive performance improved. From a teleological perspective, the linking of nutrition and reproduction allows the interaction between environmental factors which may limit a successful outcome of pregnancy. Darwin observed in 1859 that lack of food and hard living affected the fertility of free-living relatives of domesticated animals. In mammalian species, ovulatory cycles are lengthened or interrupted by inadequate energy intake or excessive energy expenditure that is not offset by increased food intake (Schneider and Wade, 2000).

The effects of poor nutrition on female reproductive function can manifest in a number of ways (Figure 2.6). At the most extreme level of amenorrhoea, reproductive cycles are suspended and anovulatory with a monophasic hormone profile. There are also variations of non-fertile cycles. Some cycles have an abbreviated luteal phase (of less than 10 days) where the follicle does not luteinize;

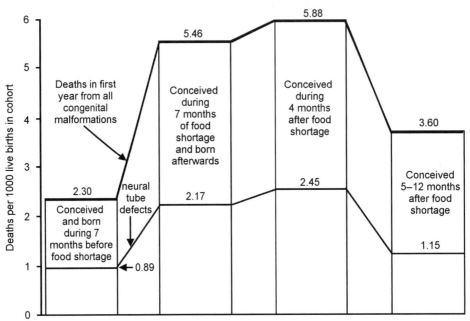

Figure 2.5 Increased incidence of congenital malformations among babies conceived during and after the Dutch Hunger Winter 1944–1945, 154 365 births, 452 deaths. [Reprinted from *The Case for Preconception Care of Men and Women*, M Wynn and A Wynn, p. 78 (1991), © AB Academic Publishers, Bicester]

usually these are anovulatory and shorter cycles. Luteal phase defects describe cycles of normal length but with abnormally low progesterone secretion. Oligomenorrhoea is irregular cycles (36–180 days). If follicular development is compromised, the cycle may be lengthened because the dominant follicle fails and another less-mature follicle takes over the dominant role and begins to develop, which extends the follicular phase, thus delaying ovulation. There may also be sub-clinical abnormalities where the cycle length is not altered, but ovulation is compromised; anovulation is often associated with oligomenorrhoea, but may also occur latently in cycles of normal length. The normal pattern of ovulatory menstrual cycles is periodically disturbed, more often immediately after menarche and preceding menopause, but also with physiological and psycho-social stresses.

Eating disorders and subnormal body weight are associated with reproductive dysfunction. Loss of a third of body fat or 10–15 per cent of normal body weight may result in abnormal reproductive function (Wentz, 1980). Severe undernutrition in anorexia nervosa results in amenorrhoea and infertility with low and non-pulsatile GnRH secretion and extremely low plasma and cerebrospinal fluid levels of leptin (Mantzoros *et al.*, 1997). The secretion of hormones reverts to a prepubertal pattern. It has been shown that the critical threshold of plasma leptin below which menstruation ceases is 1.85 ng/ml (Köpp *et al.*, 1997). Leptin values above this threshold are necessary but not solely sufficient for menstruation to resume (Audi *et al.*, 1998) so other factors, such as IGF-I, as well as increased leptin production, are needed. In bulimia nervosa, menstrual irregularities can occur,

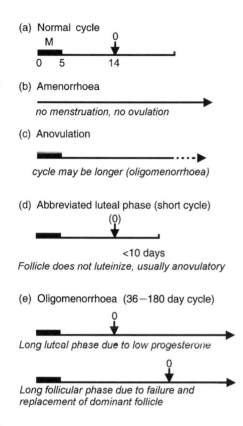

(a) Normal cycle

(b) Amenorrhoea

no menstruation, no ovulation

(c) Anovulation

cycle may be longer (oligomenorrhoea)

(d) Abbreviated luteal phase (short cycle)

<10 days
Follicle does not luteinize, usually anovulatory

(e) Oligomenorrhoea (36–180 day cycle)

Long luteal phase due to low progesterone

Long follicular phase due to failure and
replacement of dominant follicle

Figure 2.6 Disrupted menstrual cycles. (a) A typical normal menstrual cycle of 28 days with ovulation occurring at day 14; (b) amenorrhoea is the absence of menstrual cycles and ovulation; (c) anovulation is the absence of ovulation, however, menstruation may appear to be normal if follicular development and hormone synthesis occur to some extent; (d) abbreviated luteal phase results usually in a shorter than normal cycle which is usually anovulatory; (e) oligomenorrhoea is defined as a cycle longer than 36 days. The luteal phase may be lengthened because progesterone production is low; alternatively failure of the dominant follicle and subsequent recruitment of a replacement follicle can extend the follicular phase of the cycle

but as body weight is at a normal level, amenorrhoea is not usual, so bulimics are more fertile than anorexics.

In athletes and women with eating disorders or psychogenic amenorrhoea, high levels of cortisol and endogenous corticotrophin-

releasing hormone (CRH) have been observed (Villanueva *et al.*, 1986). CRH inhibits GnRH release, suppresses fasting-induced suppression of pulsatile LH secretion and increases corticosterone levels (Loucks *et al.*, 1989). It is possible that the physiological role of the increased leptin production from increasing fat stores contributes to the restoration of fertility because it is antagonistic to cortisol. Increased CRH release from the hypothalamus in response to hypoglycaemia is abrogated by leptin (Heiman *et al.*, 1997).

However, the relationship between nutrition and fecundity is not totally straightforward. Low body fat is not invariably associated with menstrual irregularity and menstrual irregularities are not always associated with low body fat. Patterns of food intake and acute fluctuations in nutrient levels can disrupt fertility in women who have a normal range of body fat. Reproductive dysfunction is more common in sports in which a thin body build is desirable, but the effect of low body fat levels may be confounded by abnormal eating patterns which are more prevalent in female athletes (Cumming *et al.*, 1994). There are also examples, in both humans and other mammals, of reduced fertility associated with chronic undernutrition being spontaneously resolved (Clarke and Henry, 1999). Indian women subject to chronic undernutrition have reduced fertility but eventually become fertile without improved dietary intake (Schneider and Wade, 2000). Conception can occur in women who are markedly below ideal body weight; pregnancy has been reported in women with a BMI of less than $15\,kg/m^2$ (Treasure and Russell, 1988). However, women who enter pregnancy in an undernourished state with limited nutrient stores are more likely to have growth-retarded, low-birth-weight babies who continue to follow a poor growth trajectory throughout childhood (Reifsnider and Gill, 2000). Undernourished women are more vulnerable to nutrient insult and are more dependent on the quality of their diet during the pregnancy as maternal stores are compromised.

Dietary fluctuations, metabolism and reproduction

A short-term increase in the provision of a high-energy diet at least one reproductive cycle before fertilization, following maintenance on a sub-optimal diet, can cause an acute increase in reproductive activity in some species, such as sheep (Foster and Nagatani, 1999). The effect, described as 'flushing', is manipulated in sheep to increase the rate of twinning. Similar responses are observed in experimental animals, where it can be demonstrated that the high energy intake in diet-restricted animals causes an increase in LH pulse frequency, reflecting increased hypothalamic GnRH secretion. Further evidence that short-term fluctuations in dietary intake affect reproductive potential comes from the observations that acute fasting, for a period of 24 h, dramatically reduces pulsatile LH secretion, which is then rapidly restored on re-feeding (Schreihofer et al., 1993). This effect of fasting can be dissociated from fasting-induced stress, indicating that it is a nutritional signal. A number of possible signals have been proposed, including glucose availability, metabolic oxidation and insulin secretion (Foster and Nagatani, 1999). Kennedy and Mitra (1963) proposed that, as the organism reaches mature size, the rate of growth slows down and basal metabolic rate falls. Developmental changes in metabolic state occur in response to altered nutrient partitioning as the animal grows (Foster and Nagatani, 1999). As the proportion of nutrients used to maintain heat falls, the brain senses the energy surfeit and its metabolic consequences. A number of contenders for the blood-borne substance(s) linking metabolism to the brain have been suggested, including glucose, insulin and amino acids (Steiner et al., 1983).

Strenuous exercise in women can also affect hypothalamic pituitary function. In athletes, amenorrhoea is associated with lack of follicular development and ovulation and a lack of phasic secretion of hormones. Asymptomatic ovulatory dysfunction may also result from exercise. This may result in prolonged follicular phases or shortened luteal phases with reduced progesterone production.

Dieting alone, without gross weight reduction, is also associated with irregular or disrupted menstrual cycles. Even mild energy reduction can cause menstrual irregularities in women of normal body weight, despite their weight not falling below 100 per cent of ideal body weight (Pirke et al., 1989). Severe dieting has more dramatic effects on ovulation (Rock et al., 1996).

Vegetarianism

It has been suggested that vegetarian diets and low energy intake might influence the menstrual cycle and fertility (Pirke et al., 1987), which would have implications for bone health as well as fertility. Pirke suggested that vegetarian diets affected the menstrual cycle more than non-vegetarian diets, even when both cause the same weight loss (Pirke et al., 1986). As vegetarian women often tend to weigh less than non-vegetarian women, it could be postulated that they are more likely to experience energy imbalances and body weight fluctuations, causing menstrual disturbances. However, although several studies suggest clinical menstrual cycle disturbances may be more common in vegetarian women than omnivorous women, a prospective study which carefully controlled for many potential confounders (such as adopting a vegetarian diet in order to lose weight) found that subclinical disturbances were less common in weight-stable healthy vegetarian women than those whose weight fluctuated (Barr, 1999).

The phases of the menstrual cycle, as well as the total length of the cycle, may be affected by diet. In vegetarian and non-vegetarian women with regular menstrual cycles, energy intakes have been shown to be higher in the luteal phase of ovulatory menstrual cycles than in the follicular phase or luteal phase of anovulatory cycles (Barr *et al.*, 1995). High dietary restraint is associated with a shortened luteal phase length (Barr *et al.*, 1994) and certain dietary components, such as fat, fibre, meat or alcohol, might affect menstrual cycles and hence fertility. Phytochemicals can affect the length of phases of the menstrual cycle: soybean isoflavones increase follicular length (Cassidy *et al.*, 1994), whereas flaxseed lignans increase luteal-phase length (Phipps *et al.*, 1993). High fibre intakes and faster intestinal transit times are associated with lower concentrations of ovarian hormones, whereas fat intake is positively associated with steroid hormone concentrations (Dorgan *et al.*, 1996). Alcohol consumption is also associated with higher levels of steroid hormone concentrations (Reichman *et al.*, 1993). The effects of diet on extending the length of the menstrual cycle or decreasing oestrogen concentration has interesting implications, as there is an association between a high dietary intake of soy products and decreased incidence of breast cancer (Whitten and Naftolin, 1998). Potentially, phytoestrogens could have a role as oestrogen replacement therapy in menopausal women.

Obesity

Obese women have lower fertility rates compared with women of lower weight, both in natural and assisted conception; they also have an increased incidence of miscarriage (Norman and Clark, 1998). Obese and overweight women are over-represented in gynaecological and fertility clinics (Friedman and Kim, 1985). The reproductive outcome in pregnant obese women is also less favourable; folic acid seems to lose its protective effect on neural tube development (Prentice and Goldberg, 1996). Pregnancy complications are greatly increased and pregnancy in obese women is associated with a higher incidence of congenital malformations and perinatal mortality, particularly that associated with preterm delivery. The distribution of fat also seems to be important, with abdominal fat having greater effects on menstrual disorders and infertility than peripheral fat (Norman and Clark, 1998).

The mechanisms by which obesity disrupts the menstrual cycle and fertility seem much more complex than those which mediate low-weight amenorrhoea. Polycystic ovary syndrome (PCOS) which is the most common cause of anovulation and is frequently associated with obesity, provides a useful model for determining the mechanism by which obesity affects fertility (Franks and Robinson, 1996). PCOS is associated with disordered energy expenditure, hyperandrogenism (hirsutism, acne, alopecia) and anovulation (amenorrhoea, oligomenorrhoea, dysfunctional uterine bleeding, infertility); obesity occurs in 35–40 per cent of affected women. The more overweight a woman with PCOS is, the more likely it is that her fertility will be affected (Franks and Robinson, 1996). Obese women with PCOS have lower levels of sex hormone-binding protein and thus higher free levels of testosterone (Kiddy *et al.*, 1990). Anovulatory women with PCOS have hyperinsulinaemia and insulin resistance (Robinson *et al.*, 1993), which seem to be responsible for anovulation. When obese women with PCOS have reduced energy intake, fasting and glucose-stimulated insulin concentrations fall, followed by a change to a more regular menstrual cycle and resumption of fertility (Kiddy *et al.*, 1989).

Weight loss

Weight loss can increase the chance of infertile overweight anovulatory women establishing ovulation and conceiving (Clark *et al.*, 1995). Over a 6-month period, a group of 13 obese PCOS and non-PCOS women on a weekly programme of behavioural change, exercise and diet, lost 6.3 kg on average. Twelve of the subjects resumed ovulation and 11 became pregnant, despite the fact that none of the women achieved their ideal weight and, in most cases, their BMI remained in the obese range. Women failing to complete the programme acted as the control group and did not achieve comparable weight loss or restored reproductive function. The group treatment approach was important for the success of this and other programmes (Galletly *et al.*, 1996), which possibly also had beneficial mood and self-esteem effects; it has been demonstrated that mood state is a predictor of treatment outcome in women undergoing *in vitro* fertilization (Thiering *et al.*, 1993). The extent of weight loss required for restored fertility in these obese women was not clear, but it may have been associated with altered body fat distribution. The weight loss had hormonal effects; levels of insulin and testosterone fell as a result of the energy restriction. As insulin stimulates ovarian androgen production, the weight loss may have restored the hormonal balance. Hyperinsulinaemia and insulin resistance occur in obese women with PCOS. Weight loss programmes, with their attendant health and economic benefits, should be the first step in treating infertile obese women to resolve ovulatory dysfunction (Galletly *et al.*, 1996).

Obese women, including those with PCOS, have high leptin levels (Havel *et al.*, 1996). Obesity appears to be a state of leptin resistance (Maffei *et al.*, 1995). High levels of leptin might lead to uncoupling of eating behaviour, to the filling of fat stores and to relative unresponsiveness of leptin receptors (Schubring *et al.*, 2000), as appears to occur in late gestation. High leptin concentrations acting at the level of the gonads have negative effects on steroidogenesis. In obese women, leptin concentrations are high enough to interfere with oestradiol production by the dominant follicle either directly or by reducing levels of androgenic precursors (Karlsson *et al.*, 1997). Follicular levels of leptin can be used as a predictor of pregnancy success both in normal and obese women with PCOS (Mantzoros *et al.*, 2000).

Optimal body mass index

Research studies clearly demonstrate that extremes of body weight limit fertility, with obese women and women with a BMI less than $21 \, kg/m^2$ being less fertile. The BMI associated with optimal fertility and best outcome of pregnancy in terms of birth-weight is approximately $24 \, kg/m^2$ (Doyle *et al.*, 1990).

Effects of Body Weight on Male Reproductive Function

Women seem more susceptible to the effects of changes in nutrient intake on reproductive function than men, but it is less easy to demonstrate effects of undernutrition on male fertility as the symptomatic changes in spermatogenesis and steroidogenesis are less easy to monitor than an altered menstrual cycle. Preconceptual nutrition in males is not a well-researched field. However, gross nutritional deficiencies or excesses have been shown to affect both conception and the outcome of pregnancy. Starvation studies have demonstrated that undernutrition affects fertility in men as well (Keys *et al.*, 1950). The first response to decreasing weight is reduced libido, followed by decreased prostatic fluid and reduced motility and viability of sperm. Sperm production ceases when weight loss rises above 25 per cent of normal body weight; refeeding restores normal reproductive function. Both general undernutrition and specific zinc deficiency delay puberty (Prasad, 1985), and low vitamin C status was associated with sperm agglutination (Dawson, 1986). As in females, undernutrition delays puberty and affects libido and sexual activity (Cumming *et al.*, 1989). Both undernutrition and obesity affect steroid hormone production; reduced fertility in obese men is associated with raised leptin levels, which have been shown to inhibit testosterone secretion (Isidori *et al.*, 1999). Obesity in men is frequently associated with decreased insulin sensitivity and reduced libido (Norman and Clark, 1998).

Quality of Diet

Although severe food deprivation is associated with impaired reproductive function and embryonic and fetal wastage, it usually does not result in a set of specific malformations following fertilization (Hirschi and Keen, 2000). With severe undernutrition, the growth rate of the fetus is reduced but maternal tissues are catabolized, which results in a release of 'balanced' nutrients into the circulation. In contrast, deficiencies of specific nutrients, such as folate, vitamins A and K, iodine, copper and manganese, have been associated with specific malformations. Poorer maternal diets are associated with increased risk of pregnancy complications. However, definitions of 'poor diets' are variable and it is often difficult to dissociate a poor diet from non-nutritional factors. It is also difficult to identify which of the nutrients present at sub-optimal level in the poor diet is responsible for the effect. Vitamin and mineral supplements are associated with a reduced risk of pregnancy complications, but the protective effects are much greater in women who consume a poor diet (Hirschi and Keen, 2000). In developed countries, primary nutrient deficiencies (insufficient level of a particular nutrient in the maternal diet) are relatively rare. However, secondary or conditional deficiencies might occur. Secondary deficiencies are where the individual

requirement for a specific nutrient is higher than normal because of a gene defect or polymorphism. Folate requirement is a good example of this (see below). A conditioned deficiency is where requirement is high, for instance because of drug–nutrient interactions or a disease process, such as a gene defect causing abnormal metabolism and increasing the risk of deficiency unless dietary intake is increased much above the levels usually required.

Poor levels of nutrition in the first trimester have been implicated in an adverse outcome, such as reduced birth-weight and shorter gestational period. However, examination of the records from the siege in Holland during World War II, when nutrient levels were progressively decreased, has suggested that undernutrition in the first trimester has much less effect than was previously believed (Lumey, 1998). The Dutch Hunger Winter 1944–1945 presents an interesting example of undernutrition in pregnancy because the population was previously well nourished and the famine was fairly short-lived, so it is possible to differentiate between the effects of undernutrition on discrete periods of pregnancy (Lumey, 1998). It is likely that, in other studies (such as Doyle *et al.*, 1990), the adverse effects of poor nutrition in the first trimester of pregnancy were also related to poor nutrition occurring prior to the pregnancy, and during the pre-conceptual period. Preconceptual undernutrition potentially leaves a woman less able to withstand any nutrient insult occurring during pregnancy, such as nausea and vomiting in pregnancy (NVP). Provided a woman is well nourished prior to the pregnancy, NVP is actually associated with a positive outcome of pregnancy (Coad *et al.*, 2001).

Protein intake

Maternal protein intake at the onset of pregnancy was found to correlate well with outcome, particularly the size of the baby at birth (Wynn and Wynn, 1988). Examination of the intake of women who delivered a healthy-sized baby led to the recommendation that 15 per cent of energy originating from protein was optimal. Similar recommendations were produced from the Institute of Medicine (1990), which recommended a protein intake above 85 g/day, in contrast to the UK RNI for pregnant women of 51 g/day (Department of Health, 1991a), a difference which may relate to the efficiency of protein utilization and the intake of other nutrients essential for protein utilization.

Studies in rats have demonstrated that maternal protein deprivation only during the preimplantation period of development causes blastocyst abnormalities with significantly reduced cell number in the inner cell mass or early blastocyst (Kwong et al., 2000) and a slower rate of cellular proliferation throughout development. This brief exposure to maternal low protein levels resulted in reduced birth-weight, overcompensatory growth post-weaning, increased systolic blood pressure and disproportionate growth of specific organs. The effects may have been mediated by a mildly hyperglycaemic maternal environment and consequent reduction in insulin levels plus reduced levels of essential amino acids. In sheep, supplementation of the diet with lupin grain had the effect of increasing the ovulation rate and subsequent reproductive performance (Nottle et al., 1997). In contrast, protein deprivation after implantation at optimal levels of protein has been shown to stimulate placental growth and have a positive effect on birth-weight in cows (Perry et al., 1999).

Micronutrients

In animals, reproductive performance has long been known to depend on nutritional status and the mechanisms underlying the effect of micronutrients on reproduction have been studied to a much greater extent (Table 2.2) than the effect of nutrition on human fertility.

In human reproduction, the emphasis has centred on recommendations for folate preconceptually and in early pregnancy. This focus has produced some useful lessons, which can be related to other aspects of health advice, particularly preconceptual nutrition. For

Table 2.2 Role of micronutrients in animal reproduction

Micronutrient	Mechanism/metabolic function	Deficiency consequences
Vitamin A	Steroidogenesis, embryonic synchrony	Delayed puberty, low conception rate, high embryonic and perinatal mortality, reduced libido in male
Vitamin E	Intramembrane free radical detoxification	Low sperm concentration and high incidence of cytoplasmic droplets, retained fetal membrane
Selenium	Component of glutathione peroxidase	Reduced sperm motility and uterine contraction, cystic ovaries, low fertility rate, retained fetal membrane
Copper	Enzyme component and catalyst involved in steroidogenesis, and prostaglandin synthesis	Low fertility, delayed/depressed oestrus, abortion/fetal resorption
Zinc	Constituent of several metalloenzymes; steroidogenesis, carbohydrate and protein metabolism	Impaired spermatogenesis and development of secondary sex organs in males, reduced fertility and litter size in multiparous species

Adapted from: Smith and Akinbamijo (2000).

instance, it is evident that a significant proportion of pregnancies are not planned and so many women, possibly a majority, are not likely to seek preconceptual counselling at all. It is evident that the earliest opportunity for health advice to be given in a pregnancy is towards the end of the first trimester at the antenatal 'booking' visit. It is also apparent that knowledge does not necessarily lead to a change of practice.

During the maturation of both the sperm and ova, DNA synthesis and cell replication are rapid, but few studies have examined the nutrient requirements necessary to support this. Theoretically, the greatest risk to the oocyte is prior to ovulation (Crisp, 1992). The ovum is also very susceptible to mutagenic agents in the period immediately after fertilization until the first cleavage is completed. Over half of human conceptions are thought to fail to implant and of those that implant, 30 per cent fail to reach term (Keen et al., 1998).

Studies of the diets of women in Hackney (Doyle et al., 1990; Wynn et al., 1991) identified 15 key nutrients of which low intake very early in pregnancy was associated with delivery of smaller babies. Ranked in order, these nutrients are: magnesium, iron, phosphorus, zinc, potassium, thiamin (vitamin B_1), niacin (vitamin B_3), copper, pantothenic acid (vitamin B_5), calcium, riboflavin (vitamin B_2), folic acid, pyridoxine (vitamin B_6) and biotin. Several of these nutrients, such as the B vitamins, are involved in energy transfer and may be implicated because a deficiency might limit the amount of nutrient oxidation and ATP turnover and, therefore, have effects on cell replication, growth and development. 'Energy transfer' nutrients are found in high concentrations in foods which themselves are germinal tissue, such as eggs, seeds and nuts, or those foods which are derived from tissues which have a high energy demand such as heart, brain, liver and kidney (Wynn and Wynn, 1995). Tetragenicity to many chemicals is increased by low nutrient intakes (Wynn and

Wynn, 1995). Wheatgerm has been used to promote fertility in farm animals and race-horses and a wholewheat loaf enriched with wheatgerm was known as 'fertility bread' in the 1930s (Wynn and Wynn, 1995). Fish eggs have also been associated with increasing fertility in South America (Price, cited in Wynn and Wynn, 1995) and are particularly high in the energy transfer nutrients identified in the Hackney studies. Interestingly, many cultures have independently incorporated wheatgerm and eggs and other foodstuffs rich in protein and micronutrients as part of a fertility diet (Wynn and Wynn, 1995).

High dietary intakes of carrots and green peppers, rich in carotene, have been associated with amenorrhoea (Kemmann et al., 1983), although it is not clear whether this was due to the very high carotene intake or to a secondary effect of manipulating the diet. Low serum ferritin levels ($<40 \, \text{ng/ml}$) have also been associated with infertility in women (Rushton, 1991). High intakes of vitamin A from dietary supplements or from therapeutic doses of retinoic acid for acne treatment around the time of conception have been associated with congenital anomalies (Hathcock et al., 1990). The UK guidelines (Chief Medical Officer letter to health professionals, Department of Health, 1991b) advise against consumption of high-dose vitamin A supplements in pregnancy, and consumption of liver and liver products, as these may contain large amounts of vitamin A. Changes in animal husbandry over the last few decades have resulted in domestic animals receiving higher doses of vitamins, so liver and liver products are richer sources of vitamin A than previously.

Folate

Periconceptual nutrition advice has focused on increased requirements for folate and recommendations for folic acid supplements. Folate is the generic name of a number of naturally occurring analogues which are essential in the diet. Folic acid refers to the synthetic form of the vitamin which is metabolized as the other forms of folate, but is more stable and biologically effective. Plasma and serum levels of folate reflect daily fluctuations, whereas red blood cell folate is relatively stable and reflects average folate status over the last 3 months (Kirke *et al.*, 1993). Folate has two important biological roles: it is a cofactor for *de novo* synthesis of purine and thymidine required for DNA and RNA synthesis. Folate deficiency inhibits nucleic acid synthesis and, therefore, DNA synthesis and mitosis or transcription of genes involved in neurulation. Folate is also required for the transfer of methyl groups in the amino acid methylation cycle and the recycling of homocysteine back to methionine. Folate deficiency of the methylation cycle results in inability to methylate proteins, lipids and myelin.

Although there is a geographical variation in incidence, neural tube defects (NTDs) are among the most prevalent congenital abnormalities with an average incidence of 1:500 births worldwide, 1:200 in the UK and 1:80 in south Wales (Department of Health, 2000). The most recent data (Department of Health, 2000) show that in 1998 there were 68 live-born babies affected by a NTD in England and Wales plus 26 NTD-affected still births and 305 NTD-affected therapeutic abortions. It is difficult to estimate the total number of affected pregnancies, but it is estimated that without antenatal screening and selective termination there would have been about 600–1200 affected births in the UK.

NTDs are caused by the failure of the neural tube to close between days 21 and 27 post-conception (Van Allen *et al.*, 1993). The mechanisms underlying the failure of the tube to close either cranially, causing anencephaly, or caudally, causing spina bifida, are not well understood. However, neural tube formation is a complex multifactorial event, associated with rapid cell proliferation and consequent high demand for precursors and co-factors required for morphogenesis that must come from the mother. Initially embryonic nutrition during the period of neurulation is via the histiotrophic uterine secretions (from the uterine glands) and then haemotrophic nutrition (diffusion of nutrients from the maternal blood) is initiated when the primitive vasculature of the developing placenta and embryo begins to circulate the embryonic blood at about 21 days after fertilization. Thus, during the critical period of closure of the neural tube, the nutrient needs of the embryo are provided both by diffusion through the cytotrophoblast from the uterine glands and by the developing fetal circulatory system. At this time the embryo is undergoing a rapid period of growth and organogenesis, so there is an excessive demand for maternally derived precursors and cofactors required for the macromolecules needed for morphogenesis.

Women in lower socio-economic groups and those who consume a diet of relatively poor quality are at increased risk of an NTD pregnancy (Wald, 1994), as are those who have already experienced an NTD pregnancy. Migrants who move from a higher-risk area to an area with a lower risk acquire the new lower risk. This environmental evidence suggested that both genetic and environmental factors, including maternal nutritional status, might be implicated. A number of randomized and non-randomized prospective and retrospective studies (reviewed by Scott and Weir, 1998) demonstrated that intake of folic acid from the preconceptual period through to the first trimester significantly reduced the incidence of NTDs. It seemed that provision of adequate folic acid allowed normal development of the fetal neural tube (Smithells *et al.*, 1980). The Medical Research Council Vitamin Study Research Group (1991) study in the UK demonstrated that folic acid (4 mg/day) supplementation significantly reduced the recurrence rate of NTDs by 71 per cent (Table 2.3).

Table 2.3 Prevention of recurrence of neural tube defects: results of the MRC Vitamin Study 1991

Group	Daily supplementation	Number of pregnancies	Number of NTD	Total number of NTD
A	4 mg folic acid	298	2	6/593 (1.0%)
B	Multivitamin preparation + 4 mg folic acid	295	4	
C	None	300	13	21/602 (3.5%)
D	Multivitamin preparation	302	8	

The study began in July 1983 and was halted in 1991. It involved women in 33 centres who had previously had a pregnancy affected with a NTD. Each participant was randomly assigned to one of four supplementation groups. All participants received ferrous sulphate and calcium phosphate in addition to the supplementation as above. Folic acid supplementation was associated with a 71% reduction in the recurrence of NTD (relative risk = 0.29; 95% confidence level = 0.12–0.71).

The recurrence rate for NTDs is about 10 times the overall incidence, but most (95 per cent) women who have babies with NTDs have not had a previously affected pregnancy. The Hungarian randomized trial (Czeizel and Dudas, 1992) demonstrated that periconceptual folic acid consumption (800 µg/day) also reduces the risk of first-time occurrence of NTDs. Following these studies, it has been UK policy (Department of Health, 1991b) to recommend that women who might become pregnant should consume a supplement of 400 µg/day of folic acid in addition to the average UK dietary intake of about 200–250 µg/day (Department of Health, 2000). The average folate intake per person in the UK is currently estimated at 240 µg/day (MAFF, 1999), which is higher since the 1980s because of increased consumption of fruit and fruit juice and fortified breakfast cereals. Women who have already had an NTD-affected pregnancy are advised to consume a daily supplement of 4 mg folic acid in addition to their dietary intake.

Initially the success of folic acid supplementation in reducing NTDs was attributed to folate deficiency in the mother affecting the closure of the neural tube. However, mothers who delivered a child with a NTD were not found to have markedly low red cell folate levels (Van der Put and Blom, 2000). NTDs affect only a small proportion of women who have a low folate intake and not all women with low red cell folate levels have fetuses with NTDs. There is no evidence that women who have had pregnancies affected by an NTD have defective folate absorption (Bower et al., 1993). Thus it is apparent that susceptibility to NTDs is not related to a primary deficiency of folate but to an increased requirement due to either defective cellular uptake of folate or altered metabolism of the folate pathways. This suggests that the mechanism is a genetic defect of folate metabolism that can be partly overcome by dietary supplementation.

The focus of research has been on genetic mutations of enzymes involved in the methylation cycle (Van der Put and Blom, 2000). A proportion of women with NTD-affected pregnancies were found to have raised homocysteine levels (Steegers-Theunissen et al., 1994). Remethylation of homocysteine to methionine by methionine synthase is folate-dependent. Hyperhomocysteinaemia can be treated by a daily dose of 0.5–1.0 mg folate (Wouters et al., 1993). Thus, rather than being directly due to a deficiency of folate, NTDs seem to be caused by a teratogenic effect of hyperhomocysteinaemia (Rosenquist et al., 1996), so the resulting methionine deficiency is implicated directly in the aetiology of NTDs (Essien and Wannberg, 1993). Women who have a high dietary methionine intake (3 months pre- to 3 months postconception) were found to have reduced risk of NTD-affected pregnancy (Shoob *et al.*, 2001). This study showed that there was a 30–55 per cent lower NTD risk among women whose average dietary intake of methionine was greater that the lowest quartile of intake (>1580 mg/day). Methionine is found in complete proteins (containing all the essential amino acids), specifically animal proteins, such as meat, fish, eggs and dairy products, which are the only important dietary sources. Polymorphisms of the methylenetetrahydrofolate reductase (MTHFR) gene can result in decreased enzyme activity. MTHFR is a regulating enzyme in the folate-dependent remethylation of homocysteine. Genetic studies have demonstrated that one of the MTHFR mutations which causes elevated homocysteinaemia is associated with an increased risk of having an NTD-affected child (Van der Put *et al.*, 1996).

During pregnancy, plasma volume expansion is proportionally greater than the expansion of red blood cell mass so haemoglobin concentration falls (described as 'physiological anaemia of pregnancy') and plasma folate and red cell folate levels progressively fall. Folate status, however, is further reduced during the latter stages of pregnancy and clinical signs of folate deficiency may become evident initially as macrocytic red cells, which may progress to megaloblastic anaemia. It has been suggested that reduced folate status may be associated with reduced intake of dietary folate due to loss of appetite (Scott and Weir, 1998). The transfer of folate to the fetus is small, but the rate of destruction of maternal folate increases in the second and third trimesters (McPartlin *et al.*, 1993), leading to a marked negative folate balance. This means that, unless a woman enters pregnancy with adequate stores to withstand this loss or receives folic acid in supplements or fortified foods during the latter stages of pregnancy, she is at risk of folate deficiency and potentially megaloblastic anaemia (Scott and Weir, 1998). This suggests that

prophylactic folic acid supplements should be recommended not just for prevention of neural tube defects but throughout pregnancy to provide for continuing red blood cell production.

There are three ways of increasing folate consumption: increasing dietary intake, advising women to take supplements, and by food fortification. It is difficult to promote such a change in diet that would allow a three-fold increase of the average folate consumption. It is problematical to achieve the required levels with an increase in dietary intake of folate-rich sources (Cuskelly *et al.*, 1996), particularly as the bioavailability and stability of naturally occurring folate is variable even in rich sources such as green leafy vegetables. Cuskelly *et al.* (1996) reported that young women who were given an extra 400 µg/day folate in the form of unfortified dietary folate had a smaller increase in their red cell folate levels than women who received 400 µg/day in the form of folic acid supplements or from fortified breakfast cereals. Folate is heat labile, particularly in neutral or alkaline solutions, and is susceptible to heavy loss during food preservation techniques; it also has low bioavailability and is not absorbed well, which may explain this finding.

Whilst folic acid supplements have been shown to be effective at reducing NTDs in the intervention trials, in practice few women actually take folic acid supplements preconceptually. Health education campaigns promoting folic acid consumption have tended to increase awareness rather than to actually change behaviour (Wild, 1997). The problem with preconceptual advice generally is that it is estimated that a large proportion of pregnancies are not planned. Women who are not planning to conceive are unlikely to take folic acid supplements. Many women who plan to become pregnant do not comply (Scott and Weir, 1998). There may be a number of reasons for this such as a reluctance to take tablets when feeling healthy, a hesitation to consume medication at all in pregnancy, particularly whilst the memory of thalidomide persists, the naming of folic acid itself and the different perceptions that a label 'acid' has compared with 'vitamin'.

The other option is fortification of food. In the UK, folic acid is voluntarily added to many breakfast cereals. Some breads and fruit juices are also fortified. Current legislation prohibits manufacturers making a health claim for a food so these fortified foods cannot be explicitly labelled as protecting against NTDs. An alternative option would be mandatory fortification of a food at an agreed concentration. The ideal target for such fortification is a dietary staple that is widely consumed but not eaten excessively. Even so, intake will vary depending on an individual's dietary pattern and members of the community other than women of reproductive age will receive larger amounts of folic acid. The preferred food for mandatory folic acid fortification in the UK is flour. Currently, manufacturers in the UK add thiamin, niacin, calcium and iron to flour at the mill. In the USA, grain has been compulsorily fortified with $140 \mu g$ folic acid per $100 g$ grain since January 1998. This is estimated to deliver an average increase of $100 \mu g$ folic acid per day to the average American diet (Allaire and Cefalo, 1998), which is lower than the recommended dose. Daly *et al.* (1997) estimated that an addition of $200 \mu g$ folic acid through fortification in the UK per day would significantly increase the protective effect without unnecessarily high exposure. The Department of Health Report (Department of Health, 2000) concluded that $240 \mu g$ of folic acid per $100 g$ flour (corresponding to a mean additional daily intake of $201 \mu g$ folic acid) was optimal. The incidence of NTDs in the USA has declined by almost 20 per cent since the mandatory fortification of grain products with folic acid (Wise, 2001), so even though the level has been criticized as being too low, the results have renewed pressure on the UK government to implement a similar policy.

Increased consumption of folic acid could potentially pose a risk in two particular circumstances. Pernicious anaemia is an auto-immune condition, usually occurring in older people, in which vitamin B_{12} is malabsorbed because of lack of intrinsic factor and the enteropathic circulation of the vitamin is interrupted. The clinical effects of vitamin B_{12} deficiency are anaemia and neuropathy. Vitamin B_{12} deficiency causes reduced activity of methionine synthase which can create a pseudo-folate-deficient state affecting purine and pyrimidine biosynthesis and thus cell division, causing anaemia. Vitamin B_{12} deficiency also results in lack of methylation of a number of cellular components including myelin basic protein, an important component of the myelin sheath. This leads to degeneration and vitamin B_{12}-associated neuropathy. Increased dietary folate consumption can mask this anaemia and complicate the diagnosis of pernicious anaemia, potentially allowing the neuropathy to progress to an advanced and irreversible state. The mathematical modelling in the Department of Health (2000) report estimated that, if flour was fortified with $240 \mu g$ per $100 g$ flour, 38 NTD-affected births per year would be prevented but approximately 0.6 per cent of people aged over 50 years would be exposed to levels of folic acid greater than $1 mg/day$. At this level of fortification, the risk of detected vitamin B_{12} deficiency increases slightly but some people in this age group are also likely to benefit from an increase in folic acid intake as their current intake is low. The report (Department of Heath, 2000) estimated that around $150 000$ people over 60 with unrecognized vitamin B_{12} deficiency could potentially be at risk if exposed to high intakes of folic acid.

The other potential vulnerable group, should mandatory fortification of flour with folic acid be adopted, are women receiving treatment for epilepsy. Anti-convulsant drugs reduce serum folate levels and may also be independently teratogenic. Pregnant women using anticonvulsant drugs have an increased risk of having a child with a birth defect including an NTD. However, folic acid increases the metabolism of anticonvulsant drugs, thus reducing their concentration and effectiveness (Labadarios *et al.*, 1978), so increased intake of folic acid can interfere with the control of epilepsy or precipitate seizures.

Increased intake of folic acid is associated with other beneficial outcomes in pregnancy, including reduced incidence of other congenital abnormalities such as urinary tract and cardiovascular defects (Czeizel, 1996), cardiotruncal and limb defects (Shaw *et al.*, 1995a) and orofacial clefts (Shaw *et al.*, 1995b). The incidence of low-birth-weight infants born to poorly nourished black women was reduced by folic acid and iron supplements (Baumslag *et al.*, 1970), and premature infants supplemented with folic acid and vitamin B_{12} had higher haemoglobin levels than infants not receiving supplementation (Worthington-White *et al.*, 1994). Prolonged use of oral contraceptives lowers folate status; the concentration of folate in plasma returns to normal levels over a 3 month period once use of oral contraceptives is ceased (Scott and Weir, 1998). There is a higher requirement for folate in multiple pregnancies and an increased requirement (additional 60 μg/day) in lactating women as folate is secreted into breast milk (Department of Health, 2000).

Fortification of flour with folic acid would provide not only a benefit in reducing the incidence of pregnancies affected by neural tube defects, but seems likely also to reduce the incidence of cardiovascular disease. There seems to be a strong association between raised levels of homocysteine and the increased risk of cardiovascular disease; increased intake of folic acid can reduce homocysteine levels (Boushey *et al.*, 1995). Evidence is also accumulating to suggest that increasing folate levels would be beneficial for patients with neurological and neuro-psychiatric disorders, including senile dementia, and may possibly reduce the incidence of some types of cancer (Department of Health, 2000).

Folate is involved in the synthesis of DNA and RNA, so one could speculate that both follicular development and spermatogenesis would be dependent on adequate folate levels. Although consumption of supplementary folic acid is recommended to support the requirements of early development, little is known about its role in fertility. The Hungarian double-blind randomized trial of periconceptional multivitamin supplementation (Czeizel, 1998) demonstrated that, as well as reducing the incidence of neural tube defects and other congenital abnormalities, a vitamin and mineral supplement also improved the fertility rate and increased the incidence of twinning. The multivitamin prepartion used in this study was Elevit Pronatal® (Roche), which contains 12 vitamins, four minerals and three trace elements, including 1200 μg vitamin A and 800 μg folic acid.* Similarly, the effects of folic acid on male fertility are not clear. No beneficial effect of folic acid supplementation for 30 days was found in sub-fertile men (Landau *et al.*, 1978), but spermatogenesis takes about 72 days so the intervention may not have been long enough for an effect to be discernable. No further studies in this area have been published. Zinc and folate interact and zinc deficiency has negative effects on the absorption and metabolism of folate in animal studies (Favier *et al.*, 1993).

Many women of reproductive age consume diets that do not provide an optimal level of nutrients. Although poorer-quality diets are often associated with lower socio-economic status, adolescents and women who are dieting

---

*Full nutritional profile of Elevit Pronatal® (Roche): vitamin A, 1200 μg; vitamin B_1, 1.6 mg; vitamin B_2, 1.8 mg; vitamin B_5, 10 mg; vitamin B_6, 2.6 mg; folic acid, 800 μg; vitamin B_{12}, 4.0 μg; vitamin C, 100 mg; vitamin D_3, 12.5 μg; vitamin E, 15 mg; biotin, 200 μg; nicotinamide, 19 mg; plus calcium, 125 mg; iron, 60 mg; magnesium, 100 mg; phosphorus, 125 mg; copper, 1.0 mg; manganese, 1.0 mg; and zinc, 7.5 mg.

to lose weight may consume markedly less than recommended levels of energy, protein, vitamins and minerals. In addition, behavioural factors such as smoking, alcohol consumption and illicit and prescribed drug use may also affect intake or requirement of essential nutrients. Use of mineral and vitamin supplements might seem to be the obvious solution. Certainly, it is almost impossible to consume the recommended level of folate from dietary sources alone. One might question whether it is appropriate to recommend a level of a nutrient that is so high relative to levels that can be achieved from the average diet. However, firstly, human societies do not want to tolerate the level of reproductive failures that occur with other species, particularly if there is an easy alternative; secondly, requirement for a vitamin may not have changed over the centuries but it may be much more difficult to achieve for individuals who have a relatively sedentary lifestyle so the total amount of food eaten is less, thus providing less total vitamins. This effect will obviously be augmented by a tendency to consume more highly processed foods of lower nutrient density, whilst at the same time possibly having a higher requirement for certain nutrients to offset the demands of the twenty-first century, such as increased pollution and levels of free radicals.

Other micronutrients

Zinc has a central role in male reproductive function, being involved in testicular development, spermatogenesis and sperm motility (Favier, 1992). It is an essential cofactor for over 80 metalloenzymes and has an important function in synthesis of DNA and RNA, protein synthesis, cell division and membrane stability. Zinc deficiency may be a result of dietary deficiency (as in vegetarianism, slimming diets and starvation), malabsorption (for instance, inflammatory bowel disease), increased requirement (as in chronic diseases,

drug use or genetic defects) or increased loss (liver and kidney diseases). Zinc concentration is very high in human semen and male genital organs compared with other tissues and organs (Wong et al., 2000). Chronic zinc deficiency is associated with growth retardation, delayed healing, compromised immune function and a number of effects on the male reproductive system. Even relatively short-term (35 days) zinc restriction (1.4–3.4 mg Zn/day) can affect andrological variables, causing oligozoospermia, impotence, hypogonadism and impaired synthesis of testosterone (Hunt et al., 1992). Limited studies have investigated the effect of oral zinc supplementation in sub-fertile men (Wong et al., 2000). Although the results were not conclusive, further investigation seems worthwhile. The sperm take up zinc in the female reproductive tract, so zinc levels in women may also be important (Matossian, 1991). The mechanisms for absorbing zinc and lead interact, so people who consume a low level of zinc absorb more lead and concentrate it in their tissues, thus the effects of zinc deficiency on fertility can be augmented by consequent increased lead levels.

Human sperm have high concentrations of polyunsaturated fatty acids and can generate significant levels of reactive oxygen species (ROS), particularly the superoxide anion and hydrogen peroxide (Wong et al., 2000). This means that the sperm are susceptible to peroxidative damage. Antioxidant nutrients such as vitamins C and E, carotenoids and selenium can protect against oxidative stress and maintain genetic integrity of sperm cell membranes and DNA. Although vitamins C and D have been shown to be important in maintaining semen quality and reproductive function in animal studies in teleost fish and male rats, respectively (Kwiecinski et al., 1989; Ciereszko and Dabrowski, 1995), it is not clear whether these findings can be extrapolated to humans. In male mammals, vitamin A deficiency causes germinal cell degeneration and affects spermatogenesis (Van Pelt and de

Rooij, 1991). Selenium supplementation (100 μg/day) in sub-fertile men with low selenium status reversibly improves sperm motility and the chance of successful conception (Scott et al., 1998).

Selenium is an essential component of glutathione peroxidase. Total selenium increases in the testes during maturation and selenium appears to be a component of the mitochondrial capsule of the sperm mid-piece (Bedwal and Bahugana, 1994). Selenium has also been identified in rat sperm (Behne et al., 1993), and is selectively incorporated into the sperm selenoprotein when administered to selenium-deficient rats. Vitamin E, like selenium, is an antioxidant that has been used to treat sub-fertile men (Suleiman et al., 1996). Over the last quarter of a century, there has been a decline in male fertility in European countries, associated with a decline in sperm concentration and motility and an increase in the proportion of morphologically abnormal sperm and a parallel increase in testicular cancer (Auger et al., 1995). The change in source of cereals from those imported from North American to European supplies was associated with a marked fall in dietary intake of selenium from 60 to 30 μg/day from 1978 to 1990 (MacPherson et al., 1993). Sperm motility is greatest when the selenium level of semen is 50–69 ng/ml and sub-fertility is associated with a semen selenium level below 36 ng/ml (Bleau et al., 1984). Although both low and high selenium status are associated with increased rates of miscarriage in women (Barrington et al., 1996; Scott et al., 1998), a recent case–control study (Al-Kunani et al., 2001) investigating selenium levels in women with a history of recurrent miscarriage found evidence of a deficiency in selenium levels in hair studies but not in serum samples, which suggests the finding may not be related to a simple nutritional deficiency.

Population studies of sub-fertile men have focused more on possible toxic factors in the environment rather than dietary deficiencies.

Concern has been raised about chemicals in the food chain with an oestrogenic effect (such as polychlorinated biphenyls, chlorinated hydrocarbons and plant phytoestrogens) causing reduced male fertility (Sharpe, 1993).

Lifestyle Choices and Fertility

Common concerns related to potentially decreased fertility include exposure to cigarette smoking, alcohol consumption and caffeine intake. Couples who are concerned about their fertility potential are advised to stop the use of tobacco products (Barbieri, 2001). Chronic alcohol abuse in women is associated with altered hepatic oestrogen receptors (Becker et al., 1989). Women with high or frequent alcohol intake have been found to have an increased frequency of menstrual irregularities (Wilsnack et al., 1984). It has been shown in animal experiments that a single administration of alcohol reduces the chance of conception (Kieffer and Ketchel, 1970). In women, even a moderate consumption of alcohol is associated with decreased fecundity (Jensen et al., 1998). The probability of conception was halved in a menstrual cycle during which women consumed any alcohol (Hakim et al., 1998). In this study, the highest conception rate was observed in women who did not drink or smoke and who consumed less than one cup of coffee per day. Pregnant women who consume alcohol also have a greater rate of pregnancy failure (Harlap and Shiono, 1980) and alcohol is known to be teratogenic in the early weeks of development causing fetal alcohol syndrome (FAS), a range of congenital malformations including growth retardation, abnormal craniofacial features and development problems (see Figure 5.1). A less severe spectrum of problems is known as Fetal Alcohol Effect (FAE). Alcohol consumption is associated with increased zinc loss and may interfere with vitamin A metabolism (Zachman and Grummer, 2001).

Intake of caffeinated beverages, predominantly coffee, has been reported to cause sub-fertility and to be linearly related to the time-to-conception (Wilcox *et al.*, 1988), however caffeine consumption is notoriously difficult to estimate from reported intake. Moderate caffeine intake (150–300 mg/day; estimated to be equivalent to one to three cups of average-strength coffee) is associated with an increased risk of infertility, fetal loss and fetal growth impairment (Dlugosz and Bracken, 1992). A dose-dependent effect has been observed; women who drank one cup of coffee per day were half as likely to conceive as women who drank less than one cup each day (Wilcox *et al.*, 1988). Studies on rats showed that exposure to caffeine during oocyte maturation prior to fertilization reduced the implantation rate and negatively affected growth rate *in utero*, possibly by affecting gene expression in the early post-fertilization period in those litters which continued development (Pollard *et al.*, 1999).

Adolescent Pregnancy

Adolescents most likely to become pregnant are frequently those with inadequate nutritional status and from a disadvantaged socio-economic background. Adolescents in more favourable environments are more likely to terminate a pregnancy. Adolescent pregnancies are associated with an increased risk of maternal pregnancy complications and an increased risk of adverse pregnancy outcomes such as failed pregnancy, low birth-weight, preterm delivery and neonatal mortality (Lenders *et al.*, 2000). Maternal skeletal maturity has not been achieved in growing adolescents and competition for nutrients between the still-growing mother and her developing fetus occurs. Despite continued maternal growth in the pregnant adolescent resulting in increased maternal weight gain, increased body fat stores and greater postpartum weight retention, growing pregnant women deliver smaller offspring than skeletally mature adolescents and older mothers (Scholl and Hediger, 1993). Pregnancy, particularly its effects on lordosis and vertebral compression, can obscure the continuing growth of adolescents. However, sensitive measurements using the knee-height measuring device suggest that about half of adolescent women are still growing 6 years after menarche (Lenders *et al.*, 2000). Adolescents are at increased risk of consuming diets low in micronutrients (such as iron, folate, zinc, calcium and vitamins A, B_6 and C) and high in energy, fat and sugar. This matter is dealt with in more detail in Chapter 11.

Conclusion

Practical advice related to preconceptual nutrition is usually only sought if there appear to be problems with fertility. Optimal fertility for both men and women is associated with a BMI in the upper end of the normal range. Obese women have both reduced fertility and a greater risk of obstetric complications. However, reducing energy and nutrient intake to adjust body weight should be done well in advance of conception. It is difficult to reduce energy intake whilst maintaining optimal levels of micronutrient and protein intake. Likewise, thin women should postpone conception until their body weight has increased because fertility is restored before optimal weight is achieved and women who conceive on the penumbra of optimal intake and body weight (Figure 2.7) continue to have a poorer prognosis (Wynn and Wynn, 1991). Behaviour which causes swings in energy balance, such as some restrictive dieting practices (erratic eating patterns and crash dieting) or high levels of sports activity, can also affect reproductive function regardless of body weight.

The timing of conception has nutritional implications: long-term use of oral contraceptives

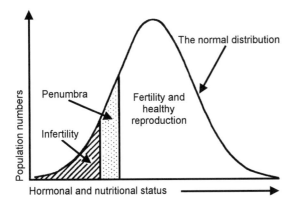

Figure 2.7 The penumbra between fertility and infertility. Hormonal and nutritional levels can be affected to a level which is above that which causes infertility. However, at this sub-optimal level of nutrition, follicular growth, hormonal secretion and embryonic development and growth may be impaired and adversely affect outcome. [Reprinted from *The Case for Preconception Care of Men and Women*, M Wynn and A Wynn, p.71 (1991), © AB Academic Publishers, Bicester]

can result in lower levels of vitamins B_6 and C and folate. Similarly a short interpregnancy interval can result in lower body stores of nutrients. An adequate and varied diet, determined from a dietary history, should be able to provide the required nutrients. However, recommendations for folate can only be met from supplements at least 3 months before conception to reduce neural tube defects. Although this recommendation is based on the need for folate for closure of the neural tube, there are some suggestions that the supplements should be taken throughout the pregnancy. There is more controversy about the need for other vitamin supplements. Certainly, the levels of vitamin A present in general vitamin and mineral supplements rather than those intended for pregnancy are higher than recommended. The studies in Hungary have supported the use of multivitamin and mineral supplements in the preconceptual period (Czeizel, 1998); however, concerns have been raised about competitive absorption between mineral

transport mechanisms (Hirschi and Keen, 2000). Hirschi and Keen (2000) promote iron supplementation but counsel that it should be augmented with zinc and copper to prevent a secondary deficiency. Other studies have associated use of supplements with an increased risk of a low-birth-weight baby (Bussell and Marlow, 2000), although this may reflect women who take supplements because they have less nutritional knowledge or because they know their diet is poor.

It is important to identify which women might be at increased risk of poor nutrition that could affect both fertility and outcome of pregnancy. Risk factors include adolescent age, those on a low income, substance abusers and those with a history of previous adverse outcome. The importance of the level of protein in the diet means that some vegetarians may need to be considered of special concern. The recent finding that an increased level of dietary methionine preconceptually and in early pregnancy is protective against NTD (Shoob *et al.*, 2001) is pertinent to vegetarians as animal proteins are a rich source of methionine. Recent research studies suggest that lifestyle factors including smoking and consumption of even small amounts of alcohol and caffeine affect not only early development but also fertility. The outcome of pregnancy appears to be established to some degree even before fertilization, so effective advice probably needs to be addressed to the population rather than just those couples who positively seek preconceptual counselling.

References

Ahmed ML (1999) Longitudinal study of leptin concentrations during puberty: sex differences and relationship to changes in body composition. *J. Clin. Endocrinol. Metab.* **84**, 899–905.

Al-Kunani AS, Knight R, Haswell SJ, Thompson JW and Lindow SW (2001) The selenium status of women with a history of recurrent miscarriage. *Br. J. Obstet. Gynaecol.* **108**, 1094–1097.

Allaire AD and Cefalo RC (1998) Preconceptional

health care model. *Eur. J. Obstet. Gynecol. Reprod. Biol.* **78**, 163–168.

Audi L, Mantzoros CS, Vidal-Puig A, Vargas D, Gussinye M and Carrascosa A (1998) Leptin in relation to resumption of menses in women with anorexia nervosa. *Mol. Psychol.* **3**, 544–547.

Auger J, Kunstmann JM, Czyglik E and Jouannet P (1995) Decline in semen quality among fertile men in Paris during the past 20 years. *New Engl. J. Med.* **332**: 281–285.

Barbieri RL (2001) The initial fertility consultation: recommendations concerning cigarette smoking, body mass index, and alcohol and caffeine consumption. *Am. J. Obstet. Gynecol.* **185**, 1168–1173.

Barr SI (1999) Vegetarianism and menstrual cycle disturbances: is there an association? *Am. J. Clin. Nutr.* **70**(Suppl.), 549S–554S.

Barr SI, Prior JC and Vigna YM (1994) Restrained eating and ovulatory disturbances: possible implications for bone health. *Am. J. Clin. Nutr.* **59**, 92–97.

Barr SI, Janelle KC and Prior JC (1995) Energy intakes are higher during luteal phase of ovulatory menstrual cycle. *Am. J. Clin. Nutr.* **61**, 39–43.

Barrington JW, Lindsay P, James D, Smith S and Robert K (1996) Selenium deficiency and miscarriage: a possible link. *Br. J. Obstet. Gynaecol.* **103**, 130–132.

Baumslag N, Edelstein T and Metz J (1970) Reduction of incidence of prematurity by folic acid supplementation in pregnancy. *Br. Med. J.* **687**, 16–17.

Becker U, Tonnesen H, Kaas-Claesson N and Gluud C (1989) Menstrual disturbances and infertility in chronic alcoholic women. *Drug Alcohol Depend* **24**, 75–82.

Bedwal RS and Bahugana A (1994) Zinc, copper and selenium in reproduction. *Experientia* **50**, 626–640.

Behne D, Duk M and Elger W (1986) Selenium content and glutathione peroxidase activity in the testis of the maturing rat. *J. Nutr.* **116**, 1442–1447.

Bleau G, Lemarbre J, Faucher G, Roberts KD and Chapdelaine A (1984) Semen selenium and human fertility. *Fertil. Steril.* **424**, 890–894.

Blum WF, Englaro P, Hanitsch S, Juul A, Hertel NT, Muller J, Skakkebaek NE, Heiman ML, Birkett M, Attanasio AM, Kiess W and Rascher W (1997) Plasma leptin levels in healthy children and adolescents: dependence on body mass index, body fat mass, gender, pubertal stage and testosterone. *J. Clin. Endocrinol. Metab.* **82**, 2904–2910.

Boushey CJ, Beresford SAA, Omenn GS and Motulsky AG (1995) A quantitative assessment of plasma homocysteine as a risk factor for vascular disease. *JAMA* **274**, 1049–1057.

Bower C, Stanley FJ, Croft M, de Klerk N, Davis RE and Nicol DJ (1993) Absorption of pteroylpolyglutamates in mothers of infants with neural tube defects. *Br. J. Nutr.* **69**, 827–834.

Bringer J, Lefebvre P, Boulet F, Clouet S and Renard E (1997) Deficiency of energy balance and ovulatory disorders. *Hum. Reprod.* **12**(Suppl. 1), 97–109.

Bronson FH (2000) Puberty and energy reserves: a walk on the wild side. In: *Reproduction in Context*, ed. Wallen K and Schneider JE, pp. 15–33. MIT Press, Cambridge, MA.

Bussell G and Marlow N (2000) The dietary beliefs and attitudes of women who have had a low birthweight baby: a retrospective preconception study. *J. Hum. Nutr. Dietet.* **13**, 29–39.

Campfield LA, Smith FJ, Guisez Y, Devos R and Burn P (1995) Recombinant mouse ob protein: evidence for a peripheral signal linking adiposity and central neural networks. *Science* **269**, 546–549.

Caprio M, Fabbrini E, Isidori AM, Aversa A and Fabbri A (2001) Leptin in reproduction. *Trends Endocrinol. Metab.* **12**, 65–72.

Cassidy A, Bingham S and Setchell KD (1994) Biological effects of a diet of soy protein rich in isoflavones on the menstrual cycle of premenopausal women. *Am. J. Clin. Nutr.* **60**, 333–340.

Chehab FF (2000) Leptin as a regulator of adipose mass and reproduction. *Trends Pharmac. Sci.* **21**, 309–314.

Chehab F, Lim M and Lu R (1996) Correction of the sterility defect in homozygous obese female mice by treatment with the human recombinant leptin. *Nat. Genet.* **12**, 318–320.

Chehab FF Mounzih K, Lu R and Lim ME (1997) Early onset of reproductive function in normal female mice treated with leptin. *Science* **275**, 88–90.

Cheung CC, Thornton JE, Kuijper JL, Weigle DS, Clifton DK and Steiner RA (1997) Leptin is a metabolic gate for the onset of puberty in the female rat. *Endocrinology* **138**(2), 855–858.

Ciereszko A and Dabrowski K (1995) Sperm quality and ascorbic acid concentration in rainbow trout semen are affected by dietary vitamin C: an across-season study. *Biol. Reprod.* **52**, 982–988.

Clark AM, Ledger W, Galletly C, Tomlinson L, Blaney F, Wang X and Norman RJ (1995) Weight loss results in significant improvement in pregnancy and ovulation rates in anovulatory obese women. *Hum. Reprod.* **10**, 2705–2712.

Clarke IJ and Henry BA (1999) Leptin and reproduction. *Rev. Reprod.* **4**, 48–55.

Coad J, Al-Rasasi B and Morgan JB (2002) Nutrient insult in early pregnancy. *Proc. Nutr. Soc.* **61**, 51–59.

Cole TJ (2000) Secular trends in growth. *Proc. Nutr. Soc.* **59**, 317–324.

Crisp TM (1992) Organisation of the ovarian follicle and events in its biology; oogenesis, ovulation or atresia. *Mutat. Res.* **296**, 89–106.

Cumming DC, Wheeler GD and McColl EM (1989) The effects of exercise on reproductive function in men. *Sports Med.* **7**, 1–17.

Cumming DC, Wheeler GD and Harber VJ (1994) Physical activity, nutrition, and reproduction. *Ann. NY Acad. Sci.* **709**, 55–76.

Cuskelly GJ, McNulty H and Scott JM (1996) Effect of increasing dietary folate on red-cell folate: implications for prevention of neural tube defects. *Lancet* **347**, 657–659.

Czeizel AE (1996) Reduction of urinary tract and cardiovascular defects by multivitamin supplementation. *Am. J. Med. Genet.* **62**, 79–183.

Czeizel AE (1998) Periconceptional folic acid containing multivitamin supplementation. *Eur. J. Obs. Gynecol. Reprod. Biol.* **78**, 151–161.

Czeizel AE and Dudas I (1992) Prevention of the first occurrence of neural-tube defects by periconceptional vitamin supplementation. *New Engl. J. Med.* **327**, 1832–1835.

Dagogo-Jack S, Fanelli C, Paramore D, Brothers J and Landt M (1996) Plasma leptin and insulin relationships in obese and non-obese humans. *Diabetes* **45**, 695–698.

Daly S, Mills JL, Molloy AM, Conley M, Lee YJ, Kirke PN, Weir DG and Scott JM (1997) Minimum effective dose of folic acid for food fortification to prevent neural tube defects. *Lancet* **350**, 1666–1669.

Darwin C (1859) *The Origin of the Species*. Penguin, London.

Dawson EB (1986) Effect of ascorbic acid on male fertility. *Ann. NY Acad. Sci.* **498**, 312–323.

Department of Health (1991a) *Dietary Reference Values for Food Energy and Nutrients for the United Kingdom*. Report on Health and Social Subjects 41. HMSO, London.

Department of Health (1991b) *Folic Acid in the Prevention of Neural Tube Defects*. Letter from Chief Medical and Nursing Officers. PL/CMO (91)11, PL/CNO (91) 6. London, 12 August 1991.

Department of Health (2000) *Folic Acid and the Prevention of Disease*. Report of the Committee on Medical Aspects of Food and Nutrition Policy. Report on Health and Social Subjects 50. The Stationery Office, London.

Dlugosz L and Bracken MB (1992) Reproductive effects of caffeine: a review and theoretical analysis. *Epidemiol. Rev.* **14**, 83–100.

Dorgan JF, Reichman ME, Judd JT, Brown C, Longcope C, Schatzkin A, Forman M, Campbell WS, Franz C, Kahle L and Taylor PR (1996) Relation of energy, fat, and fiber intakes to plasma concentrations of estrogens and androgens in premenopausal women. *Am. J. Clin. Nutr.* **64**, 25–31.

Doyle W, Crawford MA, Wynn AHA and Wynn SW. (1990) The association between maternal diet and birth dimensions. *J. Nutr. Health* **1**, 9–17.

Ellison PT (1982) Skeletal growth, fatness and menarcheal age: a comparison of two hypotheses. *Hum. Biol.* **54**, 269–281.

Essien FB and Wannberg SL (1993) Methionine but not folic acid or vitamin B-12 alters the frequency of neural tube defects in Axd mutant mice. *J. Nutr.* **123**, 27–34.

Favier AE (1992) The role of zinc in reproduction: hormonal mechanisms. *Biol. Trace Elem. Res.* **32**, 363–382.

Favier M, Faure P, Roussel AM, Coudray C, Blache D and Favier A (1993) Zinc deficiency and dietary folate metabolism in pregnant rats. *J. Trace Elem. Electrolytes Health Dis.* **7**, 19–24.

Foster DL and Nagatani S. (1999) Physiological perspectives on leptin as a regulator of reproduction: role in timing puberty. *Biol. Reprod.* **60**, 205–215.

Franks S and Robinson S (1996) Nutrition, metabolism and reproduction. In: *Scientific Essentials of Reproductive Medicine*, ed. Hillier SG, Kitchener HC and Neilson JP. Saunders, Philadelphia, PA.

Friedman CI and Kim HM (1985) Obesity and its effect on reproductive function. *Clin. Obstet. Gynecol.* **28**, 645–663.

Frische RE (1990) The right weight: body fat, menarche and ovulation. *Baillières Clin. Obstet. Gynaecol.* **4**, 419–439.

Frische RE and Arthur JW (1974) Menstrual cycle: fatness as a determinant of minimum weight necessary for their maintenance or onset. *Science* **185**, 949–951.

Galletly C, Clark A, Tomlinson L and Blaney F (1996) A group program for obese, infertile women: weight loss and improved psychological health. *J. Psychosom. Obstet. Gynecol.* **17**, 125–128.

Garcia-Mayor RV, Andrade MA, Rios M, Lage M, Dieguez C and Casanueva FF (1997) Serum leptin levels in normal children: relationship to age, gender, body mass index, pituitary-gonadal hormones, and pubertal stage. *J. Clin. Endocrinol. Metab.* **82**, 2849–2855.

Gruaz NM, Lalaoui M, Pierroz DD, Englaro P, Sizonenko PC, Blum WF and Aubert ML (1998) Chronic administration of leptin into the lateral ventricle induces sexual maturation in severely food-restricted female rats. *J. Neuroendocrinol.* **10**, 627–633.

Hakim RB, Gray RH and Zacur H (1998) Alcohol and caffeine consumption and decreased fertility. *Fertil. Steril.* **70**, 632–637.

Harlap S and Shiono PH (1980) Alcohol, smoking, and incidence of spontaneous abortions in the first and second trimester. *Lancet* **ii**, 173–176.

Hathcock JN, Hattan DG, Jenkins MY, McDonald JT, Sundaresan PR and Wilkening VL (1990) Evaluation of vitamin A toxicity. *Am. J. Clin. Nutr.* **52**, 183–202.

Havel PJ, Kasim-Karakas S, Muller W, Johnson PR, Gingerich RL and Stern JS (1996) Relationship of plasma leptin to plasma insulin and adiposity in normal weight and overweight women: effects of dietary fat content and sustained weight loss. *J. Clin. Endocrinol. Metab.* **81**, 4406–4413.

Heiman ML, Ahima RS, Craft LS, Schoner B, Stephens TW and Flier JS (1997) Leptin inhibition of the hypothalamic–pituitary–adrenal axis in response to stress. *Endocrinology* **138**, 3859–3863.

Hirschi KK and Keen CL (2000) Nutrition in embryonic and fetal development. *Nutrition* **16**, 495–499.

Hunt CD, Johnson PE, Herbel J and Mullen LK (1992) Effects of dietary zinc depletion on seminal volume and zinc loss, serum testosterone concentrations, and sperm morphology in young men. *Am. J. Clin. Nutr.* **56**, 148–157.

Institute of Medicine (1990) *Nutrition during pregnancy*. National Academy Press, Washington, DC.

Isidori AM, Caprio M, Strollo F, Moretti C, Frajese G, Isidori A and Fabbri A (1999) Leptin and androgens in male obesity: evidence for leptin contribution to reduced androgens levels. *J. Clin. Endocrinol. Metab.* **84**, 3673–3680.

Jensen TK, Hjollund NHI, Henriksen TB, Scheike T, Kolstad H, Giwercman A, Ernst E, Bonde JP, Skakkebaek NE and Olsen J (1998) Does moderate alcohol consumption affect fertility? Follow-up study among couples planning first pregnancy. *Br. Med. J.* **317**, 505–510.

Juiter A, Panhuysen G, Everaerd W, Koppesschaar H, Krabbe P and Zebssen P (1993) The paradoxical nature of sexuality in anorexia nervosa. *J. Sex. Marital. Ther.* **19**, 259–275.

Karlsson C, Lindell K, Svensson E, Bergh C, Lind P, Billig H, Carlsson LM and Carlsson B (1997) Expression of functional leptin receptors in the human ovary. *J. Clin. Endocrinol. Metab.* **82**, 4144–4148.

Keen CL, Uriu-Hare JY, Hawk SN, Janowski MA, Daston GP, Kwik-Uribe CL and Rucker RB (1998) Effect of copper deficiency on prenatal development and pregnancy outcome. *Am. J. Clin. Nutr.* **67**(Suppl.), 1003S–1011S.

Kemmann E, Pasquale SA and Skaf R (1983) Amennorrhea associated with carotenemia. *JAMA* **249**, 926–929.

Kennedy GC and Mitra J (1963) Body weight and food intake as initiating factors in the rat. *J. Physiol.* **166**, 408–418.

Keys A, Brozek J, Henschel A, Michelsen O and Taylor HL (1950) *The Biology of Starvation.* University of Minnesota Press, Minneapolis, MN.

Kiddy DS, Hamilton-Fairley D, Bush A, Short F, Anyaoku V, Reed MJ and Franks S (1989) Improvement in endocrine and ovarian function during dietary treatment of obese women with polycystic ovarian syndrome. *Clin. Endocrinol.* **36**, 105–111.

Kiddy DS, Sharp PS, White DM, Scanlon MF, Mason HD, Bray CS, Polson DW, Reed MJ and Franks S (1990) Differences in clinical and endocrine features between obese and non-obese subjects with polycystic ovary syndrome: an analysis of 263 consecutive cases. *Clin. Endocrinol.* **32**, 213–220.

Kieffer JD and Ketchel MM (1970) Blockade of ovulation in the rat by ethanol. *Acta Endocrinol.* **65**, 117–124.

Kiess W, Blum WF and Aubert ML (1997) Leptin, puberty and reproductive function: lessons from animal studies and observations in humans. *Eur. J. Endocrinol.* **138**, 26–29.

Kirke PN, Molloy AM, Daly LE, Burke H, Weir DG and Scott JM (1993) Maternal plasma folate and vitamin B_{12} are independent risk factors for neural tube defects. *Quart. J. Med.* **86**, 703–708.

Köpp W, Blum WF, von Prittwitz S, Ziegler A, Lubbert H, Emons G, Herzog W, Herpertz S, Deter HC, Remschmidt H and Hebebrand J (1997) Low leptin levels predict amenorrhea in underweight and eating disordered females. *Mol. Psychiat.* **2**, 335–340.

Kwiecinski GG, Petrie GI and DeLuca HF (1989) Vitamin D is necessary for reproductive functions of the male rat. *J. Nutr.* **119**, 741–744.

Kwong WY, Wild AE, Roberts P, Willis AC and Fleming TP (2000) Maternal undernutrition during the preimplantation period of rat development causes blastocyst abnormalities and programming of postnatal hypertension. *Development* **127**, 4195–4202.

Labadarios D, Obuwa G, Lucas EG, Dickerson JWT and Parke DV (1978) The effects of chronic drug administration on hepatic enzyme induction and folate metabolism. *Br. J. Clin. Pharmac.* **5**, 167–173.

Landau B, Singer R, Klein T and Segenreich E (1978) Folic acid levels in blood and seminal plasma of normo- and oligospermic patients prior to and following folic acid treatment. *Experientia* **34**, 1301–1302.

Lenders CM, McElrath TF and Scholl TO (2000) Nutrition in adolescent pregnancy. *Curr. Opin. Pediat.* **12**, 291–296.

Licinio J, Negrao AB, Mantzoros C, Kaklamani V, Wong ML, Bongiorno PB, Mulla A, Cearnal L, Veldhuis JD, Flier JS, McCann SM and Gold PW (1998) Synchronicity of frequently sampled, 24-h concentrations of circulating leptin, luteinizing hormone, and estradiol in healthy women. *Proc. Natl Acad. Sci. USA* **95**, 2541–2546.

Loucks AB, Mortola JF, Girton L and Yen SS (1989) Alterations in the hypothalamic–pituitary–ovarian and the hypothalamic–pituitary–adrenal axes in athletic women. *J. Clin. Endocrinol. Metab.* **68**, 402–411.

Lumey LH (1998) Reproductive outcomes in women prenatally exposed to undernutrition: a review of findings from the Dutch famine birth cohort. *Proc. Nutr. Soc.* **57**, 129–135.

MacPherson A, Barclay MNI, Dixon J, Groden BM, Scott R and Kesson E (1993) Decline in dietary selenium intake in Scotland and effect on plasma concentrations. In: *Proceedings of the 8th International Symposium on Trace Elements in Man and Animals*, ed. Anke M, Meissner D and Milss CF. Verlag Media Touriskik, Jena.

Maffei M, Halaas J, Ravussin E, Pratley RE, Lee GH, Zhang Y, Fei H, Kim S, Lallone R and Ranganathan S (1995) Leptin levels in human and rodent: measurement of plasma leptin and ob RNA in obese and weight-reduced subjects. *Nat. Med.* **1**(11), 1155–1161.

Malaisse WJ (1998) Reciprocal links between metabolic and ionic events in islet cells: their relevance to the rhythmics of insulin release. *Diabet. Metab.* **24**, 11–14.

Mantzoros C, Flier JS, Lesem MD, Brewerton TD and Jimerson DC (1997) Cerebrospinal fluid leptin in anorexia nervosa: correlation with nutritional status and potential role in resistance to weight gain. *J. Clin. Endocrinol. Metab.* **2**, 1845–1851.

Mantzoros CS, Cramer DW, Liberman RF and Barbieri RL (2000) Predictive value of serum and follicular fluid leptin concentrations during assisted reproductive cycles in normal women and in women with the polycystic ovarian syndrome. *Hum. Reprod.* **15**, 539–544.

Matossian MK (1991) Fertility decline in Europe, 1875–1913: was zinc deficiency the cause? *Perspect. Biol. Med.* **334**, 604–616.

McPartlin J, Halligan A, Scott JM, Darling M and Weir DG (1993) Accelerated folate breakdown in pregnancy. *Lancet* **341**, 148–149.

MAFF (1999) *National Food Survey 1998*. TSO, London.

Medical Research Council Vitamin Study Research Group (1991) Prevention of neural tube defects: results of the Medical Research Council Vitamin Study. *Lancet* **338**, 131–137.

Nagatani S, Guthikonda P, Thompson RC, Tsukamura H, Maeda K-I and Foster DL (1998) Evidence for GnRH regulation by leptin: leptin administration prevents reduced pulsatile LH secretion during fasting. *Neuroendocrinology* **67**, 370–376.

Norman RJ and Clark AM (1998) Obesity and reproductive disorders: a review. *Reprod. Fertil. Dev.* **10**, 55–63.

Nottle MB, Kleemann DO, Grosser TI and Seamark RF (1997) Evaluation of a nutritional strategy to increase ovulation rate in merino ewes mated in late spring–early summer. *Anim. Reprod. Sci.* **47**, 255–261.

Pasquali R, Casimirri F and Vicennati V (1997) Weight control and its beneficial effect on fertility in women with obesity and polycystic ovary syndrome. *Hum. Reprod.* **12**(Suppl. 1), 82–87.

Pelleymounter MA, Cullen MJ, Baker MB, Hecht R, Winters D, Boone T and Collins F. (1995) Effects of the obese gene product on body weight in *ob/ob* mice. *Science* **269**, 540–543.

Perry VEA, Norman ST, Owen JA, Daniel RCW and Phillips N (1999) Low dietary protein during early pregnancy alters bovine placental development. *Anim. Reprod. Sci.* **55**, 13–21.

Phipps WR, Martini MC, Lampe JW, Slavin JL and Kurzer MS (1993) Effect of flax seed ingestion on the menstrual cycle. *J. Clin. Endocrinol. Metab.* **77**, 1215–1219.

Pirke KM, Schweiger U, Laessle R, Dickhaut B, Schweiger M and Waechtler M (1986) Dieting influences the menstrual cycle: vegetarian versus non-vegetarian diet. *Fertil. Steril.* **46**, 1083–1088.

Pirke KM, Fitcher MM, Chlond C, Schweiger U, Laessle RG, Schwingenschloegel M and Hoehl C (1987) Disturbances of the menstrual cycle in bulimia nervosa. *Clin. Endocrinol.* **24**, 245–251.

Pirke KM, Fichter MM, Pirke KM, Schweiger U and Strowizki T (1989) Dieting causes menstrual irregularities in normal weight young women through impairment of episodic luteinizing hormone secretion. *Fertil. Steril.* **51**, 263–268.

Pollard I, Murray JF, Hiller R, Scaramuzzi RJ and Wilson CA (1999) Effects of preconceptual caffeine exposure on pregnancy and progeny viability. *J. Matern. Fetal Med.* **8**, 220–224.

Prasad AS (1985) Clinical manifestations of zinc deficiency. *A. Rev. Nutr.* **5**, 341–363.

Prentice A and Goldberg G (1996) Maternal obesity increases congenital malformations. *Nutr. Rev.* **54**, 146–152.

Reichman ME, Judd JT, Longcope C, Schatzkin A, Clevidence BA, Nair PP, Campbell WS and Taylor PR (1993) Effects of alcohol consumption on plasma and urinary hormone concentrations in premenopausal women. *J. Natl Cancer Inst.* **85**, 722–727.

Reifsnider E and Gill SL (2000) Nutrition for the childbearing years. *J. Obstet. Gynecol. Neonat. Nurs.* **29**, 43–55.

Robinson S, Kiddy D, Gelding SV, Willis D, Niththyananthan R, Bush A, Johnston DG and Franks S (1993) The relationship of insulin sensitivity to menstrual patterns in women with hyperandrogenism and polycystic ovaries. *Clin. Endocrinol.* **39**, 351–355.

Rock CL, Gorenflo DW, Drewnoski A and Demitrack MA (1996) Nutritional characteristics, eating pathology, and hormonal status in young women. *Am. J. Clin. Nutr.* **64**, 566–571.

Rosenquist TH, Ratashak SA and Selhub J (1996) Homocysteine induces congenital defects of the heart and neural tube: effect of folic acid. *Proc. Natl Acad. Sci.* **93**, 15 227–15 232.

Rushton DH (1991) Ferritin and fertility. *Lancet* **337**, 1554.

Saladin R, De Vos P, Guerre-Millo M, Leturque A, Girard J, Staels B and Auwern J (1995) Transient increase in obese gene expression after food intake or insulin administration. *Nature* **377**, 527–529.

Schneider JE and Wade GN (2000) Inhibition of reproduction in service of energy balance. In: *Reproduction in Context*, ed. Wallen K and Schneider JE, pp. 35–82. MIT Press, Cambridge, MA.

Scholl TO and Hediger ML (1993) A review of the epidemiology of nutrition and adolescent pregnancy: maternal growth during pregnancy and its effect on the fetus. *J. Am. Coll. Nutr.* **12**, 101–107.

Schreihofer DA, Amico JA and Cameron JL (1993) Reversal of fasting-induced suppression of luteinizing hormone (LH) secretion in male rhesus monkeys by intragastric nutrient infusion: evidence for rapid stimulation of LH by nutritional signals. *Endocrinology* **132**, 1890–1897.

Schubring C, Blum WF, Kratzsch J, Deutscher J and Kiess W (2000) Leptin, the *ob* gene product, in female health and disease. *Eur. J. Obstet. Gynecol. Reprod. Biol.* **88**, 121–127.

Schweiger U, Laessle R, Pfister H, Hoehl C, Schwingenschloegel M, Schweiger M and Pirke KM (1987) Diet-induced menstrual irregularities: effects of age and weight loss. *Fertil. Steril.* **48**, 746–751.

Scott JM and Weir DG (1998) Role of folic acid/folate in pregnancy: prevention is better than cure. *Rec. Adv. Obstet. Gynaecol.* **20**, 1–20.

Scott R, McPherson A, Yates RWS, Hussain B and Dixon J (1998) The effect of oral selenium supplementation on human sperm motility. *Br. J. Urol.* **82**, 76–80.

Sharpe RM (1993) Declining sperm counts in man – is there an endocrine cause? *J. Endocrinol.* **136**, 357–360.

Shaw GM, O'Maley CD, Wasserman CR, Tolarova MM and Lammer EJ (1995a) Maternal periconceptual use of multivitamins and reduced risk of corotruncal heart defects and limb deficiency among offspring. *Am. J. Med. Genet.* **59**, 536–545.

Shaw GM, Lammer EJ, Wasserman CR, O'Maley CD and Tolarova MM (1995b) Risks of orofacial clefts in children born to women using multivitamins containing folic acid periconceptually. *Lancet* **346**, 393–396.

Shoob HD, Sargent RG, Thompson SJ, Best RG,

Drane JW and Tocharoen A (2001) Dietary methionine is involved in the etiology of neural tube defect-affected pregnancies in humans. *J. Nutr.* **131**, 2653–2658.

Short RV (1994) Human reproduction in an evolutionary context. *Ann. NY Acad. Sci.* **709**, 416–425.

Sinning WE and Little KD (1987) Body composition and menstrual function in athletes. *Sport Med.* **4**, 34–45.

Smith OB and Akinbamijo OO (2000) Micronutrients and reproduction in farm animals. *Anim. Reprod. Sci.* **60–61**, 549–560.

Smithells RW, Sheppard S, Schorah CJ, Seller MJ, Nevin NC, Harris R, Read AP and Fielding DW (1980) Possible prevention of neural-tube defects by periconceptual vitamin supplementation. *Lancet* **i**, 339–340.

Steegers-Theunissen RP, Boers GH, Trijbels FJ, Finkelstein JD, Blom HJ, Thomas CM, Borm GF, Wouters MG and Eskes TK (1994) Maternal hyperhomocysteinemia: a risk factor for neural-tube defects? *Metab. Clin. Exp.* **43**, 1475–1480.

Stein Z and Susser M (1991) Famine and fertility. In: *Nutrition and Human Reproduction*, ed. Mosley WH. Plenum, New York.

Stein Z, Susser M, Saenger G and March F (1975) *Famine and Human Development: the Dutch Winter of 1944–45*. Oxford University Press, Oxford.

Steiner RA, Cameron JL, McNeil TH, Clifton DK and Bremner WJ (1983) Metabolic signals for the onset of puberty. In: *Neuroendocrine Aspects of Reproduction*, ed. Norman RL, pp. 183–227. Academic Press, New York.

Suleiman SA, Ali ME, Zaki ZM, el-Malik EM and Nasr MA (1996) Lipid peroxidation and human sperm motility: protective role of vitamin E. *J. Androl.* **17**, 530–537.

Suter KJ, Pohl CR and Wilson ME (2000) Circulating concentrations of nocturnal leptin, growth hormone, and insulin-like growth factor-I increase before the onset of puberty in agonal male monkeys: potential signals for the initiation of puberty. *J. Clin. Endocrinol. Metab.* **85**, 808–814.

Thiering P, Beaurepaire J, Jones M, Saunders D and Tennant C (1993) Mood state as a predictor of treatment outcome after in vitro fertilization/embryo transfer technology (IVF/ET). *J. Psychosomat. Res.* **37**, 481–491.

Treasure JL and Russell GFM (1988) Intrauterine growth and neonatal weight gain in babies of women with anorexia nervosa. *Br. Med. J.* **296**, 1038–1039.

Van Allen MI, Kalousek DK, Chernoff GF, Juriloff D, Harris M, McGillivray BC, Yong SL, Langlois S, MacLeod PM and Chitayat D (1993) Evidence for multi-site closure of the neural tube in humans. *Am. J. Med. Genet.* **47**, 723–743.

Van der Put NMJ and Blom HJ (2000) Neural tube defects and a disturbed folate dependent homocysteine metabolism. *Eur. J. Obstet. Gynecol. Reprod. Biol.* **92**, 57–61.

Van der Put NM, van den Heuvel LP, Steegers-Theunissen RP, Trijbels FJ, Eskes TK, Mariman EC, den Heyer M and Blom HJ (1996) Decreased methylene tetrahydrofolate reductase activity due to the 677C→T mutation in families with spina bifida offspring. *J. Mol. Med.* **74**, 691–694.

Van der Walt LA, Wilmsen EN and Jenkins T (1978) Unusual sex hormone patterns among desert-dwelling hunter-gatherers *J. Clin. Endocrinol. Metab.* **46**, 658–663.

Van Pelt AM and de Rooij DG (1991) Retinoic acid is able to reinitiate spermatogenesis in vitamin A-deficient rats and high replicate doses support the full development of spermatogenic cells. *Endocrinology* **128**, 697–704.

Villanueva AL, Schlosser C, Hopper B, Liu JH, Hoffman DI and Rebar RW (1986) Increased cortisol production in women runners. *J. Clin. Endocrinol. Metab.* **63**, 133–136.

Wade GN and Schneider JE (1994) Fat does not mean fertile. *J. NIH Res.* **8**, 18.

Wade GN, Schneider JE and Li HY (1996) Control of fertility by metabolic cues. *Am. J. Physiol.* **270**, E1–E19.

Wald NJ (1994) Folic acid and neural tube defects: the current evidence and implications for prevention. *Ciba Found. Symp.* **181**, 192–211.

Wentz AC (1980) Body weight and amenorrhoea. *Obstet. Gynecol.* **56**, 482–487.

Whitten PL and Naftolin F (1998) Reproductive actions of phytoestrogens. *Baillières Clin. Endocrinol. Metab.* **12(4)**, 667–690.

Wilcox A, Weinberg C and Baird D (1988) Caffeinated beverages and decreased fertility. *Lancet* **ii**, 1453–1456.

Wild J (1997) Prevention of neural tube defects. *Lancet* **350**, 30–31.

Wilsnack SC, Klassen AD and Wilsnack RW (1984) Drinking and reproductive dysfunction among women in a 1981 national survey. *Alcohol Clin Exp Res* **8**, 451–458.

Wise J (2001) Neural tube defects decline in US after folic acid is added to flour. *Br. Med. J.* **322**, 1510.

Wong WY, Thomas CMG, Merkus JMWM, Zielhuis GA and Steegers-Theunissen RPM (2000) Male factor subfertility: possible causes and the impact of nutritional factors. *Fertil. Steril.* **73**, 435–442.

Worthington-White DA, Behnke M and Gross S (1994) Premature infants require additional folate and vitamin B_{12} to reduce the severity of the anaemia of prematurity. *Am. J. Clin. Nutr.* **60**, 930–935.

Wouters MG, Boers GH, Blom HJ, Trijbels FJ, Thomas CM, Borm GF, Steegers-Theunissen RP and Eskes TK (1993) Hyperhomocysteinemia: a risk factor in women with unexplained recurrent early pregnancy loss. *Fertil. Steril.* **60**, 820–825.

Wynn AHA, Crawford MA, Doyle W and Wynn SW (1991) Nutrition of women in anticipation of pregnancy. *Nutr. Health* **7**, 69–88.

Wynn M and Wynn A (1988) Nutrition around conception and the prevention of low birthweight. *Nutr. Health* **6**, 37–52.

Wynn M and Wynn A (1991) *The Case for Preconception Care of Men and Women.* AB Academic, Bicester.

Wynn M and Wynn A (1995) A fertility diet for planning pregnancy. *Nutr. Health* **10**, 219–238.

Yura S, Ogawa Y, Sagawa N, Masuzaki H, Itoh H, Ebihara K, Aizawa-Abe M, Fujii S and Nakao K (2000) Accelerated puberty and late-onset hypothalamic hypogonadism in female transgenic skinny mice overexpressing leptin. *J. Clin. Invest.* **105**, 749–755.

Zachman RD and Grummer MA (2001) Prenatal ethanol consumption increases retinol and cellular retinol-binding protein expression in the rat fetal snout. *Biol. Neonate.* **80**, 152–157.

Zhang, Y, Proenca R, Maffei M, Barone M, Leopold L and Friedman JM (1994) Positional cloning of the mouse obese gene and its human homologue. *Nature* **372**, 425–432.

3

MATERNAL PHYSIOLOGY AND NUTRITION DURING REPRODUCTION

Elisabet Forsum

LEARNING OUTCOMES

Understanding of:

- Hormonal changes during pregnancy and lactation.

- Metabolic and physiological changes during reproduction.

- Changes in blood and circulation, kidney function and body water during pregnancy.

- Physiology of lactation.

- Changes in body weight and composition.

- Nutritional requirements during reproduction.

Introduction

The general statement that nutrition during pregnancy and lactation is important is accepted by most people. However, as this area undergoes exploration by modern research, the complexity of the subject is gradually becoming apparent. For example, the mammalian embryo and fetus cannot be thought of as a perfect parasite, and the developing organism is not attached to an unchanging maternal body. Regarding interactions between mother and foetus, it has even been suggested that 'The relationship is a complex form of symbiosis in which many aspects of physiology undergo such extensive modification that the pregnant female behaves almost as a distinct species' (Thomson and Hytten, 1973). The following chapter attempts to describe very briefly how these modifications are initiated by hormonal changes, the nature of the modifications, and their implications regarding nutritional needs during reproduction. Material in Chapters 4 and 8 should be read in relation to this chapter.

Hormonal changes

When a girl reaches puberty her ovaries contain about 400 000 oogonia. Throughout her entire reproductive life, with the exception of time periods around childbirth, a few of these oogonia will be stimulated to grow each

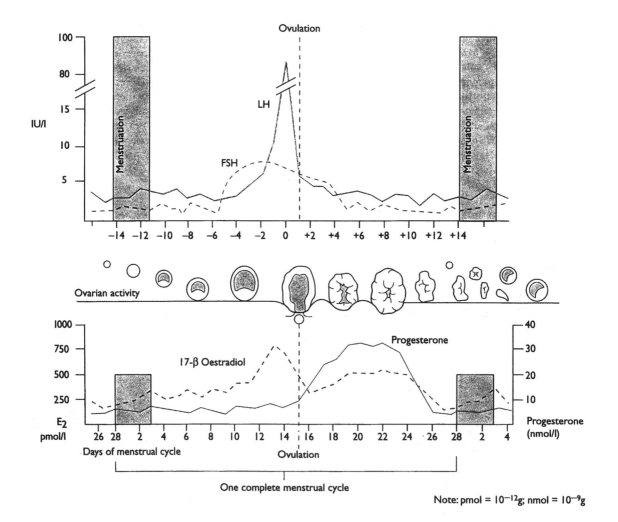

Figure 3.1 Circulatory hormone levels throughout the menstrual cycle in women. Modified from Llewellyn-Jones (1999a)

month. The hormones responsible for this stimulation are follicle-stimulating hormone (FSH) and luteinizing hormone (LH), hormones that are secreted by the anterior pituitary gland. One follicle eventually releases an ovum and, if fertilized, pregnancy follows. If the ovum is not fertilized, menstruation occurs. Figure 3.1 shows circulatory levels of important hormones during the menstrual cycle. After menstruation, oestrogen levels increase, which initially inhibits FSH release and causes a sudden increase in LH, leading to ovulation. At this stage FSH levels are also increased. The endometrial surface of the uterus proliferates considerably during this part of the menstrual cycle. This proliferation continues after ovulation in order to prepare the endometrium to receive the fertilized ovum. After having released its ovum, the follicle becomes the corpus luteum, which secretes progesterone and oestrogen. In the absence of a fertilized ovum the corpus luteum degenerates about 7 days after ovulation and hormonal secretion declines. The endometrium now becomes thinner and gradually also necrotic until menstruation begins, when the superficial layers of the endometrium are shed. A new cycle is now initiated when FSH stimulates the ovary.

If the ovum is fertilized and pregnancy occurs, the implanted embryo secretes human chorion gonadotropin (hCG), which maintains the corpus luteum, thereby allowing oestrogen and progesterone secretion to continue. Secretion of hCG, an important hormone for maternal physiology during pregnancy in general, is later taken over by the placenta, which also produces progesterone and oestrogen (Figure 3.2). The high plasma levels of these three hormones are apparently fundamental for the metabolic and physiological changes occurring in the maternal body during pregnancy.

Another important hormonal change during pregnancy is the increasing level of prolactin caused by an increased activity of the lactotrophs of the pituitary gland. This increased

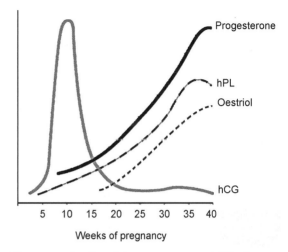

Figure 3.2 Oestriol, progesterone, hCG (human chorion gonadotropin) and hPL (human placental lactogen) plasma levels in pregnancy. Modified from Llewellyn-Jones (1999b)

activity is a result of the increased circulating levels of oestrogen and progesterone. One important function of prolactin is to prepare the mammary gland for lactation. It is capable of stimulating the mammary gland to produce milk, but this action is inhibited by the high serum levels of progesterone and oestrogen during pregnancy. Studies in women living under different nutritional circumstances have shown that circulating prolactin levels are related to the amount of food available (Lunn et al., 1980). Good nutrition is associated with lower prolactin levels and a shorter period of postpartum amenorrhoea. A possible interpretation is that prolactin helps to ensure milk synthesis when food intake is limited by preferentially channelling nutrients towards the breast, and ensures a period of nutritional recovery before a new pregnancy is established. Another hormone, also released from the pituitary, is oxytocin, which stimulates smooth muscle contraction and has a role during parturition and lactation.

During pregnancy there is also an increase in thyroid-binding globulin (TBG) owing to an increased production of this hormone in the liver in response to the increased oestrogen levels. The increased concentrations of TBG stimulate hormone production in the thyroid gland. However, the alterations in maternal thyroid function during pregnancy are intricate and far from fully understood (Glinoer *et al.*, 1990). The increased absorption of calcium in the maternal intestinal tract that is associated with pregnancy is also mediated by hormonal changes. There are increases in parathyroid hormone (PTH) secretion as well as in 1,25 dihydroxyvitamin D [1,25 (OH)$_2$D] synthesis, while the circulating concentration of calcitonin appears to be unchanged. Other important hormonal changes during pregnancy are the increases in plasma levels of aldosterone, renin substrate and angiotensin. These changes act in concert with one another and with other factors to achieve the changes in water and electrolyte balance characteristic of pregnancy. Furthermore, the hormonal changes during pregnancy affect glucose metabolism and insulin production, eventually leading to a state of insulin resistance. The hormone human placental lactogen (hPL; Figure 3.2) is of special significance in this process.

Metabolic changes

Basal metabolic rate

It is often stated that the basal metabolic rate (BMR), i.e. the energy metabolism at complete rest, increases about 20 per cent during pregnancy. However, as indicated below, the magnitude of this increase varies considerably among different women and seems to be related to their nutritional situation. The increase in BMR during pregnancy is generally considered to be an effect of increased amounts of tissues and metabolic activity. Furthermore, as discussed below, women may even decrease their BMR during early pregnancy, possibly in response to undernutrition. The physiological

mechanisms responsible for such a decrease are unknown.

Insulin and carbohydrate metabolism

During pregnancy the increased insulin secretion causes a reduction in fasting glucose levels. Insulin levels are, however, little affected during the first part of pregnancy. As pregnancy advances, maternal insulin resistance develops. This is illustrated in Figure 3.3, which shows the response of healthy women in early and late pregnancy to a 50 g oral glucose load. During early pregnancy there is a normal plasma insulin response, with plasma glucose concentrations that are even somewhat lower than in the non-pregnant state. During late pregnancy, however, plasma glucose reaches a high level despite a considerably enhanced plasma insulin response. This pattern could be explained by a relative resistance to insulin by peripheral tissues during late pregnancy. The consequence of these changes is that the glucose in the maternal blood is directed to the foetus. The insulin resistance of peripheral tissues, typical for late pregnancy, is not maintained during lactation (Neville *et al.*, 1994).

Lipid metabolism

Human pregnancy is usually associated with a substantial retention of body fat. This retention is considered to be a feature of mainly the first part of pregnancy, with the peak in body fat content occurring around gestational week 30. Plasma levels of most lipid fractions increase during pregnancy, including free fatty acids, triglycerides, cholesterol and phospholipids (Figure 3.4). These increments reflect incompletely known changes in hepatic and adipose tissue metabolism as well as in transport kinetics.

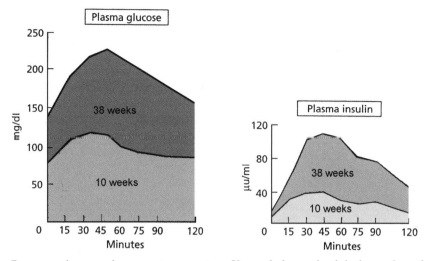

Figure 3.3 Responses in normal pregnant women to a 50 g oral glucose load during early and late pregnancy. Modified from Dunlop (1999) *Dewhurst's Textbook of Obstetrics and Gynaecology for Postgraduates*, 6th edn, pp. 76–90; reproduced by permission of Blackwell Science

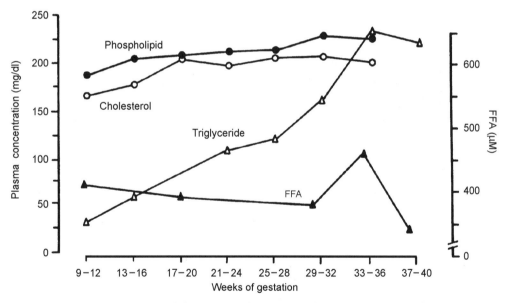

Figure 3.4 Plasma concentrations of cholesterol, triglycerides, phospholipid and free fatty acids (FFA) during normal pregnancy. Data from Kalkhoff *et al.* (1979) as modified by Rosso (1990)

Physiological changes

Blood and circulation

As shown in Table 3.1, pregnancy is associated with gradually increasing plasma and blood volumes. Red cell mass is also increased to meet the increased demand for oxygen transport. However, plasma volume expands more than red cell mass, and as a consequence there are decreased concentrations of many blood constituents, such as haemoglobin. The

Table 3.1 Plasma volume, red cell volume, total blood volume and haematocrit in pregnancy

	Non-pregnant	Gestational week 20	Gestational week 30	Gestational week 40
Plasma volume (ml)	2600	3150	3750	3850
Red cell mass (ml)	1400	1450	1550	1650
Total blood volume (ml)	4000	4600	5300	5500
Body haematocrit (%)	35.0	32.0	29.0	30.0

Modified from Llewellyn-Jones (1999c).

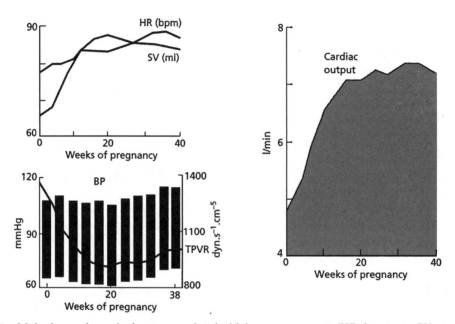

Figure 3.5 Major haemodynamic changes associated with human pregnancy (HR, heart rate; SV, stroke volume; BP, blood pressure; TPVR, total peripheral vascular resistance). Modified from Dunlop (1999) *Dewhurst's Textbook of Obstetrics and Gynaecology for Postgraduates*, 6th edn, pp. 76–90; reproduced by permission of Blackwell Science

marked circulatory changes which characterize human pregnancy are illustrated in Figure 3.5 and appear to be initiated by peripheral vasodilatation. There is obviously a marked augmentation of cardiac output resulting from increases in both heart rate and stroke volume. Despite the increases in cardiac output, blood pressure decreases for most of the duration of pregnancy, which implies that there is a very substantial reduction in total peripheral vascular resistance. If the baby is of low birthweight, increases in blood and plasma volume during pregnancy tend to be comparatively small.

Kidney function

As described above, pregnancy is associated with a decrease in peripheral vascular resistance and a systematic vasodilatation, possibly an effect of oestrogen. As a consequence, there is a marked increase in blood flow to many organs including the kidneys, which causes an

Table 3.2 Estimated amounts of extracellular and intracellular water retained during pregnancy (ml)

	Total water	Extracellular water	Intracellular water
Fetus	2414	1400	1014
Placenta	540	260	280
Amniotic fluid	792	792	0
Uterus	800	528	272
Mammary gland	304	148	156
Plasma	920	920	0
Red cells	163	0	163
Total	5933	4048	1885

Modified from Hytten FE (1980) Weight gain in pregnancy. In: *Clinical Physiology in Obstetrics*, ed. Hytten FE and Chamberlain G, pp. 193–223. Reproduced by permission of Blackwell Science.

increase in glomerular filtration rate of up to about 60 per cent of the prepregnant value. It remains at this high level until the last weeks of gestation, when it starts to decline.

Water retention

Retention of fluid always occurs during pregnancy, accounting for 6–8 kg of the average maternal weight gain. A large part of this retention is due to an increase in plasma volume. Hytten (1980) has estimated how the fluid retained during pregnancy is distributed between the extracellular and intracellular space of different organs and tissues (Table 3.2). According to this calculation about 70 per cent of the retained water is extracellular.

Breasts and lactation

During pregnancy, oestrogen, progesterone and prolactin stimulate the growth and development of the breasts. The mammary glands start to produce small amounts of milk (colostrum) 1–2 months before delivery. After parturition and the removal of the placenta, oestrogen levels drop, thereby allowing pro-lactin levels to increase. This, together with placing the infant at the breast, initiates lactation. The human breast is technically a large exocrine gland composed of 15–20 segments embedded in adipose and connective tissue (Figure 3.6). Lactation is maintained by the continuous sucking of the infant, which stimulates prolactin secretion and subsequently milk production by the mammary glands. In this way a hungry baby increases the milk production of its mother. The sucking of the nipple by the infant also stimulates the secretion of oxytocin from the pituitary. This hormone acts on the smooth muscle cells around the milk ducts in the mammary gland, causing contraction and milk ejection, the so-called let-down reflex. It should be noted that the human breast, in contrast to the mammary glands of milk-producing animals like cows and goats, can store only small quantities of milk in the so-called lactiferous sinuses (Figure 3.6). The implication is that an adequate let-down reflex is very important if the baby is to obtain sufficient milk.

Changes in Body Weight During Reproduction

Pregnancy

Figure 3.7 shows changes in weight during pregnancy in groups of women from different parts of the world. The average weight gain during gestation apparently varies between approximately 6 and 14 kg. Variations among individual women are, however, even larger. Recommendations regarding the amount of weight a woman ought to gain during pregnancy have been highly controversial throughout the past century. For a long period of time, many obstetricians favoured restricting the amount of weight gained during pregnancy to prevent toxaemia, difficult deliveries and maternal obesity. However, it was gradually

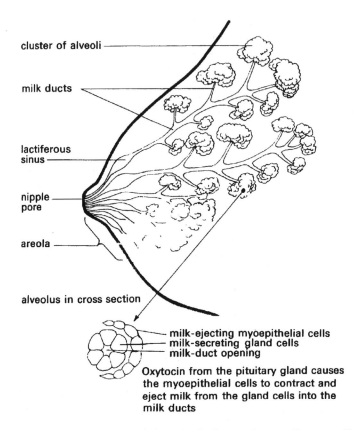

Figure 3.6 Milk-producing structures and ducts in the human breast. Courtesy, Jimmie Lynne Avery

realized that maternal weight gain is associated with infant birth weight, and that restricting maternal weight gain could result in an increased incidence of low-birth-weight infants. Hytten and Leitch (1971) established the physiological norms for total weight gain during pregnancy, the rate of weight gain during the last half of gestation, and the weight gain associated with the best reproductive performance. Using data from more than 3800 British premigravidae women who were 'eating to appetite', they concluded that the average total gain was 12.5 kg. This weight gain was associated with the best reproductive outcome in terms of infant birth-weight, infant survival and incidence of pre-eclampsia. However, Hytten and Leitch also emphasized that considerable variations in weight gain may well be consistent with good pregnancy outcomes.

Table 3.3 Recommended total weight gain in pregnant women by prepregnancy BMI (kg/m^2)

Weight-for-height category	Recommended total gain (kg)
Low (BMI <19.8)	12.5–18
Normal (BMI 19.8–26.0)	11.5–16
High (BMI 26.0–29.0)[a]	7–11.5

[a]The recommended target weight gain for obese women (BMI > 29.0) is at least 6 kg.
From Institute of Medicine (1990b) *Nutrition During Pregnancy*. Reproduced with permission by the *American Journal of Clinical Nutrition*. © *Am. J.Clin. Nutr.* American Society for Clinical Nutrition.

In 1990, an American report reassessed the relationship between pregnancy weight gain and various maternal and foetal outcomes (Institute of Medicine, 1990b). It confirmed a

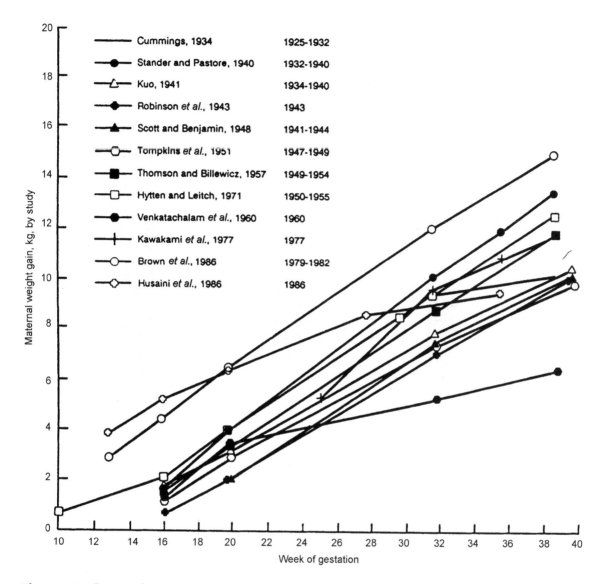

Figure 3.7 Pattern of maternal weight gain during pregnancy shown by data from 12 studies. From Institute of Medicine (1990a) *Nutrition during Pregnancy*; reproduced by permission of the National Academy of Sciences

strong relationship between pregnancy weight gain and infant size and provided target ranges for recommended weight gain according to prepregnancy body mass index (BMI; Table 3.3). These recommended weight gain ranges, known as the IOM's recommendations, have been evaluated in several studies. The results tend to show that women whose weight gain

falls within these ranges have better outcomes of pregnancy, for infants as well as for mothers, than women whose weight gain falls outside these ranges (Abrams *et al.*, 2000). Figure 3.8 illustrates how weight gains within and outside of the IOM ranges are related to pregnancy outcomes with respect to infant birth-weight and caesarean delivery.

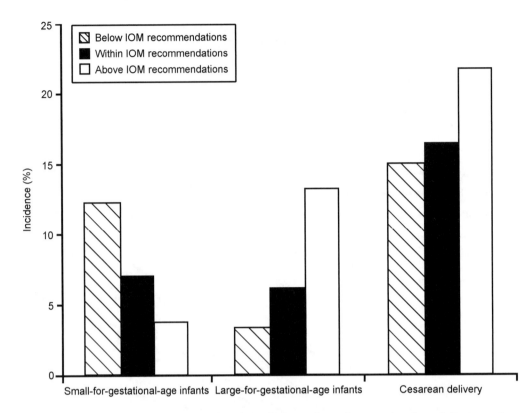

Figure 3.8 Incidence of small-for-gestational-age infants, large-for-gestational-age-infants, and caesarean delivery for women from San Fransisco with normal prepregnancy weights and pregnancy weight gains below (<12.4 kg), within (12.5–16 kg), and above (>16 kg) the weight-gain recommendations of the Institute of Medicine (IOM) in 6690 pregnancies. Data from Parker and Abrams (1992) *Obstet. Gynecol.* **79**, 664–666 as modified by Abrams *et al.* (2000) *Am. J. Clin. Nutr.* **71**(Suppl.), 1233S–1241S. Reproduced with permission by the *American Journal of Clinical Nutrition*. © *Am. J. Clin. Nutr.* American Society for Clinical Nutrition

Lactation

Many women retain significant amounts of weight after delivery. It is often stated that the fat component of this retained weight represents a physiological reserve of energy for use during lactation. However, a number of recent studies have shown that significant weight loss does not necessarily occur during lactation, especially in well-nourished, affluent women (Prentice *et al.*, 1996). However, on average, women tend to lose about 0.5 kg of body weight per month during lactation (Prentice *et al.*, 1996).

Composition of weight gained and lost during reproduction

After having established the physiological norms for total weight gain during pregnancy, Hytten also investigated the composition of the retained weight. A slight modification of his estimates is shown in Table 3.4. The figures in this table are based on the so-called reference woman (i.e. a healthy woman eating in accordance with her appetite and gaining the optimal amount of weight during pregnancy). The components of weight gain can be divided into two

Table 3.4 Site-specific protein and fat deposition during pregnancy, and energy costs involved, in a reference woman with a pregnancy weight gain of 12.4 kg delivering a baby of 3.3 kg

Site	Weight gain (g)				Energy costs (kJ)		
	Protein	Fat	Water	Total	Protein	Fat	Total
Fetus	440	440	2414	3924	12760	20240	33000
Placenta	100	4	540	644	2900	184	3084
Amniotic fluid	3	0	792	795	87	0	87
Uterus	166	4	800	970	4814	184	4998
Breasts	81	12	304	397	2349	552	2901
Blood	135	20	1287	1442	3915	920	4835
Extracellular water	0	0	1496	1496	0	0	0
Subtotal	925	480	7633	9038	26825	22080	48905
Adipose tissue	67	2676	602	3345	1943	123096	125039
Total	992	3156	8235	12383	28768	145176	173944

Modified from Prentice *et al.* (1996) *Eur. J. Clin. Nutr.* **50** (Suppl. 1), S82–S111. Reproduced by permission of Nature Publishing Group.

parts – the products of conception, and maternal tissue accretion. The latter accounts for the main part of the weight gain. An important aspect of maternal tissue accretion is fat gain which, according to Table 3.4, amounts to approximately 3 kg. This figure has been found to vary considerably among populations of women as well as among individual women within populations.

Another aspect of body fat mobilization during lactation is the fact that adipose tissue in different parts of the body has different biological functions. Figure 3.9 shows how the amount of adipose tissue in different body compartments changes postpartum in a group of well-nourished Swedish women. In women in this particular study (Sohlström and Forsum, 1995), most of the fat retained during pregnancy was on the trunk and a smaller amount on the thighs. However, fat from thigh adipose tissue seems to be more completely mobilized postpartum than fat from adipose tissue on the trunk. Furthermore, a relationship was identified between the extent and duration of lactation on the one hand and fat loss from the thighs on the other. This observation confirms previous biochemical

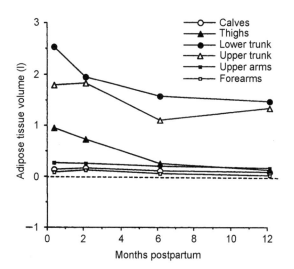

Figure 3.9 Adipose tissue volume in six body compartments throughout the first twelve months postpartum in healthy Swedish women lactating for 2–10 months. The data are averages of 10–15 women and represent values obtained postpartum minus the corresponding value obtained before pregnancy. From Sohlström (1993); reproduced by permission of Annica Sohlström

findings that the metabolism of thigh adipocytes is under hormonal control during reproduction.

Nutritional Needs During Reproduction

Assessment of human nutritional requirements

Nutritional recommendations are prepared by a number of national and international bodies. At the international level the FAO and WHO have published several reports. The European community publishes its own dietary recommendations (EC Scientific Committee for Food Reports, 1993). In Britain, the Department of Health (1991) and in the US The National Research Council, Food and Nutrition Board (1989) have prepared reports with dietary guidelines for their respective countries. Each of these reports relies on the opinion of different experts and therefore dietary recommendations may vary between countries. These recommendations are continuously revised as new knowledge becomes available. They may be designed to meet the average nutritional requirements of groups or to cover the needs of nearly all healthy individuals in a population. Recommendations are given for specific nutrients as well as for dietary composition such as the proportions of dietary energy derived from fat, protein and carbohydrate, respectively. Special consideration is usually given to the requirements of children and pregnant and lactating women.

Nutritional needs during reproduction are generally estimated as additions to the requirements of the non-pregnant, non-lactating woman. It is important to point out, however, that this approach has limitations. First, the nutritional situation that is optimal for reproduction is one where all young females (even those in the fetal state) are adequately fed. In other words, the nutritional situation before conception is as important as the nutritional situation during pregnancy and lactation. Secondly, reproduction is a biological process during which nutritional requirements are influenced by phenomena such as adaptation, storage and turnover rates. Finally, lack of a specific nutrient may be associated with permanent adverse effects when occurring at specific stages of development – so-called 'sensitive periods'.

Energy

Throughout history, special attention has been given to the diets of pregnant women. Our current understanding in the area is largely founded on the work of Hytten. As described above, he established the physiological norms for weight gain during pregnancy and conducted work aimed at separating and quantifying the different components of weight gain, thereby defining important components of gestational energy needs. Furthermore, he established the energy costs of pregnancy based on the physiological changes of the reference woman, eating according to her appetite, and gaining the 12.5 kg found to represent the optimal weight gain during pregnancy. The energy costs of forming the new tissue are shown in Table 3.4 and amount to a total of 174 MJ for the entire pregnancy. Hytten also estimated the increased BMR of the reference woman, and for the complete pregnancy this corresponded to an additional energy cost of 150 MJ, the 'energy maintenance cost of pregnancy'.

Hytten's work on the energy costs of reproduction was extended later, when investigators published measurements of the energy costs of human reproduction obtained in populations of women living under various nutritional circumstances. A compilation of these findings (Prentice and Goldberg, 2000) reveals that the energy costs of human pregnancy vary in response to the nutritional situation in which the women live (Figure 3.10). Of special interest is the observation that women may even decrease their BMR during the first part of pregnancy. Such decreases have been

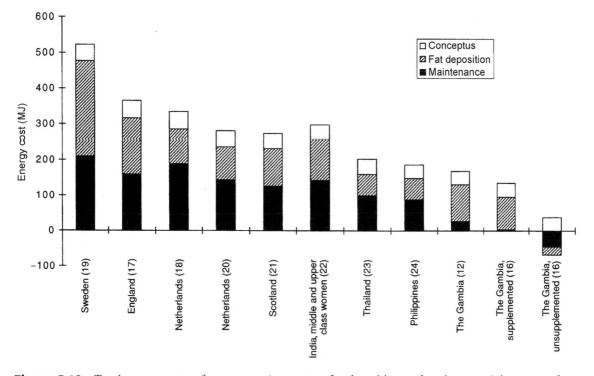

Figure 3.10 Total energy costs of pregnancy (conceptus, fat deposition and maintenance) in women from affluent and poor countries. Compiled by Prentice and Goldberg (2000) *Am. J. Clin. Nutr.* **71**(Suppl.), 1226S–1232S. Reproduced with permission by the *American Journal of Clinical Nutrition.* © *Am. J. Clin. Nutr.* American Society for Clinical Nutrition

observed in women in well-nourished populations, but are more common in women with a limited availability of food. This phenomenon has been interpreted as an energy-saving mechanism with the purpose of ensuring reproduction under circumstances of poor nutrition. Furthermore, the total energy cost of pregnancy has been found to correlate with the percentage of body fat the woman had before pregnancy as well as with her total weight gain during pregnancy (Figure 3.11). The latter relationship indicates that the apparently desirable weight gain (12.5 kg) is associated with an energy cost for maintenance of approximately 160 MJ, i.e. very close to Hytten's estimate of the energy maintenance cost of pregnancy.

During the last two decades the doubly labelled water method has given us new possibilities for the measurement of energy expenditure of humans during truly normal living conditions. As a result, a profoundly new way of looking at human energy metabolism and energy needs has developed. Thus recommendations for dietary energy are currently derived from estimates of BMR and PAL (physical activity level). PAL is a factor that ranges between approximately 1.2 and 2.5, depending on the physical activity of a subject. The total energy expenditure (TEE), equal to the dietary need for energy when body weight is constant, is the product of BMR and PAL. Prentice *et al.* suggested in 1996 that this approach for calculating dietary energy needs should also be applied to pregnant women, although available estimates of the TEE and the PAL of such women are comparatively few, and the possibility of accurately predicting

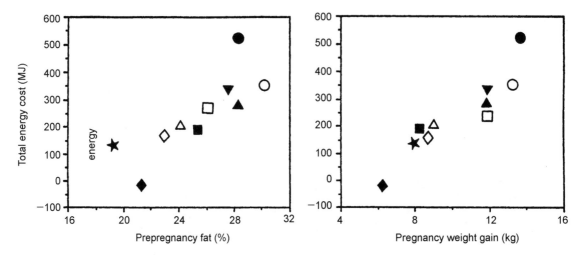

Figure 3.11 Intercountry correlations of the total energy costs of pregnancy with prepregnancy maternal fatness and pregnancy weight gain in women from Sweden (●), England (○), the Netherlands (▲▼), Scotland (□), Thailand (△), the Philippines (■) and the Gambia (★◆◇). Compiled by Prentice and Goldberg (2000) *Am. J. Clin. Nutr.* **71**(Suppl.), 1226S–1232S. Reproduced with permission by the *American Journal of Clinical Nutrition*. © *Am. J. Clin. Nutr.* American Society for Clinical Nutrition

BMR from body weight and age is not as good in pregnant as in non-pregnant women. Table 3.5 outlines how the total energy cost of pregnancy in a well-nourished woman with a PAL of 1.6 before conception can be calculated.

With respect to the energy costs of lactation, FAO/WHO/UNU recommended in 1985 that the average healthy, lactating woman needs an additional 2.09 MJ/day during the first 6 months postpartum to produce about 700–800 ml of breast milk per day containing 2.9 kJ/ml, assuming an efficiency of conversion of 80 per cent. It was then assumed that the fat deposited in the maternal body during pregnancy (equivalent on average to 150 MJ) is mobilized and used for milk production. However, when these recommendations were revised, the fact that fat loss is not a programmed component of lactation was taken into consideration (Prentice *et al.*, 1996). Thus the revised recommendations represent the full cost of lactation as well as the cost obtained when an appropriate modification for fat loss is made (Table 3.6). This table also provides figures for full as well as for partial breast-feeders. As indicated, the figures given in Table 3.6 represent the additional requirements for human lactation. The total requirement for dietary energy for a lactating woman is thus her total energy expenditure (derived from her BMR and PAL) plus an appropriate figure obtained from Table 3.6.

Protein

The increased protein requirements during pregnancy consist of an increased maintenance requirement and an allowance for the formation of new tissue. Hytten calculated the amount of protein in the different tissues synthesized during pregnancy and a slight modification of his calculation is shown in Table 3.4. During pregnancy the reference woman retains a total of 992 g protein. This figure is calculated on the basis of the amounts of new tissues formed during pregnancy and their nitrogen content. Based on such calculations, it has been

Table 3.5 Example of how to calculate energy requirements in pregnancy using estimates of the physical activity level (PAL) before and during gestation (MJ/day)

	First trimester	Second trimester	Third trimester
Non-pregnant non-lactating basal metabolic rate[a]	5.50	5.50	5.50
Pregnancy increment in basal metabolic rate	0.20	0.40	1.10
Estimated PAL[b]	1.55	1.45	1.40
Total energy expenditure	8.83	8.56	9.24
Energy deposited	0.40	0.70	0.50
Total requirement[c]	9.23	9.26	9.74
Increment over non-pregnant non-lactating energy expenditure[d]	0.43	0.46	0.94

[a]Calculated according to Schofield *et al.* (1985) on the basis of body-weight and age.
[b]This example assumes a low-activity lifestyle.
[c]The total energy cost of pregnancy (280 days) in this example is 170 MJ ($280/3 \times 0.43 + 280/3 \times 0.46 + 280/3 \times 0.94$ MJ).
[d]Non-pregnant, non-lactating PAL estimated to be 1.6.
Modified from Prentice *et al.* (1996).

Table 3.6 Calculation of energy requirements during lactation. Values represent increments to the maternal non-pregnant, non-lactating requirements[a]

Period (month)	Milk volume (g/day)	Energy requirement (kJ/day) Full costs	Energy requirement (kJ/day) Allowing for fat loss
All women			
0–1	680	2380	1730
1–2	780	2730	2080
2–3	820	2870	2220
Full breast-feeders			
3–6	820	2870	2220
6–12	650	2275	2275
12–24	600	2100	2100
Partial breast-feeders			
3–6	410	1430	780
6–12	325	1140	1140
12–24	300	1050	1050

[a]Calculated using estimates of basal metabolic rate and physical activity level.
Modified from Prentice *et al.* (1996).

the literature indicating that pregnant women store higher amounts of nitrogen, but this has been difficult to prove. The additional requirement for dietary protein during lactation is based on estimates of the amount of milk produced and its nitrogen content. According to the recommendations of the FAO/WHO/UNU Expert Consultation (1985), this figure is about 9 g per day for a woman in full lactation. This figure, as well as the figures given above for pregnancy, represent average figures and should be increased first by about 40 per cent to allow for inefficient utilisation of dietary protein (assuming 70 per cent efficiency to convert dietary protein to tissue or milk protein) and then by 25–30 per cent to allow for individual variations. The figures thus obtained should be further adjusted using an appropriate figure depending on the digestibility of the protein in the diet of the particular woman or population (FAO/WHO/UNU Expert Consultation, 1985).

Vitamins and minerals

Dietary recommendations for the fat-soluble vitamins A, D, E and K, for vitamin C,

estimated that an average of 0.6 g is stored daily during the first quarter of pregnancy, a figure which gradually increases to 6 g during the last quarter of pregnancy. There are also reports in thiamine, riboflavin, niacin, B_6, B_{12}, folic acid, sodium, potassium, chloride, calcium, phosphorous, magnesium, iron, copper, selenium, iodine and zinc have been published in the US (Institute of Medicine, 2000), in Britain (Department of Health, 1991) and for the European Community (EC Scientific Committee for Food Reports, 1993). These publications include specific recommendations for pregnant and lactating women.

The physiological requirements for iron during pregnancy and lactation are well established. The iron costs for pregnancy are obtained by adding up the iron content of the fetus, the placenta, the increased maternal red cell mass and maternal basal iron losses. Together, this amounts to about 1000 mg of iron for a complete pregnancy. During lactation the iron costs are about 1.1 mg/day as long as menstruation is absent. However, during pregnancy several indices used to assess iron status are affected. Thus haemoglobin concentration, haematocrit and red cell count decrease due to an expansion of plasma volume. Furthermore, serum-iron falls while iron-binding capacity increases. The absorption of iron from the gut is also increased during pregnancy. Serum ferritin decreases even in women taking iron supplements. So far, strict criteria defining iron deficiency during pregnancy have not been established.

During pregnancy, the growth of the fetal skeleton requires calcium and during lactation a considerable amount of this mineral is needed for milk production. These demands are met by an enhanced absorption and by mobilization from the maternal skeleton. Although calcium losses from repeated pregnancies and lactations can be significant, there are no conclusive data showing that reproduction contributes significantly to bone loss even in countries where habitual calcium intakes are low. Apparently, after the infant is weaned, compensatory mechanisms help to increase bone mineral density in the mother.

Vitamin A deficiency during pregnancy weakens the immune system, increases the risk of infections and has been linked with night-blindness as well as with poor fetal growth and premature birth. Since intakes of vitamin A are inadequate in many parts of the world, supplementation of diets consumed by women of childbearing age is sometimes considered. It is important to keep in mind that excessive intakes of vitamin A during pregnancy may be teratogenic.

Maternal vitamin D deficiency has been linked to maternal osteomalacia, and reduced birth-weight as well as to neonatal hypocalcaemia and tetany. Exclusively breast-fed infants may also be at risk for vitamin D deficiency. Low sun exposure, dark skin and living at northern latitudes are risk factors for this kind of deficiency.

Folate, folic acid or folacin deficiency during pregnancy causes megaloblastic anaemia and is linked to poor reproductive outcomes. Furthermore, it has recently been established that supplemental folic acid at the time of conception prevents the occurrence of neural tube defects, a serious malformation in the central nervous system. Therefore, it is recommended in many countries that women who have had a pregnancy affected by a neural tube defect should consume supplemental folic acid around the time of conception.

Conclusion

During her reproductive age a woman releases approximately one fertilizable ovum each month from the ovary. If fertilized this ovum is implanted in the uterine wall and develops into a fetus and finally a baby. The fetus is connected to the mother by the placenta, which is also an important endocrine organ.

The maternal physiology and metabolism adapt to the pregnant state in response to the hormones secreted by the placenta. Typical maternal changes during pregnancy are increases in blood volume and cardiac output, an increased basal metabolic rate, peripheral insulin resistance and increased blood lipid levels. Lactation is maintained by two hormones, prolactin and oxytocin, in combination with the suckling stimulus provided by the baby. Weight gain during pregnancy is highly variable between women. Averages for populations vary between 6 and 14 kg. Recent evidence suggests that the optimal weight gain of a woman is related to her prepregnant body mass index. This means that thin women should gain more weight during pregnancy than overweight and fat women.

A significant proportion of the weight gained during pregnancy is body fat. In contrast to a previously common opinion, mobilization of body fat does not seem to be a programmed component of human lactation. Recommendations for dietary energy and specific nutrients (i.e. protein, vitamins and minerals) during reproduction are issued by a number of national and international bodies. These recommendations are continuously changing as new scientific knowledge becomes available. Nutritional requirements during reproduction are often estimated as additions to the needs of the non-pregnant, non-lactating woman. However, this approach is not always appropriate. Current recommendations for energy needs during pregnancy and lactation are based on estimates of the energy costs of reproduction of a reference woman as well as on an estimate of her physical activity level.

References

Abrams B, Altman S and Pickett K (2000) Pregnancy weight gain: still controversial. *Am. J. Clin. Nutr.* **71**(Suppl.), 1233S–1241S.

Avery JL (1983) *Lact-Aid Nursing Supplementer*, revised edn. Lact-Aid International, Inc., Athens, TN.

Department of Health (1991) *Dietary Reference Values for Food Energy and Nutrients for the United Kingdom*. Report on health and social subjects 41. Committee on Medical Aspects of Food Policy. HMSO, London.

Dunlop W (1999) Normal pregnancy: physiology and endocrinology. In: *Dewhurst's Textbook of Obstetrics and Gynaecology for Postgraduates*, ed. Edmonds DK, 6th edn, pp. 76–90. Blackwell Science, London.

EC Scientific Committee for Food Reports (1993) *Nutrient and Energy Intakes for the European Community*, 31 Series. Directorate-General, Industry, Luxembourg.

FAO/WHO/UNU Expert Consultation (1985) *Energy and Protein Requirements*. World Health Organization, Geneva.

Glinoer D, De Nayer P, Bourdoux P, Lemone M, Robyn C, Van Steirteghem A, Kinthaert J and Lejeune B (1990) Regulation of maternal thyroid during pregnancy. *J. Clin. Endocrinol. Metab.* **71**, 276–287.

Hytten FE (1980) Weight gain in pregnancy. In: *Clinical Physiology in Obstetrics*, ed. Hytten FE and Chamberlain G, pp. 193–233. Blackwell Scientific, London.

Hytten FE and Leitch I (1971) The average weight gain in normal pregnancy. In: *The Physiology of Human Pregnancy*, 2nd edn, pp. 281–285. Blackwell Scientific, London,

Institute of Medicine (1990a) Total amount and pattern of weight gain: physiological and maternal determinants. In: *Nutrition during Pregnancy*, pp. 96–120. National Academy of Sciences, National Academy Press, Washington, DC.

Institute of Medicine (1990b) *Nutrition during Pregnancy*. National Academy of Sciences, National Academy Press, Washington, DC.

Institute of Medicine (2000) *Dietary Reference Intakes for Thiamine, Riboflavine, Niacin, Vitamin B$_6$, Folate, Vitamin B$_{12}$, Pantothenic Acid, Biotin and Choline*. National Academy Press, Food and Nutrition Board, Washington, DC.

Kalkhoff RK, Kissebah AH and Kim H (1979) Carbohydrate and lipid metabolism during normal pregnancy: relationship to gestational hormone action. In: *The Diabetic Pregnancy*, ed. Merkatz I and Adam PAJ, pp. 3–21. Grune and Stratton, New York.

Llewellyn-Jones D (1999a) Ovulation and the menstrual cycle. In: *Fundamentals of Obstetrics and Gynaecology*, 7th edn, pp. 9–16. Mosby International, London.

Llewellyn-Jones D (1999b) Conception and placental

development. In: *Fundamentals of Obstetrics and Gynaecology*, 7th edn, pp. 17–26. Mosby International, London.

Llewellyn-Jones D. (1999c) Physiological and anatomical changes in pregnancy. In: *Fundamentals of Obstetrics and Gynaecology*, 7th edn, pp. 31–36. Mosby International, London.

Lunn PG, Prentice AM, Austin S and Whitehead RG (1980) Influence of maternal diet on plasma prolactin levels during lactation. *Lancet* i, 623–625.

National Research Council, Food and Nutrition Board (1989) *Recommended Dietary Allowances*, 10th edn. Commission on Life Sciences, National Academy Press, Washington, DC.

Neville MC, Casey C and Hay WW (1994) Endocrine regulation of nutrient flux in the lactating woman. Do the mechanisms differ from pregnancy? In: *Nutrient Regulation during Pregnancy, Lactation and Infant Growth*, ed. Allen L, King J and Lönnerdal B. Advances in Experimental Medicine and Biology, Vol. 352, pp. 85–98. Plenum Press, New York.

Parker J and Abrams B (1992) Prenatal weight gain advice: an examination of the recent prenatal weight gain recommendations of the Institute of Medicine. *Obstet. Gynecol.* **79**, 664–669.

Prentice AM and Goldberg GR (2000) Energy adaptations in human pregnancy: limits and long-term consequences. *Am. J. Clin. Nutr.* **71** (Suppl.), 1226S–1232S.

Prentice AM, Spaaij CJK, Goldberg GR, Poppitt SD, van Raaij JMA, Totton M, Swann D and Black AE (1996) Energy requirements of pregnant and lactating women. *Eur. J. Clin. Nutr.* **50** (Suppl. 1), S82–S111.

Rosso P (1990) Lipid metabolism. In: *Nutrition and Metabolism in Pregnancy. Mother and Fetus*, pp. 47–58. Oxford University Press, Oxford.

Schofield WN, Schofield C and James WPT (1985) Basal metabolic rate. *Hum. Nutr. Clin. Nutr.* **39C**(Suppl. 1), 1–96.

Sohlström A (1993) Body fat during reproduction in a nutritional perspective. Studies in women and rats. Thesis, Karolinska Institute, Stockholm.

Sohlström A and Forsum E (1995) Changes in adipose tissue volume and distribution during reproduction in Swedish women as assessed by magnetic resonance imaging. *Am. J. Clin. Nutr.* **61**, 287–295.

Thomson AM and Hytten FE (1973) Effects of nutrition on human reproduction. *J. Reprod. Fert.* **19** (Suppl.), 581–583.

4

PHYSIOLOGICAL AND NUTRITIONAL ASPECTS OF THE PLACENTA

Michael E. Symonds, Helen Budge and Terence Stephenson

LEARNING OUTCOMES

- The importance of the placenta in mediating nutritional effects on fetal growth.

- Comparative aspects of adipose tissue, liver and skeletal muscle development in the fetus.

- The differential effects of maternal undernutrition with respect to stage of gestation on placental and fetal growth and maturation.

- The role of skeletal muscle and adipose tissue in promoting effective thermoregulatory adaptation to the extrauterine environment.

- The interaction between fetal nutrient supply and endocrine adaptations within fetal tissues.

- The use of different animal models to examine nutritional programming of fetal growth.

Introduction

The fetus and placenta together comprise the unit of reproduction of man and most mammals. The placenta not only provides the essential physical link between the fetus and its mother but, by virtue of the placental blood supply, the mother provides oxygen, nutrients,

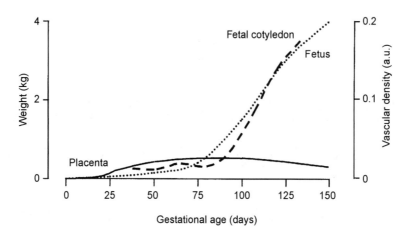

Figure 4.1   Summary of placento-fetal growth curves and changes in placental vasculature in sheep as described by Symonds *et al.* (2001) and Stegmann (1974). Solid line, placenta; dashed line, fetal cotyledonary component of placenta; dotted line, fetus

hormones and antibodies to support the life, growth and development of the fetus and removes the end-products of fetal metabolism. The actual anatomical structure of the placenta varies from one species to another but, in each species, it is so arranged that the interchange of materials can take place through the walls of the capillaries so that fetus and mother maintain their own blood supply to and from the placenta. Bearing in mind the functions of the placenta, it is easy to appreciate that abnormalities in its growth and development may have important consequences for the fetus. Understanding the nature and causes of these effects has become an important area of investigation, but there are clearly limitations to their study in man. Recourse must be made to the use of animals and this is why the bulk of this chapter appears to be animal-oriented, with most experiments having been carried out on sheep. Furthermore, because much of the work has been undertaken in the last 10–15 years, the chapter is very much in the nature of a biochemical review with some hesitancy about detailed extrapolation of the findings to man.

Normal growth and development of the placenta is critical in ensuring that a healthy, appropriately sized fetus is born at term. Maximal growth of the placenta precedes that of the fetus and this is shown for the lamb in Figure 4.1, but the nutritional exchange capacity increases with gestational age in conjunction with structural maturation of the placenta (Stegmann, 1974) as the fetus grows and its overall metabolic rate rises (Schneider, 1996). At term, placental and fetal weights are positively correlated, with placental weight normally being between 10 and 15 per cent of newborn body weight (Broughton Pipkin *et al.*, 1994).

Unsurprisingly, pathological changes in placental size occur together with alterations in fetal growth. A small placenta usually causes intrauterine growth restriction (IUGR; Owens *et al.*, 1995), whereas a large placenta, as in human pregnancy complicated by diabetes mellitus, is associated with a large fetus (Naeye, 1987). It is important that altered placental size and potential changes in placental function are identified in women as early as possible in pregnancy. This may then enable individuals to be targeted for subsequent longitudinal assessments (Table 4.1) of placental function and fetal well-being.

It has now become apparent that more modest increases or decreases in placental size

Table 4.1 Summary of potential placental measurements during pregnancy, or at time of birth, providing insight into potential physiological and/or pathological alterations in placental function contributing to altered fetal weight and development

Measurement made	Alteration following placental 'dysfunction'	Fetal adaptation/ pathology	Reference
Placental blood flow	Absent or reversed end diastolic flow as measured by Doppler flow	Intrauterine growth restriction	Kingdom, 1998
Placental relaxation and perfusion	Magnetic resonance imaging indicating reduced relaxation time	Pre-eclampsia	Duncan *et al.*, 1998
Placental weight	Decrease	Decrease in fetal weight	Owens *et al.*, 1995
	Increase	Increase in fetal weight	Naeye, 1987

which are not accompanied by gross changes in fetal weight but by altered fetal dimensions may be predictive of subsequent adult human obesity, cardiovascular disease, hypertension and Syndrome X (Table 4.2). This has led to the hypothesis that reductions in maternal nutrition at different stages of gestation can have differential effects on placental and/or fetal growth, thus offering a possible explanation of the contribution of a compromised fetal growth pattern to increased risk of adult disease (Barker, 1999). The concept that fetal physiology is programmed has become known as the 'Barker Hypothesis'. This concept has substantially added to clinical and scientific interest in placental and fetal development. Current knowledge of placental function is largely derived from animal studies in which

changes in pathologically compromised placentae are compared with age-matched, rather than nutritionally matched, controls. Material in Chapters 1, 2, 6 and 7 should be read in relation to this chapter.

Comparative Aspects of Fetal Growth and Maturation

When considering our current understanding of the interaction between placental growth and fetal organ maturation it is important that the profound differences between species in length of gestation, size and maturity at birth as well as litter size are taken into account. This is necessary if contemporary knowledge

Table 4.2 Summary of the association between altered placental weight or size, size at birth and subsequent predisposition to adult cardiovascular disease (CVD) as indicated from epidemiological studies

Change in placental weight	Change in birth-weight or dimensions	Stage of gestation at which placento-fetal adaptation occurred	Adult CVD characteristic	Reference
Increase	No change in weight	Early	Stroke	Roseboom *et al.*, 2000
	Decreased weight ± increased length	Mid	Hypertension	Barker *et al.*, 1990, 1992
Decrease	Decrease	Early/throughout?	Coronary heart disease	Martyn *et al.*, 1996
No change	Decrease ± decreased length	Late	Obesity	Barker, 1994; Osmond
			Coronary heart disease	*et al.*, 1993

of placento-fetal development is to be related to clinically important situations such as, for example, premature deliveries or small-for-gestational-age infants. Small laboratory animals (primarily rodents) are useful in gaining new insights into developmental endocrinology, but large animal models, particularly sheep, have been critical in developing our understanding of fetal physiology. It is well known that, for all studies in which animal models are used to address human-based problems, there are a number of important caveats that should be borne in mind when extrapolating the results obtained to clinical situations. When undertaking investigations with small animals it must be remembered that:

(a) Offspring are immature at birth and have an immature hypothalamic–pituitary axis. This has several major functional consequences, particularly for thermoregulation. Body temperature is normally maintained in altricial species by pups huddling together in a nest rather than as a result of active heat-producing mechanisms as in more precocial offspring such as human babies and lambs (Symonds and Lomax, 1992).

(b) Large litters are produced with variable differences in the size of offspring.

(c) The placental growth trajectory differs markedly from that of the human, peaking at the end of gestation (Langley-Evans et al., 1996) rather than in early or mid-gestation.

(d) In many studies, the number of individuals studied from the same litter is often represented as the number of fetuses, rather than considering the mother as the experimental unit (Langley-Evans et al., 1999), thereby altering the statistical power of the study.

In contrast, large animals are more comparable with humans in terms of having a long gestation and normally producing a single fetus with a mature hypothalamic–pituitary axis at birth, although they have a different placental structure. For example, sheep have what is called a syndesmochorial placenta (i.e. two maternal but three fetal layers with no maternal uterine epithelium) compared with the human placenta which is haemochorial (i.e. no maternal but three fetal layers). As we have commented above, it is unethical to conduct nutritional studies on pregnant women and certainly not possible to obtain fetal and placental samples at defined stages of gestation. In this respect, the sheep model has proved invaluable in enabling new insights into the impact of maternal nutrient restriction at different stages of gestation on fetal development. Other comparative differences between lambs and human infants, which should be noted, include the following:

(a) Lambs have very little subcutaneous adipose tissue at birth and are dependent on the rapid drying of their fleece at birth in order to reduce heat loss, whereas infants have greater total lipid stores (Mellor and Cockburn, 1986) and the amount of subcutaneous adipose tissue present at birth determines its insulatory properties.

(b) The hypothalamic–pituitary axis is more mature in lambs than in infants and this is reflected in their enhanced maturity and ability to live independently compared with infants.

The extent to which maturity and body composition impact on thermoregulatory mechanisms at birth, as well as subsequent postnatal development, is illustrated when comparing infants, lambs, piglets and rats (Table 4.3). Each species has control mechanisms, which can act to maximize heat production and/or minimize heat loss. The extent to which the ambient temperature may be either increased or decreased to enable the newborn to raise or lower its own metabolic rate is dependent on the ratio of volume to surface area plus the ability to gain an

Table 4.3 Comparison of thermoregulatory strategies after birth

	Type of thermoregulation	Strategies adopted to prevent heat loss	Mechanisms to increase heat production
Infant	Precocial	Large depots of subcutaneous adipose tissue Sleeps with parent	Non-shivering thermogenesis
Lamb	Precocial	Fully developed fleece at birth Sleeps next to ewe	Non-shivering and shivering thermogenesis
Piglet	Precocial	Sleeps next to litter mates and mother	Shivering thermogenesis
Rat pup	Altricial	Huddling in nest with litter mates	Following postnatal development of hypothalamic–pituitary axis non-shivering thermogenesis recruited

adequate milk intake. These are all factors that may act to further programme development after birth.

Placental Function and its Role in Nutrient Transfer to the Fetus

As indicated above, the placenta determines macro- and micronutrient supply to the growing fetus. Blood flow to the placenta must, therefore, be maintained together with an adequate fetal oxygen supply. Clinical emphasis has been placed on the use of non-invasive techniques to assess these aspects of placental function and includes assessment of the pattern of blood flow across the umbilical arteries (Poston, 1997) by either colour or pulsed Doppler ultrasound (Table 4.1). More recently, magnetic resonance imaging (MRI) has been utilized to further quantify placental anatomy (Duncan *et al.*, 1998). The sheep (ovine) placenta receives up to 40 per cent of cardiac output from the fetus and is one of the body's most metabolically active organs (Meschia *et al.*, 1980). Furthermore, as we have seen, it maintains fetal well-being by acting as the fetal lung, gut and kidney; it also possesses an

abundance of mitochondria, which contribute to its high metabolic rate (Carter, 2000).

Depending on the stage of gestation, oxygen consumption by the ovine placenta accounts for 40–80 per cent of the total utilization by the gravid uterus (Bell *et al.*, 1986). This occurs primarily within placental mitochondria as a result of oxidative phosphorylation associated with protein synthesis, cation transport, endocrine functions, apoptosis and proton leak (Figure 4.2). All of these processes are compromised by oxygen deficiency, although the outcome in terms of fetal compromise is dependent on the cause of the hypoxia, whose origin may be pre- or postplacental (Table 4.4). The effects of hypoxia on placental vasculature vary greatly depending on its timing and location. In preplacental hypoxia, in which intraplacental oxygen concentration is reduced, placental branching is increased (Kingdom and Kaufmann, 1997). Fetuses which are preterm and growth-restricted may have an elongated placental villous in which oxygen concentration is increased within the placental branches, possibly due to reduced extraction by the smaller fetus (i.e. postplacental hypoxia; Figure 4.3).

In order to ensure accurate diagnosis of the hypoxic location it may be necessary to measure blood flow in the uterine veins and

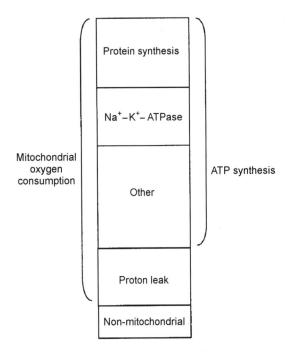

Figure 4.2 The partition of placental energy consumption between mitochondrial and non-mitochondrial metabolism as summarized by Carter (2000), based on calculations by Rolfe and Brown (1997)

umbilical arteries in conjunction with placental perfusion (Kingdom and Kaufmann, 1997). As a consequence of the necessity of defining the full extent to which fetal oxygen status may be altered under a range of pathological and/or environmental conditions, complex histological

analyses have been developed for use in the human (Bush *et al.*, 2000). These have taken into account the need to define the relative contributions from maternal and fetal components of the placenta and also its circulation (Figure 4.4; Table 4.5). Adaptations in placental structure may also determine the supply of other nutrients to the fetus.

Effect of Altered Nutrition During Pregnancy on Placental and Fetal Weight at Term

We know that in healthy mothers there are a large number of environmental, ethnic and socio-economic factors that are known to influence placental and fetal growth which will impact on maternal nutritional requirements (see Table 4.6). It is therefore important in any investigation that these variables are controlled. This is particularly the case in studies involving human subjects. In both humans and sheep, with increasing gestational age, the total metabolic requirements for fetal maintenance and growth rise as more fetal protein and lipid are deposited (Figure 4.5; Brameld *et al.*, 2000; Campbell-Brown and Hytten, 1998). It is necessary, therefore, in

Table 4.4 Summary of different types of fetal hypoxia as defined by Kingdom and Kaufmann (1997)

Source of hypoxia	Oxygen status			Examples
	Maternal	Placental	Fetal	
Preplacental	Hypoxic	Hypoxic	Hypoxic	Maternal anaemia Pregnancy at high altitude
Utero-placental	Normoxic	Hypoxic	Hypoxic	Pre-eclampsia at term Intrauterine growth restriction with preserved end-diastolic flow
Postplacental	Normoxic	Normoxic	Hypoxic	Antepartum stillbirth Feto-placental vascular obstruction, intrauterine growth restriction with absent end-diastolic flow

Table 4.5 Optimum structural and physiochemical variables required for histological examination of placentae in order to determine oxygen diffusive conductances as outlined by Bush *et al.* (2000)

Defined measurement	Sites of analysis
Blood space volumes (ml)	Maternal intervillous space
	Fetal capillary bed
Exchange surface areas (cm^2)	Maternal erythrocytes
	Upstream (maternal) aspect of trophoblast
	Downstream (fetal) aspect of trophoblast
	Luminal aspect of fetal capillaries
	Fetal erythrocytes
Oxygen–haemoglobin reaction rate (ml/ml/min/kPa)	Maternal blood
	Fetal blood
Krogh diffusion coefficient (cm^2/min/kPa)	Maternal plasma
	Trophoblast
	Stroma
	Fetal plasma

The Krogh diffusion coefficient is a measure of tissue oxygen solubility.

large animal studies for the amount of feed provided to the mother to rise as pregnancy progresses to meet these increased fetal metabolic demands. Surprisingly, in humans studied longitudinally, little change in energy intake occurs through gestation (Godfrey *et al.*, 1996).

The effects of human nutrition on weight at birth in human cohorts seem to be contradictory, as studies conducted in geographically adjacent populations indicate very different findings. For example, Godfrey *et al.* (1996) examined maternal nutrition in 538 women in Southampton, UK, and demonstrated a negative relationship between maternal carbohydrate intake and both placental and birthweights (refer to Figure 7.7). This contrasts with a subsequent publication by Mathews *et al.* (1999), who studied 693 women in the geographically adjacent city of Portsmouth and found no significant association between

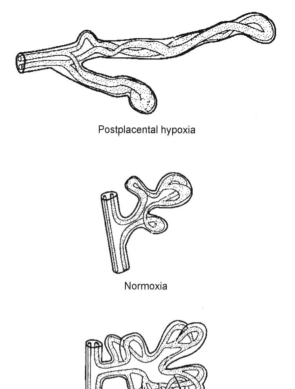

Postplacental hypoxia

Normoxia

Preplacental hypoxia

Figure 4.3 Summary of the adaptations in placental villous structure in response to altered oxygenation as described by Kingdom and Kaufmann (1997). Reproduced from Kingdom and Kaufmann (1997) *Placenta* **18**, 613–621, by permission of Harcourt Publishers Ltd

maternal nutrition and size at birth. There was a marked difference in energy intake between the mothers in these studies, which had no consistent relationship with placental or birthweights when groups were arbitrarily assigned with respect to gradations in maternal energy intake (Figure 4.6).

The extent to which apparently large differences in nutrition can have differential effects on placental or fetal growth has been well illustrated from data collected from women exposed to the Dutch famine of 1944–1945

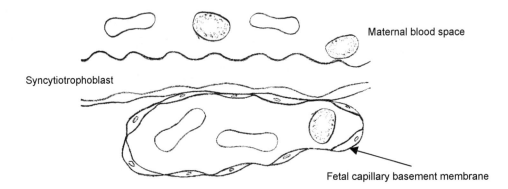

Figure 4.4 Diagram of the villous structure of a mature human placenta. Normally there is no intervention of the cytotrophoblast between the fetal capillary and syncytiotrophoblast. Consequently only one layer of trophoblast (i.e. a haemomonochorial placenta) lies between maternal and fetal blood

Table 4.6   Impact of maternal and environmental factors on birth-weight

Maternal factor	Birth outcome	Reference
Low maternal body weight	Reduced birth-weight Thinner offspring	Clarke *et al.*, 1997c; Forsen *et al.*, 1997
Low maternal birth-weight	Reduced birth-weight and higher perinatal mortality	Skjaerven *et al.*, 1997
Decrease in ambient temperature	Increased birth-weight and more adipose tissue deposition in later life	Phillips and Young, 2000; Symonds *et al.*, 1992
High altitude	Increased birth-weight	Zamudio *et al.*, 1993
Maternal smoking	Reduced birth-weight	Conter *et al.*, 1995

(Lumey, 1998). During the famine, maternal food intake was reduced by up to 50 per cent (Figure 4.7) and exposure to the famine in early gestation was associated with a large placenta at term but a normal-sized newborn. In contrast, famine exposure in late gestation resulted in less than a 10 per cent decline in birth-weight, whereas in late gestation, when maternal energy intake was increased above 2.9 MJ/day, birth-weight remained unaffected (Figure 4.8).

The effects of famine during early gestation have been proposed to be analogous to nausea

Table 4.7   Glucose and amino acids requirements for fetal growth and oxidation in the sheep

Substrate	Fetal requirement	Fraction oxidized	Reference
Glucose	7 g/day per kg body weight	0.8	Battaglia and Meschia, 1981; Hay, 1998
Nitrogen (protein/ amino acids)	1 g/day per kg body weight	0.32	Faichney and White, 1987; Marconi *et al.*, 1989

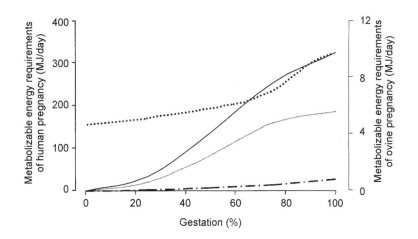

Figure 4.5 Changes in total metabolizable energy requirements (bold dotted line) according to ewe body weight (in this example for a 40 kg ewe) taking into account requirements for both ewe maintenance and growth of the conceptus on the basis of producing a 4.5 kg lamb at term (Agricultural Research Council, 1980) in relation to the increase in maternal maintenance requirements (hatched line) plus fat (dotted line) and protein (solid line) accretion in the human fetus (Campbell-Brown and Hytten, 1998).

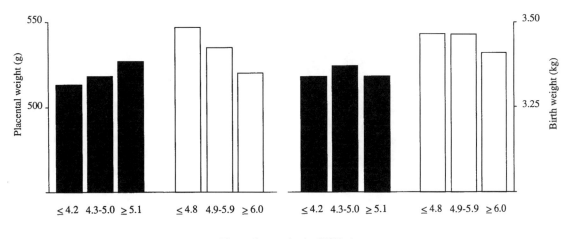

Figure 4.6 Comparison of the association between maternal energy intake in early gestation on placental and infant birth-weight at term as described in women from Southampton (Godfrey *et al.*, 1996; solid bars) and Portsmouth (Mathews *et al.*, 1999; open bars)

and vomiting in pregnancy (NVP). It is of interest that women who develop NVP in early pregnancy, with a degree of malnutrition, often have large placentas and give birth to normal-weight infants (Coad *et al.*, 2002).

These findings, together with those summarized in Table 4.2, support the concept that modest changes in maternal nutrition at specific stages of gestation can re-programme fetal development in the absence of any change

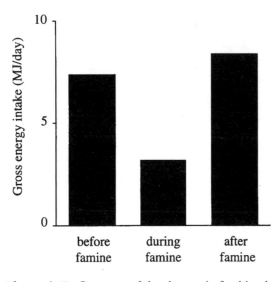

Figure 4.7 Summary of the changes in food intake during the Dutch famine of 1944–1945 as described by Roseboom *et al.* (2000)

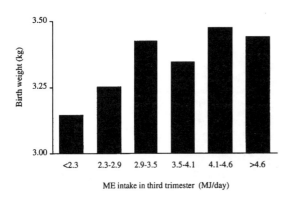

Figure 4.8 Change in birth-weight with increased maternal food intake as described during the Dutch famine of 1944–1945 (Roseboom, *et al.*, 2000)

in birth-weight. Furthermore, total energy intake, rather than other nutritional criteria such as the ratio of protein to carbohydrate intake, appear to be more important in determining outcome, as a decline in birth-weight was only observed with a very low intake of protein compared with carbohydrate (i.e. < 15 per cent) (Roseboom *et al.*, 2000).

Determination of the Nutritional Requirements of the Placenta and Fetus

The use of chronically catheterized sheep has provided accurate quantitative information regarding the developmental changes in fetal macronutrient requirements between mid- and late gestation in this species. By application of the Fick principle, which requires a combination of arterio-venous blood sampling, blood flow measurement, plus the use of radio-labelled metabolite tracer infusions, it has been possible to define the relative requirements of glucose and amino acids for oxidative metabolism and tissue growth (Table 4.7). Additional selective catheterization of fetal vessels such as, for example, the femoral or hepatic veins has enabled nutrient exchange to be determined across the hind limb or liver, respectively. These studies have primarily focused on fed and starved sheep so the impact of more subtle changes in maternal nutrition, which may also be important in programming fetal development in humans (Table 4.2), has yet to be quantified.

The development of techniques enabling fetal blood to be sampled *in utero* has resulted in additional experimental models utilizing stable isotopes (Cetin, 2001). Two different methods have been developed. One model uses non-steady-state kinetics in which a maternal bolus injection of 1-^{13}C labelled amino acid allows the measurement of unidirectional fluxes (Cetin *et al.*, 1995). Rates of placental transfer of amino acids can then be calculated from the ratio of fetal to maternal blood isotope enrichment. The second model uses steady-state kinetics as the maternal bolus is followed by a continuous maternal infusion and enables both placental permeability and feto-placental metabolism to be quantified (Marconi *et al.*, 1999). Use of these techniques has indicated that fetuses with *in utero* growth restriction but normal umbilical blood flows, heart rate,

Table 4.8 Summary of nutrient transport mechanisms across the placenta as summarized by James and Stephenson (1998)

Nutrient	Transport mechanism
Oxygen, carbon dioxide	Transcellular diffusion, flow-limited
Glucose	Transcellular carrier-mediated facilitated diffusion
Amino acids	Transcellular carrier-mediated, energy-dependent active transport
Urea	Paracellular diffusion, membrane-limited
Fatty acids[a]	Transcellular diffusion, flow-limited

[a]Placentae with maternal layers (e.g. lamb and pig) are impermeable to fatty acids.

Table 4.9 Summary of characteristics and location of placental glucose transporters (GLUT) in the human

Isoform	Function	Location	Reference
GLUT1	Basal transport for cellular metabolism	Syncytiotrophoblast and endothelial cells	Illsley, 2000; Takata *et al.*, 1992
GLUT3	High affinity, located in cells with high glucose requirements	Endothelial cells	Illsley, 2000; Jansson *et al.*, 1995

oxygenation and acid–base balance exhibit a significant reduction in fetal to maternal amino acid isotope enrichment ratio (e.g. for leucine; Pardi *et al.*, 1993). A common feature of fetal growth restriction independent of changes in oxygenation may therefore be altered placental transfer and metabolism of amino acids.

The placenta has a variety of mechanisms by which fatty acids and water-soluble nutrients are transferred to the fetus. Thus, transfer may be passive, facilitated, energy-dependent, or by pinocytosis, depending on the nutrient involved (Table 4.8).

In the case of glucose transport in fetal sheep, there is an eight-fold rise in fetal glucose requirements between mid- and late gestation. This is met by an increase in the maternal-to-fetal glucose concentration gradient, in conjunction with an enhanced placental abundance of a glucose transporter (GLUT; Figure 4.9). Two glucose transporters are present in the placenta, described as GLUT1 and GLUT3, respectively, whose function and ontogeny differ (Table 4.9; Figure 4.9). The

timing of the peak in GLUT3 abundance, in conjunction with its higher affinity for glucose compared with GLUT1, indicates a greater contribution than GLUT1 in facilitating placental glucose supply to the sheep fetus in late gestation (Ehrhardt and Bell, 1997).

In the case of amino acid transport, the extent to which gestational changes occur has not been extensively determined. This is due, in part, to the large number of different amino acid transporters (Table 4.10), some of which are sodium-dependent, whilst others are not. Only limited information on altered distribution following gross changes in placental size is currently available. The complexity of amino acid exchange is emphasized by the fact that, to date, 15 transport systems have been identified and at least 27 cDNA clones coding for mammalian amino acid transporters or transporter subunits have been identified (Jansson, 2001). It should be noted that the presence of a specific transport system within the placenta does not solely determine whether an amino acid is actively transported across the placenta

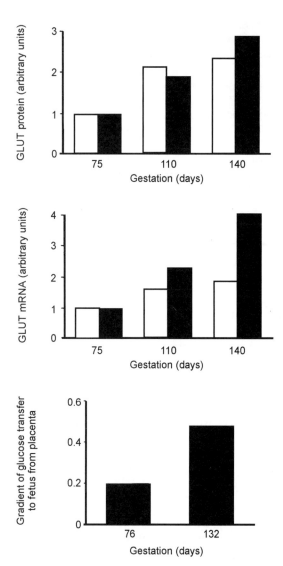

Figure 4.9 Summary of changes in maternal to fetal glucose concentration gradient and concomitant changes in placental glucose transporter (GLUT) abundance with gestational age as described by Hay (1995) and Ehrhardt and Bell (1997). GLUT1, open bars; GLUT3, solid bars

The plasma concentrations for the majority of amino acids are normally greater in fetal than in maternal plasma due to their active transfer across the placenta into the fetus (Moe, 1995). Basic amino acids are transferred to the fetus in amounts which are sufficient for tissue protein deposition. However, most amino acids are usually supplied in excess of requirements for net body nitrogen deposition. Neutral amino acids, in particular, are transferred into the fetus in excess and are used as a fetal energy source. Overall, amino acids provide half the total fetal carbon requirement in the majority of species studied to date. In addition, acidic amino acids such as glutamate and aspartate do not cross the placenta in significant amounts (Cetin, 2001). Glutamate, aspartate and serine are synthesized by the fetal liver and used by the placenta to generate glutamine, asparagine and glycine, respectively.

Hormone Secretion by the Placenta and Regulation of Fetal Growth

The placenta itself secretes a wide range of hormones which are critical for the establishment and maintenance of pregnancy as well as for the maturation of the maternal mammary gland to ensure lactation. In sheep, hormones such as noradrenaline can also be actively transported across the placenta (Bzoskie *et al.*, 1997). Anabolic hormones secreted by the placenta may modulate placental nutrient exchange capacity and thereby affect fetal growth (Table 4.11). In addition, adaptations in placental hormones can have a primary role in determining both maternal metabolic adaptation to pregnancy and fetal maturation (Zumkeller, 2000).

In vitro studies utilizing a dually perfused placenta have shown that, although the majority of placental hormone secretion enters the maternal circulation, significant amounts also

into the fetal circulation (Cetin, 2001), as placental exchange of amino acids involves: (a) direct energy-dependent transfer of amino acids; (b) placental metabolism and consumption of amino acids; and (c) placental metabolism and interconversion of amino acids.

Table 4.10 Summary of sodium-dependent and -independent amino acid transporters including additional functional characteristics as described by Boyd *et al.* (1994) and Battaglia and Regnault (2001)

Name	Amino acids transported	Other characteristics
Sodium-dependent		
A	Alanine, aminoisobutyric acid, glycine, proline, serine, threonine	Slowed by extracellular H^+
ASC	Alanine, cystine, glutamate, isoleucine, serine, threonine, valine	Insensitive to small changes in pH
N	Glutamate, histidine	Inhibited by low pH
Gly	Glycine	
X^-a,g	Aspartate, glutamate	Sensitive to pH
β	β-alanine, hypotaurine, taurine	Requires Cl^-
$B^{0,+}$	Cationic and neutral amino acids	Excludes anionic amino acids
Sodium-independent		
L	Isoleucine, leucine, methionine, phenylalanine, threonine, tryptophan, tyrosine, valine	Stimulated by low extracellular pH
T	Tyrosine, phenylalanine	Stimulated by raised pH
y^+	Arginine, lysine	Major cationic transport system (CAT1)
y^+L	Cationic amino acids	Leucine-inhibitable
$b^{0,+}$	Arginine, leucine, lysine	Higher affinity than Y^+

enter the fetal circulation (Linnemann *et al.*, 2000). Large differences exist between species in the interaction between hormone secretion and binding protein production by the placenta and mother. This makes comparisons between species very difficult, as summarized for leptin in the mouse, rat and human in Table 4.12. Furthermore, despite a much lower rate of leptin entry into fetal compared with maternal circulation, these can be positively correlated. There are also strong correlations between birth-weights and plasma hormone

Table 4.11 Summary of major metabolic hormones secreted by the placenta, proposed functions and changes associated with placental compromise

Hormone	Proposed function	Change in compromised pregnancies	Reference
Growth hormone (GH)	Regulates placental transport capacity and fetal growth	GH deficiency associated with fetal growth failure	Gluckman *et al.*, 1992; Jenkinson *et al.*, 1999
Insulin-like growth factor (IGF)-I	Regulates placental size and fetal bone growth	IGF-I secretion enhanced in diabetic pregnancies	Bhaumick *et al.*, 1992; Lok *et al.*, 1996
IGF-II	Regulates placental growth	IGF-II abundance decreased in placentae of diabetic pregnancies	Roth *et al.*, 1996; Zumkeller, 2000
Leptin	Promotes nutrient partitioning from mother to fetus	Leptin abundance increased in diabetic and pre-eclamptic pregnancies	Linnemann *et al.*, 2001; Lepercq *et al.*, 1998; McCarthy *et al.*, 1999
Placental lactogen	Promotes maternal mammary gland development	Decreased fetal intrauterine growth restriction associated with a restricted placenta	Anthony *et al.*, 1995

Table 4.12   Summary of major species differences in leptin status during pregnancy

Species	Fold increase in plasma leptin	Source of extra leptin	Change and/or source of extra binding protein	Reference
Mouse	20–40	Reduced maternal clearance	Soluble form (OB-Re) secreted by placenta	Gavrilova *et al.*, 1997
Rat	2	Maternal adipose tissue	No change	Reitman *et al.*, 2001
Human	2	Placenta	No change	Linnemann *et al.*, 2000; Masuzaki *et al.*, 1997

concentrations in cord blood, although the strength of this relationship can vary greatly (Mostyn *et al.*, 2001). This may reflect the large distribution of birth-weights within populations, the amount of fat deposition (Cetin *et al.*, 2000) as well as the number of pregnancies included, with pathological complications contributing to pronounced growth restriction.

Placental Hormone Catabolism

The placenta not only synthesizes hormones, it also promotes the catabolism of maternal hormones in order to inactivate them (Table 4.13). In this way, it is evident that the fetus can be protected from excess exposure to both

Table 4.13   Summary of placental enzyme activity critical in preventing adverse fetal exposure to maternal metabolic hormones

Enzyme	Hormone inactivated	Function	Reference
11β-Hydroxysteroid dehydrogenase type 2	Cortisol	Inactivates cortisol by conversion to cortisone	Stewart and Krozowski, 1999
5′ Monodeiodinase type III	Thyroxine, triiodothyronine	Catalyses inner ring 5′ monodeiodination to inactive metabolites	Roti *et al.*, 1981

Table 4.14   Summary of biochemical development of the major fetal organs necessary for metabolic homeostasis after birth

Organ	Biochemical development	Primary function after birth	Reference
Skeletal muscle	Appearance of uncoupling protein-3 and glycogen deposition	Heat production and mobilization of glycogen stores	Damon *et al.*, 2000
Adipose tissue	Appearance of uncoupling protein-1 and lipid storage	Rapid and large amounts of heat production from lipid	Casteilla *et al.*, 1987; Clarke *et al.*, 1997b)
Liver	Glycogen deposition and increase in activity of gluconeogenic enzymes	Glucose production and mobilization of glycogen stores	Fowden *et al.*, 1998

catabolic and anabolic hormones. Thus, it has been proposed that the reduction in placental 11β-hydroxysteroid dehydrogenase type 2, such as has been found in rats which have been fed a low-protein (9 per cent), isoenergetic diet (i.e. an abnormal protein-to-carbohydrate ratio), throughout gestation, may programme the subsequent development of hypertension (Langley-Evans et al., 1996). It has yet to be confirmed whether a persistent or transient decline in placental 11β-hydroxysteroid dehydrogenase type 2 activity actually alters fetal plasma cortisol concentration. Data in humans across a wide range of infants, including those who have IUGR, indicate a positive correlation between placental 11β-hydroxysteroid dehydrogenase type 2 activity and birth-weight (Stewart et al., 1995). Whether similar relationships are observed for body dimensions (see Table 4.2) or for normal-sized infants whose mother's nutritional status has also been recorded has yet to be demonstrated.

Transient increases in maternal cortisol secretion in early or late gestation may be sufficient to re-programme fetal cardiovascular development. Certainly, in pregnant sheep, dexamethasone treatment results in persistent hypertension, the magnitude of which increases with juvenile age (Dodic et al., 1998). Interestingly, such an effect is only observed when the ewe is treated with dexamethasone between 22 and 29 but not between 59 and 66 days of gestation. In addition, a 50 per cent decrease in maternal food intake in late gestation [from 115 days gestation until term (147–150 days)] results in raised maternal cortisol for only the first 10 days of the undernutrition, but persistently higher fetal blood pressure in the absence of any change in fetal cortisol (Edwards and McMillen, 2001).

Development of Fetal Tissues Necessary for Metabolic Homeostasis after Birth

The primary organs which enable the newborn to initiate independent metabolism once independent cardiovascular and respiration are established immediately after birth are skeletal muscle, adipose tissue and the liver (Table 4.14). Skeletal muscle and liver possess appreciable glycogen stores, which can be

Table 4.15 Summary of endocrine regulation of fetal/neonatal adipose tissue growth and maturation in lambs

Hormone	Effect on adipose tissue development	Stage of development	Reference
Cortisol	Promotes synthesis of uncoupling protein-1	Late gestation	Elmes et al., 2000
Growth hormone	Decrease in plasma concentration facilitates lipolysis	At birth	Ball et al., 1992
Insulin	Promotes lipid synthesis	Late gestation	Stevens et al., 1990
Leptin	Promotes loss of uncoupling protein-1	After birth	Mostyn et al., 2001
Norepinephrine	Acting via β-adrenergic receptor promotes initial appearance of and large increase in uncoupling protein-1	Mid-gestation/ at birth	Casteilla et al., 1989; Symonds et al., 2000
Prolactin	Increase in uncoupling protein-1	Late gestation/at birth	Symonds et al., 1998
Thyroid hormones	Large increase in uncoupling protein-1	At birth	Clarke et al., 1997b; Schermer et al., 1996

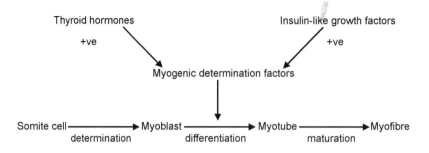

Figure 4.10 Schematic diagram of the primary stages in myogenesis and differentiation necessary for production of mature muscle myofibres plus known endocrine stimulators of myofibre synthesis. Based on Dauncey and Gilmour (1996)

mobilized and used for glucose production. In addition, adipose tissue contains energy-rich lipid that can be catabolized to release non-esterified fatty acids for use as an energy source by uncoupling proteins (UCP) in adipose tissue and muscle. Development of each tissue can be divided into four phases:

(a) differentiation of stem cells into distinct cell types which form the foundation of each organ;

(b) hyperplasia and hypertrophy as a distinct organ is formed;

(c) maturation, biochemical and enzymatic development plus appearance of hormone receptors which, when stimulated, enable effective adaptation to the extrauterine environment;

(d) adaptations to the change in nutrient supply after birth following the increase in oxygen tension and removal of the placenta.

The extent to which organ development may be irreversibly altered at any one of these stages remains to be elucidated.

Skeletal Muscle Development

Skeletal muscle growth and development is dependent on the number of muscle fibres, which is largely determined *in utero* (see Chapter 1, pp 20). Primary muscle fibres develop relatively early in gestation and fibre number is regulated by genetic rather than nutritional factors (Dwyer *et al.*, 1995) and is independent of innervation. Secondary muscle fibres constitute the major fibre population in mature muscle and form around primary fibres (Dwyer *et al.*, 1993). In large, but not small, mammals tertiary fibres are produced in late gestation and can account for a large proportion of the final number of fibres present at birth (Dauncey and Gilmour, 1996).

The developmental process by which myofibres are formed is summarized in Figure 4.10. Mesenchymal cells differentiate into myogenic precursor cells during embryonic development which then proliferate and fuse to become myotubes (Dauncey and Gilmour, 1996). Internal structural proteins are then synthesized, including the formation of the myofibrillar proteins of the sarcomere. This, in turn, leads to displacement of the cells' central nuclei to the periphery to produce a mature myofibre (see Figure 1.4). The MyoD family of nuclear proteins regulate these processes and are themselves stimulated by anabolic hormones, particularly insulin-like growth factors and thyroid hormones. Alterations in abundance of these hormones and their receptors may mediate nutritional alterations of skeletal muscle development *in utero*.

Nutritional manipulation of skeletal muscle development

In the pig, maternal nutrient restriction (e.g. energy intake reduced to 40 per cent of the level of controls) in early gestation has been found to reduce fetal muscle fibre number in the semitendinosus muscle by restricting myoblast proliferation (Dwyer *et al.*, 1994). In feed-restricted guinea-pigs, this reduction in muscle fibre number can be prevented by replenishing either the protein or carbohydrate components of the feed to normal levels (Dwyer and Stickland, 1994), and this suggests that energy restriction caused reduced myoblast proliferation. Effects of nutrition on muscle fibre development are likely to involve components of the insulin-like growth factor (IGF) axis. *In vitro* studies with spontaneously differentiating muscle cell lines that express high levels of IGF-II have shown that differentiation can be delayed if IGF-II expression is inhibited using an antisense oligonucleotide specific to IGF-II (Florini *et al.*, 1991).

In vivo studies of the double muscle syndrome, a hereditary condition in which cattle possess up to 40 per cent more muscle fibres at birth, indicate that there is an increased number of muscle cells in these animals (Swatland and Kieffer, 1974). This is associated with an increase in growth factor activity in the serum during early fetal development (Gerrard and Judge, 1993) and peak expression of IGF-II mRNA in skeletal muscle occurs later in gestation (Gerrard and Grant, 1994). A developmental delay in IGF-II expression would allow greater time for myoblast proliferation to occur as a result of muscle cell differentiation commencing later in gestation (Brameld *et al.*, 1998), hence contributing to an increase in fibre number compared with normally muscled animals. It is possible that the converse situation occurs following maternal nutrient restriction in early to mid-gestation in sheep, thereby inhibiting fetal muscle development. For

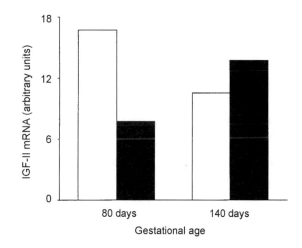

Figure 4.11 Effect of maternal nutrient restriction over the period of rapid placental growth (30–80 days gestation) followed by feeding to appetite up to term on insulin-like growth factor-II mRNA abundance in ovine fetal skeletal muscle as described by Brameld *et al.* (2000). Controls, solid bars; nutrient-restricted, open bars

example, IGF-II expression has been shown to be higher in skeletal muscle of nutrient-restricted than in well-fed fetuses at 80 days gestation, but lower relative to well-fed fetuses following refeeding up to 140 days gestation (Figure 4.11; Brameld *et al.*, 2000). This premature rise in the level of IGF-II mRNA abundance in skeletal muscle of nutrient-restricted fetuses indicates accelerated muscle differentiation, thus reducing the time when new muscle fibres could be formed. Local production of IGF-II may therefore regulate the differentiation of myoblasts and hence muscle fibre number during early fetal development, as appears to be the case in double-muscled animals (Gerrard and Grant, 1994).

The postnatal, juvenile or adult consequences of restricted muscle development *in utero* have not been studied. It is possible that this could contribute to impaired glucose disposal and a concomitant enhancement of adipose tissue deposition.

Nutritional requirements of skeletal muscle

In sheep, the fetal hind limb, which comprises 70 per cent skeletal muscle tissue, has a much higher glucose/oxygen quotient and greater rate of perfusion than that of the mother (Singh *et al.*, 1984). The uptake of 21 amino acids is significant across the hind limb, the net nitrogen uptake for which accounts for the majority of total requirements (Wilkening *et al.*, 1994). After prolonged maternal food withdrawal, although fetal glucose supply decreases by 60 per cent, umbilical uptake of free amino acids remains unaltered (Lemmons and Schreiner, 1983). As oxygen consumption remains unchanged, this indicates a doubling of amino acid catabolism. In particular, glutamine and alanine are produced, whilst uptake of branched chain amino acids, primarily leucine, is increased (Liechty and Lemmons, 1984). Not surprisingly under these conditions, growth of skeletal muscle is impaired and urea production doubled.

Adipose Tissue Development

The adipocyte lineage is derived from stem cell precursors with the potential to become brown or white adipose tissue (Smas and Sul, 1995). Both forms of adipose tissue have critical functions which are dependent the stage of development. In all species studied to date, brown adipose tissue (BAT) can rapidly generate large amounts of heat (Cannon and Nedergaard, 1985), which is used to maintain body temperature. White adipose tissue represents an endogenous energy store that secretes leptin, which has a range of biological functions in the adult, including appetite suppression (Friedman and Halaas, 1998). During late gestation, there is a parallel increase in mRNA for leptin and UCP1 in fetal adipose tissue (Stephenson *et al.*, 2001; Yuen *et al.*, 1999). The ability of BAT to generate heat is due to the possession of a unique uncoupling protein (UCP1) on the inner mitochondrial membrane (Cannon and Nedergaard, 1985). Activation of UCP1 results in proton flow across mitochondria without the need to produce ATP. Thereby, all chemical energy liberated can be used for heat production (Figure 4.12). In order to prepare the fetus for life after birth, it is critical that sufficient adipose tissue with large amounts of UCP1 and lipid is present. UCP are not exclusively expressed in adipose tissue. There are other UCPs, including UCP2 and UCP3 (Ricquier and Bouillaud, 2000). Their role in fetal development is only beginning to be addressed. UCP2 is present in spleen, lung, stomach, white adipose tissue and macrophages (Pecquer *et al.*, 2001), whilst UCP3 is found in adipose tissue and skeletal muscle (Damon *et al.*, 2000). In the fetus, the liver has a haemopoietic role and UCP2 may promote this role up to birth (Brauner *et al.*, 2001).

Endocrine regulation of adipose tissue maturation in sheep

The endocrine maturation of adipose tissue is closely linked to changes in the amount of UCP1 (Figure 4.13). Innervation commences just after mid-gestation and is followed by increases in both β-adrenoreceptor and prolactin receptor abundance, whilst UCP1 mRNA is first detected in fetal adipose tissue (Symonds and Stephenson, 1999). Thereafter, a gradual increase occurs up to term which is dependent on cortisol (Elmes *et al.*, 2000). The UCP1 level normally remains low in the fetus but can be activated by chronic cortisol or β-agonist (e.g. ritodrine) infusion (Bassett and Symonds, 1998). Within a few hours of birth, the total amount of UCP1 more than doubles in conjunction with intense stimulation of the sympathetic nervous system and the concomitant postpartum surge in thyroid

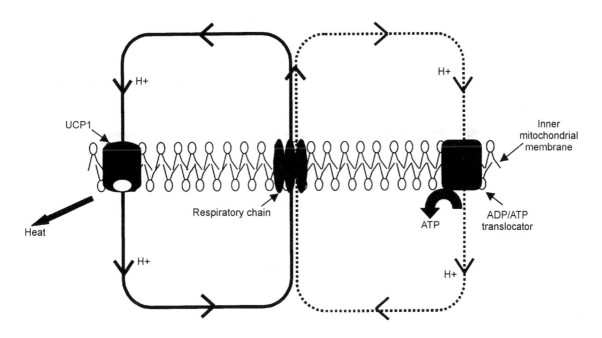

Figure 4.12 Schematic diagram of the activation of uncoupling protein-1 (UCP1), thereby resulting in rapid flow of protons (H$^+$) through UCP1 necessary for rapid production of large amounts of heat

hormones (Clarke *et al.*, 1997a). To date, a range of metabolic hormones has been shown to regulate UCP1 expression, lipid deposition and/or non-esterified fatty acid mobilization after birth (Table 4.15).

The importance of endocrine adaptations around the time of birth in maximizing UCP1 function in lambs is emphasized by the inhibitory effects of caesarean section delivery on thermoregulatory adaptation after birth (Clarke *et al.*, 1997b). In lambs born by caesarean section, the postpartum surges in catecholamines, thyroid hormones and prolactin are all greatly reduced (Table 4.16). As a consequence, UCP1 abundance is diminished and the lamb's dependence on shivering concomitantly increased. These adaptations can be prevented by exogenous administration of noradrenaline, triiodothyronine (Symonds *et al.*, 2000), or by maternal dexamethasone treatment for 2 days prepartum (Clarke *et al.*, 1998a).

Nutrient requirements for adipose tissue growth

The main metabolic precursor for lipid is glucose with small contributions from lactate and acetate (Vernon, 1986). Enhanced glucose supply to the fetus either directly, through intrafetal infusion (Stevens *et al.*, 1990), or indirectly, by promoting glucose partitioning from mother to fetus, has a direct anabolic effect on adipose tissue deposition (Symonds *et al.*, 1992). Lipid synthesis and subsequent growth of adipose tissue decreases near to term. Despite the small amount present at term in sheep, adipose tissue mass is not fixed in relation to body weight. In the fetal lamb, in which it is possible to dissect out all adipose tissue postmortem, growth restriction is accompanied by a relative maintenance in adipose tissue deposition, whereas nutritional enhancement results in a larger fetus with less

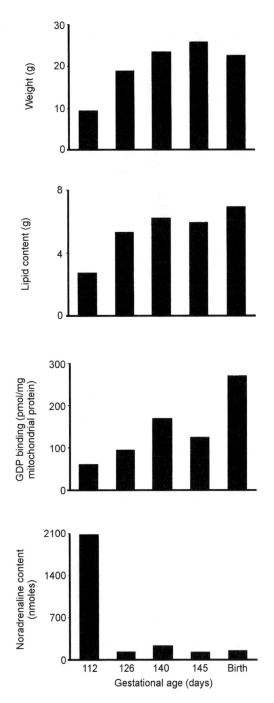

Figure 4.13 Primary developmental changes in fetal adipose tissue necessary to ensure rapid appearance and activation of uncoupling protein-1 immediately after birth in the lamb. Based on Symonds and Stephenson (1999)

adipose tissue, either total or per kg body weight (Table 4.17).

Adipose tissue growth in fetuses adapted to nutritional restriction or enhancement

Growth and maturation of adipose tissue can be significantly influenced by maternal nutrition (Table 4.17). The overall endocrine response of the fetus to altered maternal nutrition will determine whether organ size, sensitivity and function is subsequently enhanced or compromised after birth. In general, fetuses whose growth is restricted or increased (usually due to maternal diabetes) have more adipose tissue (either per kg body weight, or in total) at birth. This may act to maximize their ability to maintain body temperature immediately after birth (Symonds et al., 1992), but may be at the long-term expense of an increased predisposition to obesity in later life. Fetal endocrine adaptations to placental insufficiency in lambs, which can act to re-programme not only adipose tissue but potentially all fetal tissues, are summarized in Figure 4.14. Overall there is decreased abundance of fetal anabolic hormones and an increase in catabolic hormones, although it is not only the magnitude of adaptations that can be critical, but also the timing. The extent to which fetal endocrine status is altered during more modest and chronic nutritional challenges has yet to be examined in such detail. Importantly, fetal adaptations to maternal nutrient restriction are not usually linked to fetal hypoxia (Edwards and McMillen, 2001), which accompanies fetal growth restriction following placental restriction (Owens et al., 1995).

Adipose tissue development can be altered in the absence of any changes in the weight of tissue, in conjunction with an altered placental growth trajectory (Figure 4.15). For example, when sheep are underfed between early and

Table 4.16 Summary of the effect of caesarean section delivery of lambs on the endocrine adaptation to birth

Hormone	Effect of caesarean section delivery	Functional significance of hormone	Reference
Cortisol	Increases	Promotes recruitment of shivering thermogenesis	Alexander and Bell, 1982; Clarke et al., 1997a
Norepinephrine	Decreases	Promotes non-shivering thermogenesis	Symonds et al., 2000
Prolactin	Decreases	Promotes lipid mobilization	Yang et al., 2001
Thyroid hormones	Decreases	Promote non-shivering thermogenesis	Clarke et al., 1997; Schermer et al., 1996

Table 4.17 Effect of altered maternal nutrition on fetal weight and adipose tissue deposition in lambs

Change in maternal nutrition	Period of gestation	Effect on fetal weight	Effect on fetal adipose tissue weight	Effect on fetal adipose tissue as fraction of fetal weight	Reference
Decrease	Early to mid	None	None	None	Heasman et al., 1998
Decrease	Late	None	Decrease	None	Symonds et al., 1998
Decrease	Throughout[a]	Decrease	Decrease	None	Symonds et al., 1998
Increase	Late	Increase	Increase	Decrease	Budge et al., 2000

[a] Mediated by restricted placental growth following maternal carunclectomy prior to mating.

mid-gestation, effects on placental weight ensue (Heasman et al., 1998) and these are consistent with those reported from the Dutch famine (Lumey, 1998). Feeding singleton-bearing ewes between 50 and 60 per cent of their metabolizable energy requirements for maternal metabolism and growth of the conceptus (in order to achieve a 4.5 kg lamb), between 30 and 80 days of gestation (term = 148 days gestation), results in two major differences when compared with the well-fed controls:

(a) At 80 days gestation, the mean weight of individual placentomes and the total weight of the cotyledonary (i.e. fetal) component of the placenta are reduced without any effect on fetal weight (Clarke et al., 1998b).

(b) When 80-day-nutrient-restricted ewes are subsequently refed to fully meet their

metabolizable energy requirements for the remainder of pregnancy (i.e. 100 per cent), they have a larger placenta at term than control ewes without any effect on fetal weight (Heasman et al., 1998).

At term, fetuses of nutrient restricted ewes have a longer crown–rump length, height and thoracic circumference (Heasman et al., 1998). Adipose tissue sampled at term from previously nutrient-restricted fetuses exhibits programmed increases in the expression of glucocorticoid receptor and 11β-hydroxysteroid dehydrogenase type 1 mRNA and 11-oxoreductase enzyme activity (Whorwood et al., 2001). The sensitivity of adipose tissue to glucocorticoids may, therefore, be reset. These results are in accord with findings in adult humans, in which abdominal fat depots have been shown to express high levels of

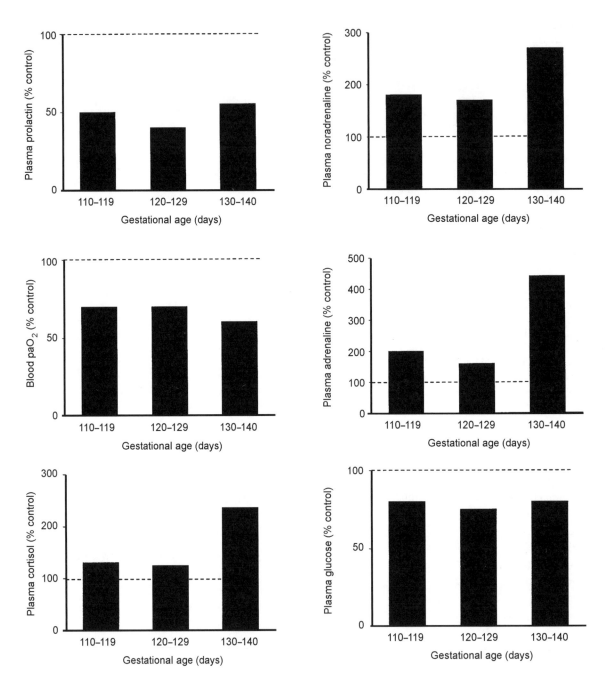

Figure 4.14 Summary of relative differences in plasma concentrations of fetal metabolic hormones between control and growth-retarded, placentally restricted fetuses with gestational age as described by Owens *et al.* (1994), Phillips *et al.* (1996, 2001) and Simonetta *et al.* (1997)

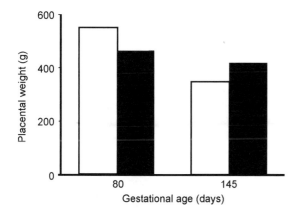

glucocorticoid receptor (Pedersen *et al.*, 1994) and 11β-hydroxysteroid dehydrogenase type 1 (which acts as 11-oxoreductase catalysing the conversion of cortisone to bio-active cortisol; Stewart and Krozowski, 1999). Programming of increased levels of glucocorticoid receptor and 11β-hydroxysteroid dehydrogenase type 1 expression in central fat depots by nutrient restriction could contribute to mechanisms linking gestational undernutrition and adult obesity in human populations (Figure 4.16).

Figure 4.15 Adaptations in placental growth following maternal nutrient restriction between early to mid-gestation in sheep, as described by Clarke *et al.* (1998a) and Heasman *et al.* (1998). Controls, solid bars; nutrient-restricted, open bars

Liver Development

In sheep, growth and maturation of the fetal liver continue up to term, with the greatest

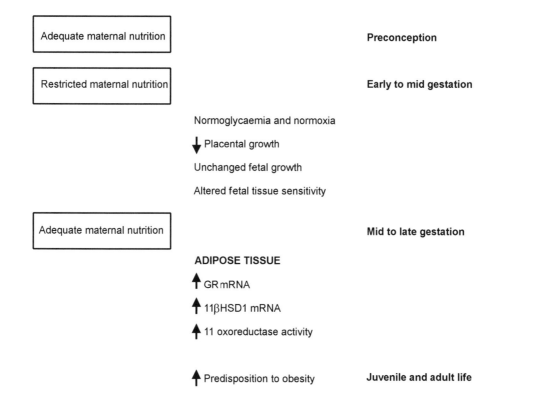

Figure 4.16 Summary of proposed mechanism by which fetal adipose tissue sensitivity may be reprogrammed following maternal nutrient restriction between early and mid-gestation in sheep, as described by Whorwood *et al.* (2001). ↑, increase; ↓, decrease; GR, glucocorticoid receptor; 11β-HSD1, 11β-hydroxysteroid dehydrogenase type 1

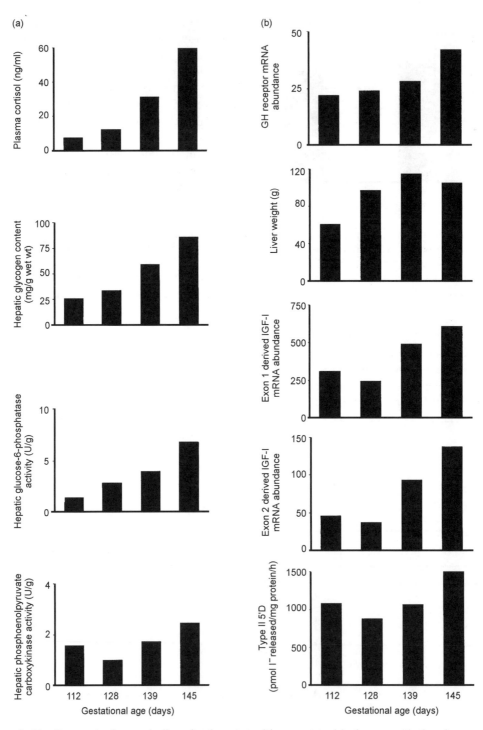

Figure 4.17   Ontogenic changes in liver development with respect to (a) plasma cortisol and enzymatic activity and (b) liver weight and receptor abundance over the final month of gestation as described by Fowden *et al*. (1998), Clarke *et al*. (1997a) and Li *et al*. (1996)

changes occurring over the final 2 weeks of gestation. These are dependent on an intact fetal adrenal gland and coincident with the gradual increase in plasma cortisol concentration (Fowden *et al.*, 1998). During this short time period there is a 3–4-fold increase in hepatic glycogen concentration plus gluconeogenic enzyme activity [Figure 4.17(a)]. Gluconeogenesis does not normally occur *in utero*. At the same time, the abundance of members of the class I cytokine receptor superfamily increases, which may be critical in priming the postnatal switch from fetal to adult modes of somatotrophic growth regulation. Near to term, class 2 transcript for IGF-I therefore becomes more abundant [Figure 4.17(b)] in conjunction with the first appearance of the adult form of the growth hormone receptor (Li *et al.*, 1999). These two genes may be more nutritionally sensitive than other exons for IGF-I and the growth hormone receptor and become abundant as nutritional supply with respect to demands becomes limiting in late gestation. At the same time hepatic IGF-II mRNA expression, for which the greatest expression throughout life is during fetal development, decreases (Forhead *et al.*, 1998). The extent to which these are direct effects of cortisol or mediated through an increase in local triiodothyronine production (the metabolically active thyroid hormone) is unclear. These changes all coincide with an increase in hepatic 5′ monodeiodinase activity, the enzyme which stimulates outer-ring deiodination of thyroxine to triiodothyronine (Clarke *et al.*, 1997a).

Liver development in fetuses adapted to nutritional restriction or enhancement

Fetal nutrient restriction in sheep, as a result of either severe maternal undernutrition (i.e. 14 days of feeding 25 per cent of *ad libitum*; Bauer *et al.*, 1995) or placental restriction, results in a smaller liver (Kind *et al.*, 1995) and reduced plasma and tissue IGF-I, whereas IGF-II is unchanged (Owens *et al.*, 1994). The decline in plasma IGF-I cannot be entirely explained by a decrease in hepatic mRNA abundance because, in contrast to the adult in which the liver is the primary source of IGF-I, other tissues including skeletal muscle and kidney contribute to the IGF-I pool (Kind *et al.*, 1995). Conversely, increasing maternal nutrition does not enhance liver weight (Budge *et al.*, 2000). The abundance of IGF-I and growth hormone receptor mRNA can be enhanced near to term in fetuses of ewes previously nutrient-restricted between early to mid-gestation (Brameld *et al.*, 2000). These adaptations, in conjunction with an increase in hepatic glucocorticoid receptor mRNA expression (Whorwood *et al.*, 2001), may act to substantially alter hepatic function after birth, thereby contributing to glucose intolerance as an adult.

Conclusion

It is now clear from studies largely in sheep, that subtle alterations in maternal energy intake throughout pregnancy can affect placental development and/or function. These have the potential to substantially alter fetal physiology in the absence of any change in fetal weight. As a result, growth, development and/or maturation of a range of fetal tissues in the human infant such as skeletal muscle, adipose tissue and liver may be re-programmed. The consequences in terms of adult health and disease may not manifest themselves until much later in life.

References

Agricultural Research Council (1980) Requirements for energy. In: *The Nutritional Requirements of*

Ruminant Livestock, pp. 115–119. Commonwealth Agricultural Bureau, Slough, UK.

Alexander G and Bell AW (1982) The role of the adrenal in the metabolic response of young lambs to the cold. *J. Devl. Physiol.* **4**, 53–73.

Anthony RV, Liang R, Kayl EP and Pratt SL (1995) The growth hormone/prolactin gene family in ruminant placentae. *J. Reprod. Fertil. Suppl.* **49**, 83–95.

Ball KT, Power GG, Gunn TR, Johnston BM and Gluckman PD (1992) Modulation of growth hormone secretion by thermogenically derived free fatty acids in the perinatal lamb. *Endocrinology* **131**, 337–343.

Barker DJP (1994) *Mothers, Babies and Disease in Later Life*. BMJ Publishing Group, London.

Barker DJP (1999) Fetal programming and public health. In: *Fetal Programming: Influences on Development and Disease in Later Life*, ed. Wheeler T and Barker DJP, pp. 3–11. RCOG Press, London.

Barker DJP, Bull AR, Osmond C and Simmonds SJ (1990) Fetal and placental size and risk of hypertension in adult life. *Br. Med. J.* **301**, 259–262.

Barker DJP, Godfrey KM, Osmond C and Bull A (1992) The relation of fetal length, ponderal index and head circumferences to blood pressure and the risk of hypertension in adult life. *Paediatr. Perinat. Epidemiol.* **6**, 35–44.

Bassett JM and Symonds ME (1998) β_2-Agonist ritodrine, unlike natural catecholamines, activates thermogenesis prematurely *in utero* in fetal sheep. *Am. J. Physiol.* **275**, R112–R119.

Battaglia FC and Meschia G (1981) Foetal and placental metabolisms: their interrelationship and impact upon maternal metabolism. *Proc. Nutr. Soc.* **40**, 99–113.

Battaglia FC and Regnault TRH (2001) Placental transport and metabolism of amino acids. *Placenta* **22**, 145–161.

Bauer MK, Breier BH, Harding J, Veldhuis JD and Gluckman PD (1995) The fetal somatotrophic axis during long term maternal undernutrition in sheep; evidence of nutritional regulation *in utero*. *Endocrinology* **136**, 1250–1257.

Bell AW, Kennaugh JM, Battaglia FC, Makowski EL and Meschia G (1986) Metabolic and circulatory studies of fetal lamb at midgestation. *Am. J. Physiol.* **250**, E538–E544.

Bhaumick B, George D and Bala RM (1992) Potential of epidermal growth factor-induced differentiation of cultured human placental cells by insulin-like growth factor-I. *J. Clin. Endocrinol. Metab.* **74**, 1005–1011.

Boyd RDH, D'Souza SW and Sibley CP (1994) Placental transfer. In: *Early Fetal Growth and Development*, ed. Ward RHT, Smith SK and Donnai D, pp. 211–221. RCOG Press, London.

Brameld JM, Buttery PJ, Dawson JM and Harper JMM (1998) Nutritional and hormonal control of skeletal muscle cell growth and differentiation. *Proc. Nutr. Soc.* **57**, 207–217.

Brameld JM, Mostyn A, Dandrea J, Stephenson TJ, Dawson J, Buttery PJ and Symonds ME (2000) Maternal nutrition alters the expression of insulin-like growth factors in fetal sheep liver and skeletal muscle. *J. Endocrinol.* **167**, 429–437.

Brauner P, Nibbelink M, Flachs P, Vitkova I, Kopecky P, Mertelikova I, Janderova L, Penicuad L, Casteilla L, Plavka R and Kopecky J (2001) Fast decline of hematopoiesis and uncoupling protein 2 content in human liver after birth: location of the protein in Kupffer cells. *Pediatr. Res.* **49**, 440–447.

Broughton Pipkin F, Hull D and Stephenson TJ (1994) Fetal physiology. In: *Marshall's Physiology of Reproduction*, 4th edn, Vol. 3, *Pregnancy and Lactation, Part Two, Fetal Physiology, Parturition and Lactation*, ed. Lamming GE, pp. 767–861. Chapman & Hall, London.

Budge H, Bispham J, Dandrea J, Evans L, Heasman L, Ingleton P, Sullivan C, Wilson V, Stephenson T and Symonds ME (2000) Effect of maternal nutrition on brown adipose tissue and prolactin receptor status in the fetal lamb. *Pediatr. Res.* **47**, 781–786.

Bush PG, Mayhew TM, Abramovich DR, Aggett PJ, Burke MD and Page KR (2000) Maternal cigarette smoking and oxygen diffusion across the placenta. *Placenta* **21**, 824–833.

Bzoskie I, Blount I, Kahiwai K, Humme J and Padbury JF (1997) Placental norepinephrine transporter development in the ovine foetus. *Placenta* **18**, 65–70.

Campbell-Brown M and Hytten FE (1998) Nutrition. In: *Clinical Physiology in Obstetrics*, ed. Chamberlain G and Broughton Pipkin F, pp. 165–191. Blackwell Science, Oxford.

Cannon B and Nedergaard J (1985) The biochemistry of an inefficient brown adipose tissue. *Essays Biochem.* **20**, 110–164.

Carter AM (2000) Placental oxygen consumption. Part I: in vivo studies – a review. *Placenta* **21** (Suppl. A, Trophoblast Research 14), S31–S37.

Casteilla L, Forest C, Robelin J, Ricquier D, Lombert A and Ailand G (1987) Characterisation of mitochondrial-uncoupling protein in bovine fetus and newborn calf. *Am. J. Physiol.* **254**, E627–E636.

Casteilla L, Champigny O, Bouillaud F, Robelin J and Ricquier D (1989) Sequential changes in the expression of mitochondrial protein mRNA during the development of brown adipose tissue in bovine and ovine species. *Biochem. J.* **257**, 665–671.

Cetin I (2001) Amino acid interconversions in the fetal–placental unit: the animal model and human studies *in vivo*. *Pediatr. Res.* **49**, 148–154.

Cetin I, Marconi AM, Baggiani AM, Buscalia M, Fennessey PV and Battaglia FC (1995) *In vivo* placental transport of glycine and leucine in human pregnancies. *Pediatr. Res.* **37**, 571–575.

Cetin I, Morpurga PS, Radaelli T, Taricco E, Cortelazzi D, Bellotti M, Pardi G and Beck-Peccoz P (2000) Fetal plasma leptin concentrations: relationship with different intrauterine growth patterns from 19 weeks to term. *Pediatr. Res.* **48**, 646–651.

Clarke L, Bryant MJ, Lomax MA and Symonds ME (1997a) Maternal manipulation of brown adipose tissue and liver development in the ovine fetus during late gestation. *Br. J. Nutr.* **77**, 871–883.

Clarke L, Heasman L, Firth K and Symonds ME (1997b) Influence of route of delivery and ambient temperature on thermoregulation in newborn lambs. *Am. J. Physiol.* **272**, R1931–R1939.

Clarke L, Heasman L and Symonds ME (1997c) Influence of maternal body weight on adaptation after birth in near-term lambs delivered by caesarean section. *Reprod. Fertil. Devl.* **10**, 333–339.

Clarke L, Heasman L and Symonds ME (1998a) Influence of maternal dexamethasone administration on thermoregulation in lambs delivered by caesarean section. *J. Endocrinol.* **156**, 307–314.

Clarke L, Heasman L, Juniper DT and Symonds ME (1998b) Maternal nutrition in early-mid gestation and placental size in sheep. *Br. J. Nutr.* **79**, 359–364.

Coad J, Al-Rasasi B and Morgan J (2002) Nutrient insult in pregnancy. *Proc. Nutr. Soc.* **61**, 51–59.

Conter V, Cortinovis I, Rogari P and Riva L (1995) Weight gain in infants born to mothers who smoked during pregnancy. *Br. Med. J.* **310**, 768–771.

Damon M, Vincent A, Lombardi A and Herpin P (2000) First evidence of uncoupling protein-2 (UCP-2) and -3 (UCP-3) gene expression in piglet skeletal muscle and adipose tissue. *Gene* **246**, 133–141.

Dauncey MJ and Gilmour RS (1996) Regulatory factors in the control of muscle development. *Proc. Nutr. Soc.* **55**, 543–559.

Dodic M, May CN, Wintour EM and Coghlan JP (1998) An early prenatal exposure to excess glucocorticoid leads to hypertensive offspring in sheep. *Clin. Sci.* **94**, 149–155.

Duncan KR, Gowland P, Francis S, Moore R, Baker PN and Johnson I (1998) The investigation of placental relaxation and estimation of placental perfusion using echo-plannar magnetic resonance imaging. *Placenta* **19**, 539–544.

Dwyer CM and Stickland NC (1994) Supplementation of a restricted maternal diet with protein or carbohydrate alone prevents a reduction in fetal muscle fibre number in the guinea-pig. *Br. J. Nutr.* **72**, 173–180.

Dwyer CM, Fletcher JM and Stickland NC (1993) Muscle cellularity and postnatal growth in the pig. *J. Animal Sci.* **71**, 3339–3343.

Dwyer CM, Stickland NC and Fletcher JM (1994) The influence of maternal nutrition on muscle fiber number development in the porcine fetus and on subsequent postnatal growth. *J. Animal Sci.* **72**, 911–917.

Dwyer CM, Madgwick AJA, Ward SS and Stickland NC (1995) Effect of maternal undernutrition in early gestation on the development of fetal myofibres in the guinea-pig. *Reprod. Fertil. Devl.* **7**, 1285–1292.

Edwards LJ and McMillen IC (2001) Maternal undernutrition increases arterial blood pressure in the sheep fetus during late gestation. *J. Physiol.* **533**, 561–570.

Ehrhardt RA and Bell AW (1997) Developmental increases in glucose transporter concentration in the sheep placenta. *Am. J. Physiol.* **273**, R1132–R1141.

Elmes M, Mostyn A, Forhead A, Stephenson T, Fowden AL and Symonds ME (2000) Influence of cortisol on uncoupling protein-1 (UCP1) abundance and activity in the late gestation sheep fetus. *J. Physiol.* **523**, P181P.

Faichney GJ and White GA (1987) Effect of maternal nutritional status on fetal and placental growth and on fetal urea synthesis. *Aust. J. Biol. Sci.* **40**, 365–377.

Florini JR, Magri KA, Ewton DZ, James PL, Grindstaff K and Rotwein PS (1991) 'Spontaneous' differentiation of skeletal myoblasts is dependent upon autocrine secretion of insulin-like growth factor-II. *J. Biol. Chem.* **266**, 15 917–15 923.

Forhead AJ, Li J, Gilmour RS and Fowden AL (1998) Control of hepatic insulin-like growth factor II gene expression by thyroid hormones in the fetal sheep near term. *Am. J. Physiol.* **275**, E149–E156.

Forsen T, Eriksson JG, Tuomilehto J, Teramo K, Osmond C and Barker DJP (1997) Mother's weight in pregnancy and coronary heart disease in a cohort of Finnish men: follow up study. *Br. Med. J.* **315**, 837–840.

Fowden AL, Li J and Forhead AJ (1998) Glucocorticoids and the preparation for life after birth: are there long-term consequences of the life insurance? *Proc. Nutr. Soc.* **57**, 113–122.

Friedman JM and Halaas JL (1998) Leptin and the regulation of body weight in mammals. *Nature* **395**, 763–770.

Gavrilova O, Barr V, Marcus-Samuels B and Reitman M (1997) Hyperleptinemia of pregnancy associated with the appearance of a circulating form of the leptin receptor. *J. Biol. Chem.* **272**, 30 546–30 551.

Gerrard DE and Grant AL (1994) Insulin-like growth factor-II expression in developing skeletal muscle of double muscled and normal cattle. *Dom. Animal Endocrinol.* **11**, 339–347.

Gerrard DE and Judge MD (1993) Induction of myoblast proliferation in L6 myoblast cultures by fetal serum of double muscled and normal cattle. *J. Animal Sci.* **71**, 1464–1470.

Gluckman PD, Gunn AJ, Cutfield WS, Guilbaud O and Wilton P (1992) Congenital idiopathic growth hormone deficiency associated with prenatal and early postnatal growth failure. *J. Pediatr.* **121**, 920–923.

Godfrey K, Robinson S, Barker DJP, Osmond C and Cox V (1996) Maternal nutrition in early and late pregnancy in relation to placental and fetal growth. *Br. Med. J.* **312**, 410–414.

Hay WW (1995) Current topic: metabolic interrelationships of placenta and fetus. *Placenta* **16**, 19–30.

Hay WW (1998) Nutrient and metabolic needs of the fetus and a very small infant: a comparative approach. *Biochem. Soc. Trans.* **26**, 75–78.

Heasman L, Clarke L, Firth K, Stephenson T and Symonds ME (1998) Influence of restricted maternal nutrition in early to mid gestation on placental and fetal development at term. *Pediatr. Res.* **44**, 546–551.

Illsley NP (2000) Glucose transporters in the human placenta. *Placenta* **21**, 14–22.

James DK and Stephenson TJ (1998) Fetal nutrition and growth. In: *Clinical Physiology in Obstetrics*, ed. Chamberlain G and Broughton Pipkin F, pp. 467–497. Blackwell Science, Oxford.

Jansson T (2001) Amino acid transporters across the placenta. *Pediatr. Res.* **49**, 141–147.

Jansson T, Wennergren M and Illsley NP (1995) Cellular localization of glucose transporter messenger RNA in human placenta. *Reprod. Fertil. Devl.* **7**, 1425–1430.

Jenkinson CM, Min SH, Mackenzie DD, McCutheon SN, Brier BH and Gluckman PD (1999) Placental development and fetal growth in growth hormone-treated ewes. *Growth Hormone IGF Res.* **9**, 11–17.

Kind KL, Owens JA, Robinson JS, Quinn KJ, Grant PA, Walton PE, Gilmour RS and Owens PC (1995) Effect of restriction of placental growth on expression of IGFs in foetal sheep – relationship to fetal growth, circulating IGFs and binding-proteins. *J. Endocrinol.* **146**, 23–24.

Kingdom J (1998) Placental pathology in obstetrics: adaptation or failure of the villous tree? *Placenta* **19**, 347–351.

Kingdom JCP and Kaufmann P (1997) Oxygen and placental villous development: origins of fetal hypoxia. *Placenta* **18**, 613–621.

Langley-Evans SC, Phillips GJ, Benediktsson R, Gardner DS, Edwards CRW, Jackson AA and Seckl JR (1996) Protein intake in pregnancy, placental glucocorticoid metabolism and the programming of hypertension. *Placenta* **17**, 169–172.

Langley-Evans SC, Welham SJM and Jackson AA (1999) Fetal exposure to a maternal low protein diet impairs nephrogenesis and promotes hypertension in the rat. *Life Sci.* **64**, 965–974.

Lemmons JA and Schreiner RL (1983) Amino acid metabolism in the ovine fetus. *Am. J. Physiol.* **244**, E459–E466.

Lepercq J, Caucaz M, Lahlou N, Timsit J, Girard J, Auwerx J and de Mouzan SH (1998) Overexpression of placental leptin in diabetic pregnancy. *Diabetes* **47**, 847–850.

Li J, Owens PC, Owens JC, Saunders JC, Gilmour RS and Fowden AL (1996) The ontogeny of hepatic growth hormone receptor and insulin-like growth factor I gene expression in the sheep fetus during late gestation: developmental regulation by cortisol. *Endocrinology* **137**, 1650–1657.

Li J, Gilmour RS, Saunders JC, Dauncey MJ and Fowden AL (1999) Activation of the adult mode of ovine growth hormone receptor gene expression by cortisol during late fetal development. *FASEB J.* **13**, 545–552.

Liechty EA and Lemmons JA (1984) Changes in ovine fetal hindlimb amino acid metabolism during maternal fasting. *Am. J. Physiol.* **246**, E430–E435.

Linnemann K, Malek A, Sager R, Blum WF, Schneider H and Frusch C (2000) Leptin production and release in the dually in vitro perfused human placenta. *J. Clin. Endocrinol. Metab.* **85**, 4298–4301.

Linnemann K, Malek A, Schneider H and Fusch C (2001) Physiological and pathological regulation of feto/placentao/maternal leptin expression. *Biochem. Soc. Trans.* **29**, 86–90.

Lok F, Owens JA, Mundy L, Robinson JS and Owens PC (1996) Insulin-like growth factor I promotes growth selectively in fetal sheep in late gestation. *Am. J. Physiol.* **270**, R1148–R1155.

Lumey LH (1998) Compensatory placental growth after restricted nutrition in early pregnancy. *Placenta* **19**, 105–112.

Marconi AM, Battaglia FC, Meschia G and Sparks JW (1989) A comparison of amino acid arteriovenous differences across the placenta and liver in the fetal lamb. *Am. J. Physiol.* **257**, E909–E915.

Marconi AM, Paolini CL, Stramare L, Cetin I, Fennessey PV, Pardi G and Battaglia FC (1999) The steady state maternal-fetal leucine enrichments in normal and growth restricted pregnancies. *Pediatr. Res.* **46**, 114–119.

Martyn CN, Barker DJP and Osmond C (1996) Mothers pelvic size, fetal growth and death from stroke and CHD in men. *Lancet* **348**, 1264–1268.

Masuzaki H, Ogawa Y, Sagawa N, Hosoda K, Matsumoto T, Mise H, Nishimura H, Yoshimasa Y, Tanaka I, Mori T and Nakao K (1997) Nonadipose tissue production of leptin: leptin as a novel placenta-derived hormone in humans. *Nat Med.* **3**, 1029–1033.

Mathews F, Yudkin P and Neil A (1999) Influence of maternal nutrition on outcome of pregnancy: prospective cohort study. *Br. Med. J.* **319**, 339–343.

McCarthy JF, Misra DN and Roberts JM (1999) Maternal plasma leptin is increased in preeclampsia and positively correlates with foetal cord concentration. *Am. J. Obstet. Gynecol.* **180**, 731–736.

Mellor DJ and Cockburn F (1986) A comparison of energy metabolism in the new-born infant, piglet and lamb. *Q. J. Exp. Physiol.* **71**, 361–379.

Meschia G, Battaglia FC, Hay WW and Sparks JW (1980) Utilization of substrates by the ovine placenta. *Fed. Proc.* **39**, 245–249.

Moe AJ (1995) Placental amino acid transport. *Am. J. Physiol.* **268**, C1321–C1331.

Mostyn A, Keisler DH, Webb R, Stephenson T and Symonds ME (2001) The role of leptin in the transition from fetus to neonate. *Proc. Nutr. Soc.* **60**, 187–194.

Naeye RL (1987) Do placental weights have clinical significance? *Hum. Pathol.* **18**, 387–391.

Osmond C, Barker DJP, Winter PD, Fall CHD and Simmonds SJ (1993) Early growth and cardiovascular disease in women. *Br. Med. J.* **307**, 1519–1524.

Owens JA, Kind KL, Carbone F, Robinson JS and Owens PC (1994) Circulating insulin-like growth factors-I and -II and substrates in fetal sheep following restriction of placental growth. *J. Endocrinol.* **140**, 5–13.

Owens JA, Owens PC and Robinson JS (1995) Experimental restriction of growth. In: *The Fetus and Neonate*, Vol. 3, *Growth*, ed. Hanson MA, Spencer JAD and Rodeck CH, pp. 139–175. Cambridge University Press, Cambridge.

Pardi G, Cetin I, Marconi AM, Lanfranchi A, Bozzetti P, Ferrazzi E and Battaglia FC (1993) Diagnostic value of blood sampling in fetuses with growth retardation. *New Engl. J. Med.* **328**, 692–696.

Pecquer C, Alves-Guerra M-C, Gelly C, Lévi-Meyrueis C, Couplan E, Collins S, Ricquier D, Bouillaud F and Miroux B (2001) Uncoupling protein-2: *in vivo* distribution, induction upon oxidative stress and evidence for translational regulation. *J. Biol. Chem.* **276**, 8705–8712.

Pedersen SB, Jonler M and Richelsen B (1994) Characterization of regional and gender differences in glucocorticoid receptors and lipoprotein lipase activity in human adipose tissue. *J. Clin. Endocrinol. Metab.* **78**, 1354–1359.

Phillips DIW and Young JB (2000) Birth weight, climate at birth and risk of obesity in adult life. *Int. J. Obes. Relat. Metab. Disord.* **24**, 281–287.

Phillips ID, Simonetta G, Owens JS, Robinson JS, Clarke IJ and McMillen IC (1996) Placental restriction alters the functional development of the pituitary–adrenal axis in the sheep fetus during late gestation. *Pediatr. Res.* **40**, 861–866.

Phillips ID, Anthony RV, Simonetta G, Owens JA, Robinson JS and McMillen IC (2001) Restriction of fetal growth has a differential impact on fetal prolactin and prolactin receptor mRNA expression. *J. Neuroendocrinol.* **13**, 175–181.

Poston L (1997) The control of blood flow to the placenta. *Exp. Physiol.* **82**, 377–387.

Reitman ML, Bi S, Marcus-Samuels B and Gavrilova O (2001) Leptin and its role in pregnancy and fetal development – an overview. *Biochem. Soc. Trans.* **29**, 68–72.

Ricquier D and Bouillaud F (2000) The uncoupling protein homologues: UCP1, UCP2, UCP3, StUCP and AtUCP. *Biochem. J.* **345**, 161–179.

Rolfe DFS and Brown GC (1997) Cellular energy utilization and molecular origin of standard metabolic rate in mammals. *Physiol. Rev.* **77**, 731–758.

Roseboom TJ, van der Meulen JHP, Osmond C, Barker DJP, Ravelli ACJ, von Montfrans S-T, Michels RPJ and Blecker OP (2000) Coronary heart disease in adults after perinatal exposure to famine. *Heart* **84**, 595–598.

Roth S, Abernathy MP, Lee WH, Pratt L, Denne S, Golichowski A and Pescovitz OH (1996) Insulin-like growth factors I and II peptide and messenger RNA levels in macrosomic infants of diabetic pregnancies. *J. Soc. Gynecol. Invest.* **3**, 78–84.

Roti E, Fang SL, Green K, Emerson CH and Braverman LE (1981) Human placenta is an active site of thyroxine and 3,3′,5-triiodothyronine tyrosol ring deiodination. *J. Clin. Endocrinol. Metab.* **53**, 498–501.

Schermer SJ, Bird JA, Lomax MA, Shepherd DAL and Symonds ME (1996) Effect of fetal thyroid-ectomy on brown adipose tissue and thermo-regulation in newborn lambs. *Reprod. Fertil. Devl.* **8**, 995–1002.

Schneider H (1996) Ontogenic changes in the nutritive function of the placenta. *Placenta* **17**, 15–26.

Simonetta G, Rourke AK, Owens JS, Robinson JS and McMillen IC (1997) Impact of placental restriction on the development of the sympathoadrenal system. *Pediatr. Res.* **42**, 805–811.

Singh S, Sparks JW, Meschia G, Battaglia FC and Makowski EL (1984) Comparison of fetal and maternal hindlimb metabolic quotients in sheep. *Am. J. Obstet. Gynecol.* **149**, 441–449.

Skjaerven R, Wilcox AJ, Oyen N and Magnus P (1997) Mother's birth weight and survival of their off-spring: population based study. *Br. Med. J.* **314**, 1376–1380.

Smas CM and Sul HS (1995) Control of adipocyte differentiation. *Biochem. J.* **309**, 697–710.

Stegmann JHJ (1974) Placental development in sheep. *Bijdragen tot de Dierkunde* **44**, 4–72.

Stephenson T, Budge H, Mostyn A, Pearce S, Webb R and Symonds ME (2001) Fetal and neonatal adipose tissue maturation: a primary site of

cytokine and cytokine-receptor action. *Biochem. Soc. Trans.* **29**, 80–85.

Stevens D, Alexander G and Bell AW (1990) Effects of prolonged glucose infusion into fetal sheep on body growth, fat deposition and gestation length. *J. Devl. Physiol.* **13**, 277–281.

Stewart PM and Krozowski ZS (1999) 11b-Hydroxysteroid dehydrogenase. *Vitam. Horm.* **57**, 249–324.

Stewart PM, Rogerson FM and Mason JL (1995) Type 2 11b-hydroxysteroid dehydrogenase messenger ribonucleic acid and activity in human placenta and fetal membranes: its relationship to birth weight and putative role in fetal adrenal sterio-dogenesis. *J. Clin. Endocrinol. Metab.* **80**, 885–890.

Swatland HJ and Kieffer NM (1974) Fetal develop-ment of the double muscled condition in cattle. *J. Animal Sci.* **38**, 752–757.

Symonds ME and Lomax MA (1992) Maternal and environmental influences on thermoregulation in the neonate. *Proc. Nutr. Soc.* **51**, 165–172.

Symonds ME and Stephenson T (1999) Maternal nutrient restriction and endocrine programming of fetal adipose tissue development. *Biochem. Soc. Trans.* **27**, 97–103.

Symonds ME, Bryant MJ, Clarke L, Darby CJ and Lomax MA (1992) Effect of maternal cold exposure on brown adipose tissue and thermogenesis in the neonatal lamb. *J. Physiol. Lond.* **455**, 487–502.

Symonds ME, Phillips ID, Anthony RV, Owens JA and McMillen IC (1998) Prolactin receptor gene expression and foetal adipose tissue. *J. Neuroendocrinol.* **10**, 885–890.

Symonds ME, Bird JA, Sullivan C, Wilson V, Clarke L and Stephenson T (2000) Effect of delivery temperature on endocrine stimulation of thermo-regulation in lambs born by cesarean section. *J. Appl. Physiol.* **88**, 47–53.

Symonds ME, Budge H, Stephenson T and McMillen IC (2001) Fetal endocrinology and development – manipulation and adaptation to long term nutri-tional and environmental challenges. *Reproduction* **29**, 33–37.

Takata K, Kasahara T, Kasahara M, Ezaki O and Hirano H (1992) Localization of erthrocyte/HepG2-type glucose transporter (GLUT1) in human placental villi. *Cell Tissue Research* **267**, 407–412.

Vernon RG (1986) The growth and metabolism of adipocytes. In: *Control and Manipulation of Animal Growth*, ed. Buttery PJ, Haynes NB and Lindsay DB, pp. 67–83. Butterworths, London.

Whorwood CB, Firth KM, Budge H and Symonds ME (2001) Maternal undernutrition during early- to mid-gestation programmes tissue-specific alterations in the expression of the glucocorticoid receptor, 11b-hydroxysteroid dehydrogenase isoforms and type 1 angiotensin II receptor in neonatal sheep *Endocrinology* **142**, 2854–2864.

Wilkening RB, Boyle DW, Teng C, Meschia G and Battaglia FC (1994) Amino acid uptake by the fetal ovine hindlimb under normal and euglycemic hyperinsulinemic states. *Am. J. Physiol.* **266**, E72–E78.

Yang L, Kuo CB, Liu Y, Coss D, Xu X, Chen C, Oster-Granite ML and Walker AM (2001) Administration of unmodified prolactin (U-PRL) and a molecular mimic of phosphorylated prolactin (PP-PRL) during rat pregnancy provides evidence that the U-PRL:PP-PRL ratio is crucial to the normal development of pup tissues. *J. Endocrinol.* **168**, 227–238.

Yuen BSJ, McMillen IC, Symonds ME and Owens JA (1999) Abundance of leptin messenger ribonucleic acid in fetal adipose tissue is related to fetal body weight. *J. Endocrinol.* **163**, R1–R4.

Zamudio S, Droma T, Norkyel KY, Acharya G, Zamudio JA, Niermeyer SN and Moore LG (1993) Protection from intrauterine growth retardation in tibetans at high altitude. *Am. J. Phys. Anthropol.* **91**, 215–224.

Zumkeller W (2000) The role of growth hormone and insulin-like growth factors for placental growth and development. *Placenta* **21**, 451–467.

5

LIFESTYLE AND MATERNAL HEALTH INTERACTIONS BETWEEN MOTHER AND FETUS

Mohammed Ibrahim and J. Stewart Forsyth

LEARNING OUTCOMES

- Maternal and fetal non-nutritional interactions can influence the course of the pregnancy, fetal development and health during childhood and adult life. The impact of these interactions on outcomes depends primarily on the time of the insult during pregnancy.

- Lifestyle, including smoking, alcohol and prescribed and recreational drugs, can affect pregnancy outcome and the effect of these should be addressed antenatally.

- Social and maternal health factors can determine the nature of the fetal environment and this will influence the health and well-being of the infant at birth.

Introduction

The health and well-being of a newborn infant is related to a multitude of genetic, biological and environmental factors. Within this complex developmental network, a key influence on the growth and development of the infant is the nutritional and non-nutritional interaction that takes place between the mother and the fetus during the period of conception and throughout the remainder of pregnancy. If a mother has a specific nutritional deficiency, e.g. macronutrient, mineral or vitamin, this will have a direct impact on the fetus. However, the normal nutritional interaction between mother and fetus can also be disturbed by the mother having a medical condition which influences fetal metabolism, e.g. diabetes mellitus, or by the mother developing a pregnancy-related disorder which adversely affects fetal growth and nutrition, e.g. pre-eclampsia. Moreover, the fetus can be affected by non-nutritional interactions that relate to maternal social and lifestyle factors including alcohol intake, smoking and drug administration.

This chapter will consider the lifestyle and maternal health factors that can impact on fetal environment and influence the growth, health and well-being of the infant. Material in Chapters 2 and 3 should be read in relation to this chapter.

Lifestyle Interactions Between Mother and Fetus

Diet

Health status differs by social class and race, with differences existing even between the most affluent sectors of the population (Gorski, 1998). Even when maternity care is provided free of charge, perinatal complications are more frequent in lower socio-economic status areas (Gudmundsson et al., 1997).

The relationship of maternal social class to adverse pregnancy outcome is independent of maternal age, parity and adverse reproductive history (de Sanjose and Roman, 1991). However social class is closely related to maternal diet (Morrison et al., 1989), and dietary factors can significantly influence perinatal outcome. For example the intakes of the essential fatty acids (EFA) and their long-chain poly-

unsaturated fatty acid derivatives, arachidonic acid (AA) and docosahexaenoic acid (DHA; Fulton et al., 1988) are significantly related to socio-economic status. The long-chain polyunsaturated fatty acids (LCPUFAs) are important components of cell membranes, especially those in the brain and the eyes (Crawford, 2000). During pregnancy there is active transport of DHA across the placenta (Hay, 1994). The LCPUFA status of women during pregnancy is dependent upon dietary intake, especially oily fish. Oily fish intake is significantly lower in women from lower socio-economic groups (JS Forsyth, unpublished data) and therefore their infants maybe at risk from a relative deficiency of these fatty acids. Women who do not include oily fish in their diet have lower plasma DHA levels and this effect is exacerbated if the mother is multiparous. It has been estimated that maternal DHA levels may take more than 6 months after delivery to reach full functional recovery. There is increasing evidence that LCPUFA deficiency may be associated with impaired visual (Carlson et al., 1993, 1996) and cognitive development (Agostoni et al., 1995; Willatts et al., 1998). Dietary interactions before and during pregnancy need to be directed at the socially disadvantaged, although previous strategies have not met with great success. These issues are also discussed in Chapter 10.

Overweight and obesity

There is no agreed definition of overweight in pregnancy. However a pregravid body mass index [BMI, defined as weight (kg)/height (m)^2] of >25 was the criterion used in a Swedish study (Cnattingius et al., 1998) for definition of obesity, while a pregravid BMI >35 has been used in the USA to define obesity (Bianco et al., 1998). In the UK a BMI >30 is defined as obesity while a BMI of 25–30 is regarded as overweight. In 1993 almost 40 per cent of women between the ages of 16 and 64 were either overweight or obese (Department of Health, 1994).

Overweight (even if it is moderate) is a risk factor for gestational diabetes mellitus and hypertensive disorders (Abrams and Parker, 1988; Naeye, 1990; Perlow et al., 1992). Obese pregnant women have higher arterial blood pressure and their haemoglobin is more concentrated than that in non-obese pregnant women. Obesity also alters cardiac function (Tomoda et al., 1996). The incidence of hypertension is 2.2–21.4 times higher in obese pregnant women compared with controls; the incidence of pre-eclampsia is 1.22–9.7 times more common in obese women than in controls (Edwards et al., 1978, 1996; Gross et al., 1980; Calandra et al., 1981; Naeye, 1990; Galtier-Dereure et al., 1995).

Obesity during pregnancy is associated with a slightly higher risk of urinary tract infections and thromboembolic disorders (Garbaciak et al., 1985); however anaemia is less frequent in obese pregnant women (Garbaciak et al., 1985; Abrams and Parker, 1988).

The relation between maternal obesity and preterm delivery is controversial (Galtier-Dereure et al., 2000), but most authors report a higher frequency of labour induction in obese pregnant women, whereas no differences have been reported in the duration of labour (Gross et al., 1980; Le Thai et al., 1992; Galtier-Dereure et al., 1995) and the percentage of instrumental delivery (corrected for other illnesses including diabetes mellitus; Edwards et al., 1978; Gross et al., 1980; Johnson et al., 1987; Le Thai et al., 1992). The rate of caesarean section is significantly higher in obese women than controls (1.15–3 times; Edwards et al., 1978; Gross et al., 1980; Calandra et al., 1981; Garbaciak et al., 1985; Galtier-Dereure et al., 1995; Bianco et al., 1998). For each one-unit increase of BMI in the pregravid weight there is a 7 per cent increase in the risk of caesarean section (Brost et al., 1997). Reasons for caesarean section are fetal macrosomia, cephalopelvic dispro-

portion, fetal distress and failed induction (Galtier-Dereure et al., 2000). Anaesthetic and postoperative risks are also higher in obese patients, and with massive increases in perioperative and total operative time, blood loss and endometritis (Perlow and Morgan, 1994).

Infants of overweight mothers have a higher incidence of congenital malformations. It has been reported that if the mother is overweight there is a 35 per cent increase in the risk of major congenital malformation and if the mother is obese the incidence of such malformations is up to 37.5 per cent higher (Naeye, 1990). The most frequently reported congenital malformation is neural tube defect (NTD; Waller et al., 1994; Shaw et al., 1997; Watkins et al., 1996). This higher incidence persists even after correction for confounding factors including age, smoking, socioeconomic status and folate intake (Galtier-Dereure et al., 2000). Other abnormalities include cryptorchism (Berkowitz et al., 1995) and increased risk of fluctuating dental asymmetry, which might indicate developmental destabilization (Kieser et al., 1997). Several studies have indicated a higher incidence of neonatal mortality in relation to excess maternal pregravid weight. The incidence of perinatal death is 1.15–2.5 times higher with high maternal weight. Maternal complications and preterm deliveries contribute to this increase in mortality. Apgar scores are significantly lower in infants of obese mothers than in infants of normal-weight mothers (Calandra et al., 1981; Mancuso et al., 1991; Perlow et al., 1992).

Pregravid maternal BMI is a strong predictor of birth-weight; obese mothers deliver large-for-gestational age infants 1.4–18 times more frequently than non-obese pregnant women (Edwards et al., 1978; Gross et al., 1980; Calandra et al., 1981; Johnson et al., 1987; Mancuso et al., 1991; Le Thai et al., 1992; Galtier-Dereure et al., 1995). Neonatal skinfold thickness is significantly higher in infants born to obese pregnant women than in infants born to lean mothers (Whitelaw, 1976). Macrosomia (macrosomic infants are infants with high birth-weight due to increased body fat and enlarged viscera) increases the risk of birth-related injuries and thus perinatal morbidity and mortality (Spellacy et al., 1985). Caesarean section might reduce the risk of birth-related injuries, but does not alter the perinatal death rate (Okun et al., 1997).

Maternal obesity has long-term effects on the mother as well as the infant. After delivery obese mothers are more likely to suffer from urinary symptoms such as stress incontinence and urgency (Rasmussen et al., 1997). These effects persist after correction for other factors like diabetes mellitus. Weight gain during pregnancy is a strong predictor for sustained weight retention (Greene et al., 1988). Weight gain during pregnancy is discussed in more detail in Chapter 3.

Infants of obese mothers, especially infants who are macrosomic at delivery, are more likely to be overweight at the age of 1 year. However this may not be a cause and effect relation as other factors, including genetic predisposition, play an important role in the development of obesity (Edwards et al., 1978).

Tobacco smoking

Prevalence studies in the 1990s showed that between one in five and one in three pregnant women in developed countries smoke during pregnancy (Dodds, 1995; Tappin et al., 1997; Cnattingius and Haglund, 1997). Tobacco smoking during pregnancy has been associated with physical (intrauterine growth retardation; Fielding, 1978; Conter et al., 1995), cognitive and behavioural effects in offspring (Sexton et al., 1990). Smokers also in general have a poorer dietary intake of micronutrients and, interestingly, even when the intakes are equivalent to those of non-smokers the circulatory concentrations of antioxidant nutrients, including vitamins A, E and C, of smokers are lower than those of non-smokers (McArdle and Ashworth, 1999).

Pregnant smokers have a higher incidence of abruptio placentae (Odendaal et al., 2001), placenta previa (Castles et al., 1999), spontaneous abortions (Mishra et al., 2000), stillbirths (Pollack et al., 2000), preterm births (Cuk et al., 2000; Odendaal et al., 2001), premature rupture of the membranes (Castles et al., 1999) and amnionitis. Anencephaly (To and Tang, 1999), congenital heart defects (Kallen, 1999), and oro-facial clefts (Lorente et al., 2000; Chung et al., 2000) are more common in the newborns of smokers than in those of non-smokers.

Alcohol

Lemoinne et al. (1968) first recognized the multiple effects that alcohol can have on the developing fetus. Alcohol is now appreciated as the most common major teratogen to which the fetus may be exposed and fetal alcohol syndrome (FAS) is currently a leading cause of mental retardation in the Western world (Murphy-Brennan and Oei, 1999). From various studies, the incidence of FAS ranges from 0.2 to 3.0 affected infants per 1000 live births (West et al., 1998). It is also estimated that 10–20 per cent of moderate mental deficiency (IQ in the 50–80 range) is a result of fetal alcohol exposure (Streissguth et al., 1990). Current evidence would suggest that the average daily consumption of as little as two drinks per day or periodic binge drinking in early pregnancy might be associated with recognizable abnormalities (Jacobson et al., 1994).

FAS is often an unrecognized diagnosis and is based on clinical signs alone. FAS is characterized by pre- and/or postnatal growth deficiency, CNS dysfunction and typical facial features (short palpebral fissures, short, upturned nose, hypoplastic philtrum, hypoplastic maxilla). Malocclusion and a disturbed facial growth may occur (Figure 5.1). The

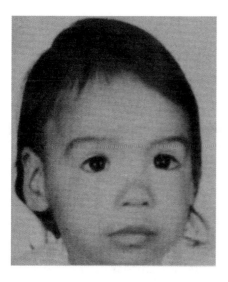

Figure 5.1 Fetal alcohol syndrome [reproduced from Lyons (1997) *Smith's Recognizable Patterns of Human Malformations*, p. 557, by permission of WB Saunders]

cognitive and behavioural disturbances (CNS dysfunction) have a great influence on the children's ability to learn and on their adult life. FAS is to a large extent found in areas with less than satisfactory socio-economic conditions. Prenatal alcohol exposure can also lead to changes in retinal function as evidenced by an abnormal electroretinogram (ERG) response. The ERG can therefore be a tool with which to identify suspected alcohol embryopathy. More recent magnetic resonance imaging studies (MRI), particularly when combined with quantitative analysis, have indicated that specific brain areas such as the basal ganglia, the corpus callosum, and parts of the cerebellum might be especially susceptible to the teratogenic effects of alcohol (Roebuck *et al.*, 1998).

Prevention is essential since the brain damage prevails, despite comprehensive medical, social and educational supportive efforts being made during childhood.

Progress has been slow in developing animal models for studying the underlying mechanisms; however it has recently been shown that, during the synaptogenesis period, also known as the brain growth spurt period, ethanol has the potential to trigger massive neuronal apoptosis in the *in vivo* mammalian brain (Olney *et al.*, 2000).

The brain growth spurt period in humans spans the last trimester of pregnancy and the first years of life (see Chapter 1). The *n*-methyl-D-aspartate (NMDA) antagonist and γ-amino-butyric acid (GABA) mimetic properties of ethanol may be responsible for its apoptogenic action, in that other drugs with either NMDA antagonist or GABA mimetic actions also trigger apoptotic neuro-degeneration in the developing brain. Furthermore, NMDA antagonist and GABA mimetic drugs are sometimes abused by pregnant women and are also used as anti-convulsants, sedatives or anaesthetics in pediatric medicine. In addition, the observation that ethanol and several other drugs (e.g. methamphetamine) trigger massive neuronal apoptosis in the developing brain provides an unprecedented opportunity to study both neuro-pathological aspects and molecular mechanisms of apoptotic neuro-degeneration in the *in vivo* mammalian brain (Olney *et al.*, 2000).

Drug therapy during pregnancy

The thalidomide disaster has made the public aware of the potential for drugs to produce fetal abnormalities. However few drugs have been proven to be teratogenic in humans.

In general, drugs should be avoided if possible, especially during organogenesis (during the first trimester) as they may have teratogenic effects. Table 5.1 shows known teratogenic drugs for the human embryo. Otherwise only drugs known to be safe should be used. Drugs given after organogenesis will not produce a major anatomical defect but may affect the growth and development of the fetus. Most drugs can cross the placenta and

Table 5.1   Known teratogenic drugs for the human embryo

Acitretin
Alcohol
Altertamine
Androgens
Anticoagulants (oral)
Anti-convulsants:
    Carbamazepine
    Ethosuximide
    Oxcarbazepine
    Phenobarbital
    Phenytoin
    Sodium valproate
    There is insufficient information about the
    teratogenicity of the newer anti-convulsants in
    humans. Risk of teratogenicity is greater if more
    than one drug is used
Co-trimoxazole – theoretical risk as trimethprim
   (Bactrim) is a folate antagonist
Cytotoxics
Isotretioin
Lithium
Methyl mercury
Penicillamine
Podaphyllum resin
Pyrimethamine
Ribavirin
Statins
Tamoxifen
Thioquanine
Tretinoin

Source: *British National Formulary*, Issue 41, March 2001.

expose the developing embryo and fetus to their pharmacological effects.

In the UK the Monthly Index of Medical Specialities (MIMS) serves as a suitable reference for the prescription of drugs to pregnant women.

Drug–nutrient interactions

Drugs interact with nutrition in a variety of ways (Dickerson, 1988), as food may affect the absorption and metabolism of drugs, and drugs may affect the metabolism of and requirement for nutrients. Drugs are metabolized in the body by a two-stage enzymatic process involving a non-specific mixed function oxidase system which is located primarily but not exclusively in hepatic microsomes. This system has very low activity in the fetus and newborn infant. The activity of the enzymes involved may be modified by deficiencies of energy, protein, vitamins or minerals. The activity of the system is substrate-induced and drugs that are given over long periods, such as those given for the treatment of epilepsy, may induce a deficiency of folic acid; this vitamin is required for the synthesis of a vital component of the system, cytochrome P450 (Labadarios *et al.*, 1978).

Epilepsy and antiepileptic drugs during pregnancy

Pregnant women with epilepsy constitute 0.5 per cent of all pregnancies (Nulman *et al.*, 1999). Factors such as epilepsy, anti-convulsant-induced teratogenicity, a patient's genetic predisposition and the severity of the convulsive disorder may contribute to adverse pregnancy outcome for the children of women with epilepsy. Although 90 per cent of patients using anti-convulsant drugs can expect a favourable pregnancy result, this outcome can be maximized by careful preconceptional, antepartum and postpartum management. There is no clear-cut agreement that any one of the four major drugs used for the treatment of seizure disorders (phenytoin, phenobarbital, valproic acid and carbamazepine) is more teratogenic than others. Preconceptional counselling should include patient education to ensure a clear understanding of the risks of uncontrolled seizures and the possible teratogenicity of anti-convulsants (Malone and D'Alton, 1997).

Anti-epileptic drug therapy with valproic acid (VPA) during early pregnancy can result in a 1–2 per cent incidence of spina bifida, a closure defect of the posterior neural tube in the human (Nau *et al.*, 1991). This is probably due to folic acid deficiency induced by the drug. Folic acid, 5 mg/day, should be administered 3 months before conception and during the first trimester to prevent folic acid deficiency-induced malformations (Nulman *et al.*, 1999). Antenatal management in these patients should also include regular assessment of patients for anti-convulsant-associated birth defects through detailed ultrasound examination and levels of maternal serum α-feto-proteins (Nau, 1994). Anti-convulsant therapy can cause osteomalacia, despite an apparently adequate vitamin D intake (Stamp *et al.*, 1978).

Anti-convulsant interaction with phytomenadione (vitamin K) metabolism may lead to an increased risk for neural tube defect and early neonatal bleeding. If phenobarbital, carbamazepine or phenytoin is administered, maternal phytomenadione supplementation should begin 4 weeks before the expected date of delivery (Nulman *et al.*, 1999).

Narcotic drug addiction during pregnancy

Drug abuse is a general public health problem, and involves a growing number of pregnant women. Five per cent of pregnant women who gave birth in the USA in 1992 used illegal drugs while they were pregnant (Mathias, 1995). Therefore, withdrawal syndromes in the newborn have also increased. Pregnancy in a narcotic drug addict is a high-risk condition. The prevention of neonatal and paediatric complications involving both physical and psychological conditions requires early individual medical, psychological and social support adapted to each pregnant addict.

Neonatal abstinence syndrome (NAS) is the most striking effect of fetal exposure to drugs and symptoms are easily recognized. Pharmacological treatment can consist of either seda-

tives or replacement drugs and the dosage depends on the severity of the withdrawal symptoms which are evaluated using a score system. NAS symptoms usually resolve within a few days, although some signs, especially irritability and tremors, may persist until 3 months of age. In addition to the long-term developmental and cognitive risks, these infants are subject to considerable social adverse factors. In one study, in over 50 per cent of cases parental authority was suspended by the juvenile court (Fabris *et al.*, 1998).

Heroin alone or in association with methadone now represents the drug used by approximately 80 per cent of addicted mothers in Western countries. The main effect of heroin is NAS, which might be prolonged (up to 6 months in animals studied) as heroin clearance from neonatal tissues is slow and prolonged (Hutchings, 1982). Studies have so far failed to show long-term neurologic or cognitive deficits directly associated with heroin use during pregnancy.

Cocaine abuse is a significant problem not only in the general population but also among pregnant women. Since cocaine readily crosses the placenta and is metabolized slowly by the fetus, infants can be exposed to significant levels of cocaine for long periods. In humans the most common consequences of cocaine abuse during pregnancy include premature birth, lower birth-weight, respiratory distress, bowel infarctions, cerebral infarctions, reduced head circumference, and increased risk of seizures. Behaviourally these newborns show an increased degree of 'tremulousness', crying and irritability, and are over-reactive to environmental stimuli. Within a month these behaviours have recovered dramatically, but not to normal levels. Thus, while there are a number of abnormalities associated with cocaine-exposed neonates, they are not imminently debilitating or life-threatening. However, the long-term consequences of this prenatal cocaine exposure remain to be elucidated (Keller and Snyder-Keller, 2000).

Fetuses exposed *in utero* to cocaine are at risk of long-term neuro-behavioural damage, not just because of the drug itself, but also because of clustering of other health determinants, including low socio-economic status, low maternal education and maternal addiction. One methodological approach to separating the direct neuro-toxic effects of cocaine from these synergistic insults is to follow up a cohort of children exposed *in utero* to cocaine and then adopted by middle–upper class families. The Toronto Adoption Study, supported by Health Canada, has demonstrated the direct neuro-toxic effects of cocaine on IQ and language. These effects are mild to moderate compared with those measured in fetuses exposed *in utero* to cocaine and reared by their natural mothers (Koren *et al.*, 1998).

Based on findings in humans and the confirmation of prenatal exposures in animals, amphetamines and methamphetamines increase the risk of an adverse outcome when abused during pregnancy. Clefting, cardiac anomalies and fetal growth deficits that have been seen in infants exposed to amphetamines during pregnancy have all been reproduced in animal studies involving prenatal exposures to amphetamines. The differential effects of amphetamines between genetic strains of mice and between species demonstrate that pharmacokinetics and the genetic disposition of the mother and developing embryo can have an enormous influence on enhancing or reducing these potential risks. The effects of prenatal exposure to amphetamines in producing altered behaviour in humans appear less compelling when one considers other confounding variables of human environment, genetics and polydrug abuse. In view of the animal data concerning altered behaviour and learning tasks in comparison with learning deficits observed in humans, the influence of the confounding variables in humans may serve to increase the sensitivity of the developing embryo/fetus to prenatal exposure to amphetamines. These factors and others may predispose the developing conceptus to the damaging effects of amphetamines by actually lowering the threshold of susceptibility at the sites where damage occurs. Knowledge of the effects of prenatal exposure of the fetus and the mother to designer amphetamines is lacking. In the few studies in which designer drugs have been examined in animal models, more questions have been raised than answered. Possible reasons why no malformations or significant fetal effects were found in the study by St Omer include the genetic strain of rat used, the conservative exposure profile, or the fact that the placenta metabolized methylenedioxymethamphetamine (MDMA) before it reached the embryo. These questions underscore the need for further investigations concerning the prenatal exposure effects of designer compounds and the effects of amphetamine and methamphetamine in general (Plessinger, 1998).

The risks for the mother and the fetus warrant prescription of substitution therapy during pregnancy. Published results concerning pregnancies in women on substitution therapy have been encouraging and clearly show a decrease in maternal and fetal complications. These studies are, however, difficult to conduct and subject to a number of biases relating to social and economical factors and also the type of substance abuse (smoking, alcohol, drug; Cayol *et al.*, 2000).

Methadone maintenance was introduced in 1964 as a medical response to the post-World War II heroin epidemic in New York City. The principal effects of methadone maintenance are to relieve narcotic craving and suppress the abstinence syndrome. A majority of patients require 80–120 mg/day of methadone or more to achieve these effects and require treatment for an indefinite period of time, since methadone maintenance is a corrective but not a curative treatment (Joseph *et al.*, 2000). Methadone maintenance is indicated for pregnant women addicted to heroin, however animal studies have shown that birth-weights are significantly lower in the methadone-treated animals.

Prescribing drugs during pregnancy requires a careful balance of risk and benefit. Under-treatment of any maternal illness might be harmful to both the mother and the growing fetus, but conversely drugs may adversely influence organogenesis and this risk will depend on several factors, including the nature of the drug, time of exposure, dose, genetic factors and the mother's previous obstetric history (see Table 5.3 for the common terato-genic drugs).

Caffeine

Caffeine is a methylated xanthine that acts as a mild central nervous system stimulant (CNS). It is present in many beverages, including coffee, tea and cola, as well as chocolate (Christian and Brent, 2001). Caffeine constitutes 1–2 per cent of roasted coffee beans and 3.5 per cent of fresh tea leaves (Spiller, 1984).

Many over-the-counter medications, such as cold and allergy tablets, headache medicines and stimulants also contain caffeine, although the concentration of caffeine in these medicines is small. Consumption of caffeinated beverages during pregnancy is quite common (Hill et al., 1977), with an estimated intake of 144 mg/day in the USA (Morris and Weinstein, 1981).

A number of adverse clinical consequences have been reported to be related to caffeine intake during pregnancy, including the occur-rence of congenital malformations, fetal growth retardation, small-for-date babies (Eskenazi et al., 1999; Fernandes et al., 1998), miscarriages (spontaneous abortions) (Cnattingius et al., 2000; Fernandes et al., 1998); behavioural effects and maternal fertility problems (Curtis et al., 1997). Animal studies are needed to substantiate these epi-demiological associations (Christian and Brent, 2001).

Maternal Health Interactions Between Mother and Fetus

Anaemia

Anaemia is one of the most frequent compli-cations of pregnancy. Normal physiologic changes in pregnancy affect haemoglobin, and there is a relative (due to disproportionate increase of plasma volume) or absolute reduc-tion in haemoglobin concentration. The most common true anomalies during pregnancy are iron-deficiency anaemia (approximately 75 per cent) and folate-deficiency megaloblastic anaemia, which are more common in women who have inadequate diets and who are not receiving prenatal iron and folate supplements. Severe anaemia may have adverse effects on the mother and the fetus. Anaemia with haemoglobin levels less than 6 g/dl is associated with poor pregnancy outcome (Cuervo and Mahomed, 2001; Sifakis and Pharmakides, 2000).

Prematurity, spontaneous abortions, low birth-weight, and fetal deaths are complications of severe maternal anaemia. Nevertheless, a mild to moderate iron deficiency (haemoglobin level of 10–12 g/dl) does not appear to have a significant effect on fetal haemoglobin concen-tration (Sifakis and Pharmakides, 2000). A haemoglobin level of 11 g/dl in the late first trimester and also of 10 g/dl in the second and third trimesters are considered as lower limits for haemoglobin concentration. In an iron-deficient state, iron supplementation must be given and follow-up is indicated to diagnose iron-unresponsive anaemia.

Maternal anaemia diagnosed before mid-pregnancy has been associated with an increased risk of preterm delivery. Maternal anaemia detected during the later stages of pregnancy, especially the third trimester, often reflects the expected (and necessary) expansion of maternal plasma volume. However, all have been associated with an increased incidence of preterm delivery (Yip, 2000). This increased risk may reflect in part the failure to expand maternal plasma volume adequately, thus diminishing appropriate placental perfusion. Although controlled trials of iron supplementation during pregnancy have consistently demonstrated positive effects on maternal iron status at delivery, they have not demonstrated reductions in factors that are associated with maternal anaemia, i.e. increased risk of preterm delivery and infant low birth-weight.

Recently, concerns have been voiced about harmful effects of iron supplementation during pregnancy (Scholl and Reilly, 2000). Questions about the efficacy of iron supplementation during pregnancy in reducing adverse outcomes such as preterm delivery and side effects from iron supplementation, including the potential for oxidation of lipids and DNA, require further research in iron-deficient women.

Hypertension

Hypertension in pregnancy is defined as a systolic blood pressure $\geqslant 140\,mmHg$ and a diastolic blood pressure of $\geqslant 90\,mmHg$, or by a rise in blood pressure from the non-pregnant state of systolic $\geqslant 30\,mmHg$ and diastolic $\geqslant 15\,mmHg$ (Atallah et al., 2002).

Hypertensive diseases in pregnancy comprise various disorders from transient hypertension to the dangerous pre-eclampsia/eclampsia. Diagnosis of these diseases requires an understanding of the normal physiological adaptations during pregnancy. High blood pressure with or without proteinuria is a major cause of maternal and infant mortality and morbidity worldwide, and perinatal morbidity and mortality. Hypertension during pregnancy is common, with 1 in 10 women having high blood pressure.

Pre-eclampsia is a multisystemic disorder that usually consists of hypertension, significant proteinurea (at least $300\,mg/24\,h$) and oedema, but when severe can involve the liver, kidneys, clotting system and the brain (Duley et al., 2000). Pre-eclampsia affects 2–8 per cent of pregnancies (Zhang and Ding, 1994) and can occur at any time during the second half of pregnancy. The only definitive treatment for pre-eclampsia is to deliver the fetus and the placenta.

Eclampsia is the occurrence of one or more convulsions in association with the syndrome of pre-eclampsia; it is a rare but serious complication. In developed countries it complicates 1 in 2000 deliveries (Douglas and Redman, 1994), while in developing countries it affects 1 in 100 to 1 in 1700 pregnancies (Crowther, 1985). Eclampsia probably accounts for 50 000 maternal deaths a year worldwide, which is about 10 per cent of direct maternal deaths during pregnancy (Duley, 1992).

The 'HELLP syndrome' consists of maternal haemolysis, elevated liver enzymes and a low platelet count. It has different pathophysiologic characteristics from pre-eclampsia and eclampsia, but it complicates severe eclampsia. It is associated with high maternal and fetal morbidity and mortality (Vigil-de Gracia et al., 1996). It is recommended that such pregnancies are dealt with in tertiary centres (Ben Letaifa et al., 2000).

Diabetes mellitus

Diabetes mellitus complicates around 2.6 per cent of pregnancies (Cunningham et al., 1997), 90 per cent of which is gestational diabetes. Gestational diabetes mellitus (GDM) is defined as carbohydrate intolerance of variable severity with onset or first recognition during the present pregnancy (ACOG, 1995). GDM is a heterogeneous disorder in which age, obesity and genetic background contribute to the severity of the disease. Women with GDM are at risk of later development of type 2 diabetes mellitus. GDM is accompanied by alterations in fasting, postprandial and integrated 24 h plasma amino acids, glucose and lipids (Metzger *et al.*, 1980). The pathophysiology of GDM remains controversial; it may reflect a predisposition to type 2 diabetes expressed under the metabolic condition of pregnancy or it may represent the extreme manifestation of metabolic alterations that normally occur in pregnancy (Kuhl, 1991). GDM causes a state of dyslipidaemia consistent with insulin resistance. During pregnancy, women with GDM have higher serum triglyceride concentrations but a lower level of LDL-cholesterol concentration than normal pregnant women (Koukkou *et al.*, 1996). Total cholesterol, HDL cholesterol and apolipoprotein concentrations are not significantly different between GDM and normal pregnancies (Butte, 2000).

Pregestational diabetes mellitus is a well-recognized high-risk condition in modern obstetrics with maternal as well as fetal complications being closely related to the severity of the diabetes. In prepregnancy diabetes mellitus, a major concern is fetal death (stillbirth) during the third trimester and, although this is associated with poorly controlled diabetes, the underlying mechanism is poorly understood (Hanson and Persson, 1993). Other obstetric complications include pre-eclampsia and polyhydramnios, both of which may necessitate preterm delivery with its possible complications. Moreover, fetal macrosomia (Figure 5.2) increases the chance of operative delivery and the risk of related birth trauma including shoulder dystocia, Erb's palsy, fractures and subconjunctival haemorrhages (Cousins, 1987; Johnstone *et al.*, 1990; Hanson and Persson, 1993).

Infant hypoglycaemia

A rapid fall in infant plasma glucose concentration (usually soon after birth but may develop after 24 h) is characteristic of infants of diabetic mothers. The severity of this

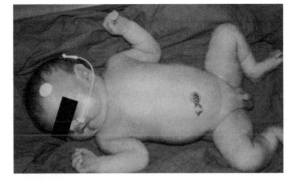

Figure 5.2 Macrosomic infant of a diabetic mother [reproduced from Candy *et al.* (2001) *Clinical Paediatrics and Child Health*, p. 10, by permission of WB Saunders]

hypoglycaemia depends on many factors, which may include the maternal glucose level during pregnancy as well as glucose homeostasis during the delivery.

Fetal hyperglycaemia

Fetal hyperglycaemia, which is the direct effect of maternal high blood sugar (Light *et al.*, 1972), suppresses fetal plasma free fatty acids and diminishes hepatic glucose output. Other contributing factors to this hypoglycaemia may include defective compensatory mechanisms, which involve catecholamine and glucagon. Maternal hypoglycaemia may also cause fetal/infant adrenal medullary exhaustion, which results from long-standing hypoglycaemia during fetal life and neonatal hypoglycaemia (Stern *et al.*, 1968; Keenan *et al.*, 1972; Artal *et al.*, 1982).

Hypocalcaemia

Up to 50 per cent of infants born to diabetic mothers will have a degree of hypocalcaemia (Mimouni *et al.*, 1986b), the incidence and severity of which is directly related to maternal glucose homeostasis during pregnancy and labour (Tsang *et al.*, 1972). It usually appears during the very early hours of life and changes little after 24 h. The pathogenesis of hypocalcaemia in infants of diabetic mothers remains unclear. Hypocalcaemia is usually associated with a degree of hyperphosphataemia and less frequently with hypomagnesaemia. Hypocalcaemia is usually mild (total serum calcium above 2 mmol/l) and requires no treatment. However, symptomatic hypocalcaemia requires active treatment as it might cause neonatal convulsions. The bone mass of infants of diabetic mothers is significantly higher than that of normal infants and this is probably a direct effect of the hyperinsulinaemic status and the effect of insulin and insulin-like growth factor-1 on bone formation.

Polycythaemia, jaundice and hyperviscosity

Infants of diabetic mothers have increased risk of polycythaemia (venous haematocrit more than 65 per cent) and this will increase whole blood viscosity (Mimouni *et al.*, 1986a). Polycythaemic infants have an increased tendency for diminished blood flow, especially in the hepatic, cerebral, renal and mesenteric circulations. Lysis of the red cell mass will exaggerate and prolong physiological jaundice (Peevy *et al.*, 1980; Miodovnik *et al.*, 1987). Polycythaemia in infants of diabetic mothers is thought to be secondary to a relative cellular hypoxia, which in turn is due to higher metabolic rates in the hyperinsulinaemic status. Hypoxia will stimulate erythropoietin secretion and a high erythropoietin level has been well documented in cord blood of polycythemic infants ($>4 \mu U/ml$; Widness *et al.*, 1981).

Congenital malformation

Infants of diabetic mothers are at increased risk of congenital malformations, which could probably be addressed by better preconceptional care. Overall, the risk of congenital malformation is 2–3-fold that of a normal pregnancy and this increase is directly related to the level of glycosylated haemoglobin at the time of conception (McElvy *et al.*, 2000). These complications are more common in type 1 diabetes mellitus. Malformations include caudal regression syndrome, spina bifida, hydrocephalus, sacral agenesis and anomalies of the heart and urogenital system (Roberton, 1999).

Allergy

Immunological development occurs before birth and at birth an infant has an immune system similar to that of adults although he or she has not developed responses to specific allergens. In the normal course of events 'tolerance' develops and the capacity of an individual to react to a normally effective allergen stimulus (e.g. a food protein) is established. Development of oral tolerance is associated with specific T cells and is affected by specifically activated T suppressor cells. Hypersensitivity occurs when the secondary boosting of the immune response to an allergen is excessive and leads to gross tissue damage manifested as eczema (often seen in infants), asthma, oedema or urticaria. In normal circumstances T-cells are able to evaluate the threat posed by an allergen and can distinguish between harmless and harmful allergens. When, however, the system breaks down, harmless substances are recognized as harmful, thereby provoking an immune response.

Prevalence of food hypersensitivity

It is generally accepted that there has been an increased prevalence of food hypersensitivities in the developed world; 30 per cent of the population experience one or more episodes of food intolerance in his or her lifetime. The problem of chronicity of some hypersensitivities is increasing. These facts represent a major public health problem in terms of morbidity and expense to the National Health Service. There is a known association between atopic eczema in infancy and childhood asthma, which has food allergy implications (Kjellman and Nilsson, 1998).

Approximately 48 per cent of all adult patients presenting with an adverse response involving the immune system suffer from type 1 immediate hypersensitivity and this is commonly described as atopic disease (Table 5.2). The strongest predisposing factor to the development of allergy is a family history, with a risk of developing allergy of 10 per cent if neither parent is atopic, 50 per cent if one parent is atopic and 66 per cent if both parents are atopic. Atopic disease is also related to other risk factors including race, gender, maternal age, family structure, lifestyle and environmental factors, in particular early feeding history. Table 5.3 outlines biochemical markers for the prediction of the development of allergy.

The prevalence of allergy to a given food depends on the age of the subject and the course of food allergy depends on the nature of the allergens and the onset of sensitivity. Those with allergies to peanuts, nuts, fish and shellfish rarely become tolerant, whereas tolerance is often developed in early childhood for milk and eggs. The prevalence of true allergy differs depending on the test used for diagnosis

Table 5.3 Prediction of allergy and prevention strategies

1. *Prediction*
   Family history of atopy
   High cord blood IgE
   Reduced $CD8^+$ T cells, particularly those bearing $\gamma\delta$-TCR
   Other possible markers of atopy: proliferative response to food antigens, cytokine production, T cell subsets

2. *Prevention Programme*
Strategies
   Breast-feeding
   Maternal diet restriction during pregnancy and lactation
   Hydrolysed infant formula
   Late introduction of common allergenic foods
Essential
   Good test for prediction of high-risk infants
   An effective intervention strategy implemented in existing health-care infrastructure
   The intervention should be acceptable to health-care authorities and to the parents
   It should be cost-effective

From Samartin *et al.* (2001).

(Samartin *et al.*, 2001): 6–8 per cent of infants, 1–5 per cent of adults (Metcalf, 1995), 2–8 per cent of children and 1 per cent adults (Sampson, 1997), and 1.4 per cent children and 0.3 per cent adults (Chandra, 1997) in the presence of food allergy confirmed by double-blind placebo-controlled challenges (see pp 338 & 358).

Table 5.2 Immunologic mechanisms in adult patients with atopic eczema and food allergy

Immunologic mechanisms	Percentage of patients
Type I immediate hypersensitivity	48%
Type II antibody-mediated cytotoxicity	6%
Type III immune complex	10%
Type IV delayed hypersensitivity	18%
More than one type of reaction	28%

From Chandra (1993), cited by Samartin *et al.* (2001).

Early dietary modulators

A statement of the European Society for Paediatric Allerogology and Clinical Immunology (ESPACI) Committee on Hypoallergenic Formulas and the European Society for Paediatric Gastroenterology, Hepatology and Nutrition (ESPGHAN) Committee on Nutrition comments on current unresolved issues in the treatment and prevention of food allergy in infants and children (Host *et al.*, 1999). There is very limited evidenced-based research where trials are randomized and controlled for confounding variables that is designed to establish appropriate weaning practices for infants (full-term and preterm) to prevent food allergy development. The results from a 7 year follow-up study from Dundee indicated that breast-feeding in the full-term infant, together with the delayed introduction (15 weeks) of solid foods, may benefit later childhood health, including prevention of respiratory disease (Wilson *et al.*, 1998). There is very limited evidence that exclusion diets (cow's milk, eggs, wheat) during pregnancy delay or prevent the onset of allergy in high-atopic-risk infants and the definitive study is still to be carried out (Warner *et al.*, 2000).

Because it has been known for some time that certain food proteins (cow's milk, eggs) are detectable in breast milk, the exclusion of these proteins from the mother's diet might protect infants with a family history of atopic disease from developing eczema (Table 5.2). In fact maternal exclusion diets (e.g. cow's milk, eggs) during lactation seems to benefit some breast-fed (high-atopic-risk) infants with eczema (Cant *et al.*, 1986; Sigurs *et al.*, 1992; Arshad *et al.*, 1992). There is also evidence that maternal exclusion diets during late gestation and lactation benefit the high-risk infant (Lilja *et al.*, 1989; Lovegrove *et al.*, 1994; Marini *et al.*, 1996). An impressive 7 year follow-up study has reported on combined maternal and infant avoidance (Zeiger and Heller, 1995). In this study mothers avoided cow's milk, eggs and peanuts in the last trimester and during lactation. In addition, in the diet of their full-term infants cow's milk was avoided to 12 months, eggs until 2 years and peanuts until 3 years old. The study represented the largest cohort of high-risk infants followed for the longest period in a randomized control design. However, perinatal maternal/infant food allergy avoidance compared with standard infant feeding practices failed to modify atopic disease at 7 years. In addition, benefits of

intervention were limited because of frequent remission of food sensitization and food allergy in early childhood. The diet intervention was probably too stringent and impractical for many mothers. Male gender, parental asthma, ethnicity, parental smoking and dust mites all contributed to the predisposition to allergy development and all but one of these factors can be modified. Table 5.3 outlines the essential elements that are required for a successful prevention programme.

Earlier studies modulating food intakes of the mother, the infant or both mother and infant provided some hope that allergy development could be at least delayed or even prevented, but many authors were also right to be cautious regarding the long-term benefits. 'Food as medicine' in the treatment of food allergy during the developmental period must be viewed with caution. Results from intervention studies are often disappointing and there is concern about delayed tolerance and the problem of spontaneous remission. Clearly there is a need to target those at greatest risk, i.e. those with a family history of allergy.

Asthma

Maternal asthma is a risk factor for preterm and post-term births and increases the risk of some pregnancy complications such as pre-eclampsia (Stenius-Aarniala *et al.*, 1988; Schatz, 1999b). Although about 1–4 per cent of pregnant women have asthma, it is often underdiagnosed (as in the rest of the population) and sub-optimally treated (Liccardi *et al.*, 1998). The course of asthma during pregnancy varies; it improves, remains stable or worsens in similar proportions of women (Schatz, 1999a).

Undertreatment of pregnant asthmatics, which might be due to unfounded fears of adverse pharmacological effects on the developing fetus, remains a major problem. Three reasons have been given for the increasing complications associated with maternal asthma. These are hypoxia, other physiological consequences of poorly controlled asthma and medicines used for asthma treatment (Schatz, 1999b). Few studies support the hypothesis that better controlled asthma will improve the perinatal outcome. The risk of an asthma exacerbation is high immediately postpartum, but the severity of asthma usually returns to the preconception level after delivery and often follows a similar course during subsequent pregnancies. Changes in β (2)-adrenoceptor responsiveness and changes in airway inflammation induced by high levels of circulating progesterone have been proposed as possible explanations for the effects of pregnancy on asthma. Good control of asthma is essential for maternal and fetal well-being. Acute asthmatic attacks can result in dangerously low fetal oxygenation. Chronically poor control is associated with pregnancy-induced hypertension, pre-eclampsia and uterine haemorrhage, as well as greater rates of caesarean section, preterm delivery, intrauterine growth retardation, low birth-weight and congenital malformation. Women with well-controlled asthma during pregnancy, however, have outcomes as good as those in their non-asthmatic counterparts (Schatz et al., 1995).

Inhaled therapies remain the cornerstone of treatment. It is generally better than systemic treatment as it reduces the risk of systemic side effects and the likelihood of fetal penetration. Oral corticosteroids have been associated with risk of pre-eclampsia (Stenius-Aarniala et al., 1988; Schatz, 1997; Alexander et al., 1998). Whether this represents the severity of asthma or the effect of the drug is difficult to ascertain from the currently available data. Oral steroid in the first trimester is associated with increasing incidence of cleft lip and palate (Rodriguez-Pinilla and Martinez-Frias, 1998).

Cystic fibrosis and pregnancy

In women with cystic fibrosis there is higher risk of maternal illness and death during pregnancy, which is a consequence of deteriorating pulmonary function. Prematurity is a risk for infants of mothers with cystic fibrosis, contributing to a high rate of perinatal death. Attention to dietary intake and the prevention of malabsorption together with monitoring of the pulmonary function are important aspects of managing cystic fibrosis during pregnancy (Kent and Farquharson, 1993).

Systemic lupus erythematosus and pregnancy

Recurrent spontaneous abortion is a well-recognized complication of maternal systemic lupus erythematosus (SLE; Hayslett, 1982) and is associated with antiphospholipid antibodies. Antiphospholipid syndrome where there is no associated clinical illness is also associated with higher than normal pregnancy loss. In severe forms where there is renal involvement and high antiphospholipid antibodies, the fetal mortality is >25 per cent. Prematurity, pre-eclampsia and IUGR are also common features in lupus pregnancy especially with antiphospholipid antibodies (Lima et al., 1995). Remission and exacerbation can occur during pregnancy with frequent exacerbation during the postpartum period (Wechsler et al., 1999).

The main manifestations in the neonate are cardiac, dermatological, haemolytic anaemia and thrombocytopenia, i.e. neonatal lupus erythematosus (NLE), which is related to antibodies crossing the placenta at different stages of the pregnancy (Dorner et al., 2000). The major morbidity and mortality is from complete congenital heart block and this is due to maternal anti-Ro (an anticytoplasmic antibody) antibodies which cross the placenta and are deposited in the fetal heart, initiating immune inflammatory responses which cause fibrosis and calcification of the aterioventricular node and bundle of His (Wechsler et al.,

1999). Anti-Ro antibodies are found in 20 per cent of patients with SLE (Reichlin, 1998).

Conclusion

The delivery of a healthy normally formed infant is the culmination of complex nutritional and non-nutritional interactions occurring between the mother and fetus over a period of 40 weeks. The nature of the non-nutritional interaction is varied and for many interactions the underlying mechanism and the clinical consequence is uncertain.

References

Abrams B and Parker J (1998) Overweight and pregnancy complications. *Int. J. Obes.* **12**, 293–303.

ACOG (1995) Technical bulletin. Diabetes and pregnancy. Number 200 – December 1994 (replaces no. 92, May 1986). Committee on Technical Bulletins of the American College of Obstetricians and Gynecologists. *Int. J. Gynaecol. Obstet.* **48**(3), 331–339.

Agostoni C, Trojan S, Bellu R, Riva E and Giovannini M (1995). Neurodevelopmental quotient of healthy term infants at 4 months and feeding practice: the role of long-chain polyunsaturated fatty acids. *Pediatr. Res.* **38**, 262–266.

Alexander S, Dodds L and Armson BA (1998) Perinatal outcomes in women with asthma during pregnancy. *Obstet. Gynecol.* **92**, 435–440.

Arshad SH, Matthews S, Gant C and Hide DW (1992) Effect of allergy avoidance on development of allergic disorders in infancy. *Lancet* **339**, 1494–1497.

Artal R, Platt LD, Kammula RK, Strassner HT, Gratacos J and Golde SH (1982) Sympathoadrenal activity in infants of diabetic mothers. *Am. J. Obstet. Gynecol.* **142**, 436–439.

Atallah AN, Hofmeyr GJ and Duley L (2002) Calcium supplementation during pregnancy for preventing hypertensive disorders and related problems. *The Cochrane Library* Issue 3, updated software, Oxford.

Ben Letaifa D, Ben Hamada S, Salem N, Ben Jazia K, Slama A, Mansali L and Jegham H (2000) Maternal and perinatal morbidity and mortality associated with HELLP syndrome. *Ann. Franc. Anesthes. Reanimation* **19**, 712–718.

Berkowitz GS, Lapinski RH, Godbold JH, Dolgin SE and Holzman IR (1995) Maternal and neonatal risk factors for cryptorchidism. *Epidemiology* **6**, 127–131.

Bianco AT, Smilen SW, Davis Y, Lopez S, Lapinski R and Lockwood CJ (1998) Pregnancy outcome and weight gain recommendations for the morbidly obese woman. *Obstet. Gynecol.* **91**, 97–102.

Brost BC, Goldenberg RL, Mercer BM, Iams JD, Meis PJ, Moawad AH, Newman RB, Miodovnik M, Caritis SN, Thurnau GR, Bottoms SF, Das A and McNellis D (1997) The Preterm Prediction Study: association of cesarean delivery with increases in maternal weight and body mass index. *Am. J. Obstet. Gynecol.* **177**, 333–337; discussion 337–341.

Butte NF (2000) Carbohydrate and lipid metabolism in pregnancy: normal compared with gestational diabetes mellitus. *Am. J. Clin. Nutr.* **71**, 1256S–1261S.

Calandra C, Abell DA and Beischer NA (1981) Maternal obesity in pregnancy. *Obstet. Gynecol.* **57**, 8–12.

Candy D, Davies G and Ross E (2001) *Clinical Paediatrics and Child Health*, 1st edn, p. 10. WB Saunders, Philadelphia, PA.

Cant AJ, Bailes JA, Marsden RA, Hewitt D (1986) Effect of maternal dietary exclusion on breast fed infants with eczema: two controlled studies. *Br. Med. J.* **293**, 231–233.

Carlson SE, Werkman SH *et al.* (1993) Visual acuity development in healthy preterm infants: effect of marine-oil supplementation. *Am. J. Clin. Nutr.* **58**, 35–42.

Carlson SE, Ford AJ, Werkman SH, Peeples JM and Koo WW (1996) Visual-acuity development in healthy preterm infants: effect of marine-oil supplementation. *Pediatr. Res.* **39**, 882–888.

Castles A, Adams EK, Melvin CL, Kelsch C and Boulton ML (1999) Effects of smoking during pregnancy. Five meta-analyses. *Am. J. Prev. Med.* **16**, 208–215.

Cayol V, Corcos M, Clervoy P and Speranza M (2000) Pregnancy and drug abuse: current situation and therapeutic strategies. *Ann. Med. Interne* (*Paris*), **151** (Suppl B), B20–26.

Chandra RK (1997) Food hypersensitivity and allergic disease: a selective review. *Am. J. Clin. Nutr.* **66**, 526–529.

Christian MS and Brent RL (2001) Teratogen update: evaluation of the reproductive and developmental risks of caffeine. *Teratology* **64**, 51–78.

Chung KC, Kowalski CP, Kim HM and Buchman SR (2000) Maternal cigarette smoking during pregnancy and the risk of having a child with cleft lip/palate. *Plast. Reconstruct. Surg.* **105**, 485–491.

Cnattingius S and Haglund B (1997) Decreasing smoking prevalence during pregnancy in Sweden: the effect on small-for-gestational-age births. *Am. J. Public Health* **87**, 410–413.

Cnattingius S, Bergstrom R, Lipworth L and Kramer MS (1998) Pre pregnancy weight and the risk of adverse pregnancy outcomes. *New Engl. J. Med.* **338**, 147–152.

Cnattingius S, Signorello LB, Anneren G, Clausson B, Ekbom A, Ljunger E, Blot WJ, McLaughlin JK, Petersson G, Rane A and Granath F (2000) Caffeine intake and the risk of first-trimester spontaneous abortion. *New Engl. J. Med.* **343**, 1839–1845.

Conter V, Cortinovis I, Rogari P and Riva L (1995) Weight growth in infants born to mothers who smoked during pregnancy. *Br. Med. J.* **310**, 768–771.

Cousins L (1987) Pregnancy complications among diabetic women: review 1965–1985. *Obstet. Gynecol. Surv.* **42**, 140–149.

Crawford M (2000) Placental delivery of archidonic and decosahexinoic acids: implications for the lipid nutrition of the preterm infant. *Am. J. Clin. Nutr.* **71**, 275S–284S.

Crowther C (1985) Eclampsia at Harare Maternity Hospital. An epidemiological study. *S. Afr. Med. J.* **68**, 927–929.

Cuervo LG and Mahomed K (2001) Treatments for iron deficiency anaemia in pregnancy. *Cochrane Database Systematic Review* **2**.

Cuk D, Mamula O and Frkovic A (2000) The effect of maternal smoking on pregnancy outcome. *Lijecnicki Vjesnik* **122**, 103–110.

Cunningham FG, MacDonald P, Gant NF, Leveno KJ and Gilstrap LC (1997) *Williams Obstetrics*, 20th edn. Prentice-Hall, London.

Curtis KM, Savitz DA and Arbuckle TE (1997) Effects of cigarette smoking, caffeine consumption, and alcohol intake on fecundability. *Am. J. Epidemiol.* **146**, 32–41.

Department of Health (1994) *Health Survey for England*. Available from: www.doh.gov.uk/public/sum94.htm#

de Sanjose S and Roman E (1991) Low birthweight, preterm, and small for gestational age babies in Scotland. *J. Epidemiol. Community Health* **45**, 207–210.

Dickerson JWT (1988) The interrelationship of nutrition and drugs. In: *Nutrition in the Management of Diseases*, 2nd edn, ed. Dickerson JWT and Lee H, pp. 392–421. Arnold, London.

Dodds L (1995) Prevalence of smoking among pregnant women in Nova Scotia from 1988 to 1992. *Can. Med. Assoc. J.* **152**, 185–190.

Dorner T and Feist E (2000) Significance of auto antibodies in neonatal lupus erythematosus. *Int. Arch. Allergy Immunol.* **123**(1), 58–66.

Douglas KA and Redman CW (1994) Eclampsia in the United Kingdom. *Br. Med. J.* **309**, 1395–1400.

Duley L (1992) Maternal mortality associated with hypertensive disorders of pregnancy in Africa, Asia, Latin America and the Caribbean. *Br. J. Obstet. Gynaecol.* **99**, 547–553.

Duley L, Gulmezoglu AM and Henderson-Smart DJ (2000) Anticonvulsants for women with pre-eclampsia. *The Cochrane Library*, Issue 2, updated software, Oxford.

Edwards LE, Dickes WF, Alton IR and Hakanson EY (1978) Pregnancy in the massively obese: course, outcome, and obesity prognosis of the infant. *Am. J. Obst. Gynecol.* **131**, 479–483.

Edwards LE, Hellerstedt WL, Alton IR, Story M and Himes JH (1996) Pregnancy complications and birth outcomes in obese and normal-weight women: effects of gestational weight change. *Obstet Gynecol.* **87**, 389–394.

Eskenazi B, Stapleton AL, Kharrazi M and Chee WY (1999) Associations between maternal decaffeinated and caffeinated coffee consumption and fetal growth and gestational duration. *Epidemiology* **10**, 242–249.

Fabris C, Prandi G, Perathoner C and Soldi A (1998) Neonatal drug addiction. *Panminerva Med.* **40**, 239–243.

Fernandes O, Sabharwal M, Smiley T, Pastuszak A, Koren G and Einarson T (1998) Moderate to heavy caffeine consumption during pregnancy and relationship to spontaneous abortion and abnormal fetal growth: a meta-analysis. *Reprod. Toxicol.* **12**, 435–444.

Fielding JE (1978) Smoking and pregnancy. *New Engl. J. Med.* **298**, 337–339.

Fulton M, Thomson M, Elton RA, Brown S, Wood DA and Oliver MF (1998) Cigarette smoking, social class and nutrient intake: relevance to coronary heart disease. *Eur. J. Clin. Nutr.* **42**, 797–803.

Galtier-Dereure F, Montpeyroux F, Boulot P, Bringer J and Jaffiol C (1995) Weight excess before pregnancy: complications and cost. *Int. J. Obes. Relat. Metab. Disord.* **19**, 443–448.

Galtier-Dereure F, Boegner C and Bringer J (2000) Obesity and pregnancy: complications and cost. *Am. J. Clin. Nutr.* **71**, 1242S–1248S.

Garbaciak JA Jr, Richter M, Miller S and Barton JJ (1985) Maternal weight and pregnancy complications. *Am. J. Obstet. Gynecol.* **152**, 238–345.

Gorski PA (1998) Perinatal outcome and the social contract – interrelationships between health and humanity. *J. Perinatol.* **18**, 297–301.

Greene GW, Smiciklas-Wright H, Scholl TO and Karp RJ (1988) Postpartum weight change: how much of the weight gained in pregnancy will be lost after delivery? *Obstet. Gynecol.* **71**, 701–707.

Gross T, Sokol RJ and King KC (1980) Obesity in pregnancy: risks and outcome. *Obstet. Gynecol.* **56**, 446–450.

Gudmundsson S, Bjorgvinsdottir L, Molin J, Gunnarsson G and Marsal K (1997) Socio-economic status and perinatal outcome according to residence area in the city of Malmo. *Acta Obstet. Gynecol. Scand.* **76**, 318–323.

Hanson U and Persson B (1993) Outcome of pregnancies complicated by type 1 insulin-dependent diabetes in Sweden: acute pregnancy complications, neonatal mortality and morbidity. *Am. J. Perinatol.* **10**, 330–333.

Hay WW (1994) Placental transport of nutrients to the fetus. *Hormone Res.* **42**, 215–222.

Hayslett JP (1982) Effect of pregnancy in patients with SLE. *Am. J. Kidney Dis.* **2**, 223–228.

Hill RM, Craig JP, Chaney MD, Tennyson LM and McCulley LB (1977) Utilization of over-the-counter drugs during pregnancy. *Clin. Obstet. Gynecol.* **20**, 381–394.

Host A, Koletzko B and Dreborg S (1999) Dietary products used in infants for treatment and prevention of food allergy. *Arch. Dis. Child.* **81**, 80–84.

Hutchings DE (1982) Methadone and heroin during pregnancy: a review of behavioral effects in human and animal offspring. *Neurobehav. Toxicol. Teratol.* **4**, 429–434.

Jacobson JL, Jacobson SW and Sokol RJ (1994) Effects of prenatal exposure to alcohol, smoking, and illicit drugs on postpartum somatic growth. *Alcohol. Clin. Exp. Res.* **18**, 317–323.

Johnson SR, Kolberg BH, Varner MW and Railsback LD (1987) Maternal obesity and pregnancy. *Surg. Gynecol. Obstet.* **164**, 431–437.

Johnstone FD, Nasrat AA and Prescott RJ (1990) The effect of established and gestational diabetes on pregnancy outcome. *Br. J. Obstet. Gynaecol.* **97**, 1009–1015.

Joseph H, Stancliff S and Langrod J (2000) Methadone maintenance treatment (MMT): a review of historical and clinical issues. *Mount Sinai J. Med.* **67**, 347–364.

Kallen K (1999) Maternal smoking and congenital heart defects. *Eur. J. Epidemiol.* **15**, 731–737.

Keenan WJ, Light IJ and Sutherland JM (1972) Effects of exogenous epinephrine on glucose and insulin levels in infants of diabetic mothers. *Biol. Neonate* **21**, 44–53.

Keller RW Jr and Snyder-Keller A (2000) Prenatal cocaine exposure. *Ann. NY Acad. Sci.* **909**, 217–232.

Kent NE and Farquharson DF (1993) Cystic fibrosis in pregnancy *Can. Med. Assoc. J.* **149**, 809–813.

Kieser JA, Groeneveld HT and Da Silva PC (1997) Dental asymmetry, maternal obesity, and smoking. *Am. J. Phys. Anthropol.* **102**, 133–139.

Kjellman NIM and Nilsson L (1998) From food allergy and atopic dermatitis to respiratory allergy. *Pediatr. Allergy Immunol.* **9**(Suppl. 11), 13–17.

Koren G, Nulman I, Rovet J, Greenbaum R, Loebstein M and Einarson T (1998) Long-term neurodevelopmental risks in children exposed *in utero* to cocaine. *Ann. NY Acad. Sci.* **846**, 306–313.

Koukkou E, Watts GF and Lowy C (1996) Serum lipid, lipoprotein and apolipoprotein changes in gestational diabetes mellitus: a cross-sectional and prospective study. *J. Clin. Pathol.* **49**, 634–637.

Kuhl C (1991) Aetiology of gestational diabetes. *Baillière's Clin. Obstet. Gynaecol.* **5**, 279–292.

Labadarios D, Obuwa G, Lucas EG, Dickerson JWT and Parke DV (1978) The effects of chronic drug administration on hepatic enzyme induction and folate metabolism. *Br. J. Clin. Pharmacol.* **5**, 167–173.

Lemoine P, Harrousean H and Borteym JP (1968) Les enfants de parents alcooliques: anomalies observées: à propos de 127 cas. *Quest. Med.* **25**, 477–482.

Le Thai N, Lefebvre G, Stella V, Vauthier D, Sfoggia D, Goulon V and Darbois Y (1992) Pregnancy and obesity. A case control study of 140 cases. *J. Gynecol. Obstet. Biol. Reprod.* **21**, 563–567.

Liccardi G, D'Amato M and D'Amato G (1998) Asthma in pregnant patients: pathophysiology and management. *Monaldi Arch. Chest Dis.* **53**, 151–159.

Light IJ, Keenan WJ and Sutherland JM (1972) Maternal intravenous glucose administration as a cause of hypoglycemia in the infant of the diabetic mother. *Am. J. Obstet. Gynecol.* **113**, 345–350.

Lilja G, Dannaeus A, Foucard T, Graff LV, Johansson SG and Oman H (1989) Effects of maternal diet during late pregnancy and lactation on the development of atopic disease in infants up to 18 months of age – in vivo results. *Clin. Exp. Allergy* **19**, 473–479.

Lima F, Buchanan NM, Khamashta MA, Kerslake S and Hughes GR (1995) Obstetric outcome in systemic lupus erythematosus. *Sem. Arthrit. Rheumatol.* **25**, 184–192.

Lorente C, Cordier S, Goujard J, Ayme S, Bianchi F, Calzolari E, De Walle HE and Knill-Jones R (2000) Tobacco and alcohol use during pregnancy and risk of oral clefts. Occupational Exposure and Congenital Malformation Working Group. *Am. J. Public Health* **90**, 415–419.

Lovegrove JA, Hampton SM and Morgan JB (1994) The immunological and long term atopic outcome in infants born to women following a milk-free diet during late pregnancy and lactation: a pilot study. *Br. J. Nutr.* **71**, 223–238.

Lyons K (1997) *Smith's Recognizable Patterns of Human Malformations*, 5th edn, p. 557. WB Saunders, Philadelphia, PA.

Malone FD and D'Alton ME (1997) Drugs in pregnancy: anticonvulsants. *Sem. Perinatol.* **21**, 114–123.

Mancuso A, D'Anna R and Leonardi R (1991) Pregnancy in the obese patient. *Eur. J. Obstet. Gynecol. Reprod. Biol.* **39**, 83–86.

Marini A, Agosti M, Motta G and Mosca F (1996) Effects of a dietary and environmental prevention programme on the incidence of allergy symptoms in high atopic risk infants: three year follow-up. *Acta Paediatr.* **414**(Suppl.), 1–22.

Mathias R (1995) NIDA Survey, first national data on drug use during pregnancy. *Women and Drug Abuse* **10**, 1.

McArdle HJ and Ashworth CJ (1999) Micronutrients in fetal growth and development. *Br. Med. Bull.* **55**, 499–510.

McElvy SS, Miodovnik M, Rosenn B, Khoury JC, Siddiqi T, Dignan PS and Tsang RC (2000) A focused preconceptional and early pregnancy program in women with type 1 diabetes reduces perinatal mortality and malformation rates to general population levels. *J. Maternal–Fetal Med.* **9**, 14–20.

Metcalf DD (1995) Allergic gastrointestinal diseases. In: *Clinical Immunology: Principles and Practice.* ed. Rich RR, Fleisher TA, Schartz BD, Shearer WT, Strober W, pp. 966–975. Mosby Year Book, St Louis, MO.

Metzger BE, Phelps RL, Freinkel N and Navickas IA (1980) Effects of gestational diabetes on diurnal profiles of plasma glucose, lipids, and individual amino acids. *Diabetes Care* **3**, 402–409.

Mimouni F, Miodovnik M, Siddiqi TA, Butler JB, Holroyde J and Tsang RC (1986a) Neonatal polycythemia in infants of insulin-dependent diabetic mothers. *Obstet. Gynecol.* **68**, 370–372.

Mimouni F, Tsang RC, Hertzberg VS and Miodovnik M (1986b) Polycythemia, hypomagnesemia, and hypocalcemia in infants of diabetic mothers. *Am. J. Dis. Child.* **140**, 798–800.

Miodovnik M, Mimouni F, Tsang RC, Skillman C, Siddiqi TA, Butler JB and Holroyde J (1987) Management of the insulin-dependent diabetic during labor and delivery. Influences on neonatal outcome. *Am. J. Perinatol.* **4**, 106–114.

Mishra GD, Dobson AJ and Schofield MJ (2000) Cigarette smoking, menstrual symptoms and miscarriage among young women. *Aust. NZ J. Public Health* **24**, 413–420.

Morris MB and Weinstein L (1981) Caffeine and the fetus: is trouble brewing? *Am. J. Obstet. Gynecol.* **140**, 607–610.

Morrison J, Najman JM, Williams GM, Keeping JD and Andersen MJ (1989) Socioeconomic status and pregnancy outcome. *Br. J. Obstet. Gynaecol.* **96**, 298–307.

Murphy-Brennan MG and Oei TP (1999) Is there evidence to show that fetal alcohol syndrome can be prevented? *J. Drug Educ.* **29**, 5–24.

Naeye RL (1990) Maternal body weight and pregnancy outcome. *Am. J. Clin. Nutr.* **52**, 273–279.

Nau H (1994) Valproic acid-induced neural tube defects. *Ciba Found. Symp.* **181**, 144–152.

Nau H, Hauck RS and Ehlers K (1991) Valproic acid-induced neural tube defects in mouse and human: aspects of chirality, alternative drug development, pharmacokinetics and possible mechanisms. *Pharmacol. Toxicol.* **69**, 310–321.

Nulman I, Laslo D and Koren G (1999) Treatment of epilepsy in pregnancy. *Drugs* **57**, 535–544.

Odendaal HJ, van Schie DL and de Jeu RM (2001) Adverse effects of maternal cigarette smoking on preterm labor and abruptio placentae. *Int. J. Gynaecol. Obstet.* **74**, 287–288.

Okun N, Verma A, Mitchell BF and Flowerdew G (1997) Relative importance of maternal constitutional factors and glucose intolerance of pregnancy in the development of newborn macrosomia. *J. Maternal–Fetal Med.* **6**, 285–290.

Olney JW, Ishimaru MJ, Bittigau P and Ikonomidou C (2000) Ethanol-induced apoptotic neurodegeneration in the developing brain. *Apoptosis* **5**, 515–521.

Peevy KJ, Landaw SA and Gross SJ (1980) Hyperbilirubinemia in infants of diabetic mothers. *Pediatrics* **66**, 417–419.

Perlow JH and Morgan MA (1994) Massive maternal obesity and perioperative cesarean morbidity. *Am. J. Obstet. Gynecol.* **170**, 560–565.

Perlow JH, Morgan MA, Montgomery D, Towers CV and Porto M (1992) Perinatal outcome in pregnancy complicated by massive obesity. *Am. J. Obstet. Gynecol.* **167**, 958–962.

Plessinger MA (1998) Prenatal exposure to amphetamines. Risks and adverse outcomes in pregnancy. *Obstet. Gynecol. Clin. N. Am.* **25**, 119–138.

Pollack H, Lantz PM and Frohna JG (2000) Maternal smoking and adverse birth outcomes among singletons and twins. *Am. J. Public Health* **90**, 395–400.

Rasmussen KL, Krue S, Johansson LE, Knudsen HJ and Agger AO (1997) Obesity as a predictor of postpartum urinary symptoms. *Acta Obstet. Gynecol. Scand.* **76**, 359–362.

Reichlin M (1998) Antibodies to Ro and La. *Ann. Med. Interne* (*Paris*) **149**, 34–41.

Roberton NR (1999) Infant of diabetic mother. In: *Textbook of Neonatology*, ed. Rennie JM, pp. 138–140. Churchill Livingstone, London.

Rodriguez-Pinilla E and Martinez-Frias ML (1998) Corticosteroids during pregnancy and oral clefts: a case-control study. *Teratology* **58**, 2–5.

Roebuck TM, Mattson SN and Riley EP (1998) A review of the neuroanatomical findings in children with fetal alcohol syndrome or prenatal exposure to alcohol. *Alcohol. Clin. Exp. Res.* **22**, 339–344.

Samartin S, Marcos A and Chandra RK (2001) Food hypersensitivity. *Nutr. Res.* **21**, 473–497.

Sampson HA (1997) Food Allergy. *JAMA* **278**, 1888–1894.

Schatz M (1997) Asthma treatment during pregnancy. What can be safely taken? *Drug Safety* **16**, 342–350.

Schatz M (1999a) Asthma and pregnancy. *Lancet* **353**, 1202–1204.

Schatz M (1999b) Asthma and pregnancy: background, recommendations, and issues. Introduction to the workshop. *J. Allergy Clin. Immunol.* **103**, S329.

Schatz M, Zeiger RS, Hoffman CP, Harden K, Forsythe A, Chilingar L, Saunders B, Porreco R, Sperling W, Kagnoff M *et al.* (1995) Perinatal outcomes in the pregnancies of asthmatic women: a prospective controlled analysis. *Am. J. Respir. Crit. Care Med.* **151**, 1170–1174.

Scholl TO and Reilly T (2000) Anemia, iron and pregnancy outcome. *J. Nutr.* **130**, 443S–447S.

Sexton M, Fox NL and Hebel JR (1990) Prenatal exposure to tobacco: II. Effects on cognitive functioning at age three. *Int. J. Epidemiol.* **19**, 72–77.

Shaw GM, Velie EM and Wasserman CR (1997) Risk for neural tube defect-affected pregnancies among women of Mexican descent and white women in California. *Am. J. Public Health* **87**, 1467–1471.

Sifakis S and Pharmakides G. (2000) Anemia in pregnancy. *Ann. NY Acad. Sci.* **900**, 125–136.

Sigurs N, Hattevig G and Kjellman B (1992) Maternal avoidance, cow's milk and fish during lactation: effect on allergic manifestations, skin prick tests and specific IgE antibodies in children at age 4 years. *Pediatrics* **89**, 735–739.

Spellacy WN, Miller S, Winegar A and Peterson PQ (1985) Macrosomia – maternal characteristics and infant complications. *Obstet. Gynecol.* **66**, 158–161.

Spiller MA (1984) The coffee plant and its processing. *Prog. Clin. Biol. Res.* **158**, 75–89.

Stamp TCB, Flanagan RJ, Richens A, Round JM, Thomas M, Jackson M, Dupre P and Twigg CA (1978) Anticonvulsant osteomalacia. In: *Endocrinology of Calcium Metabolism*, International Congress Series no. 421, ed. Copp DH and Talmage RV, pp. 16–22. Exepta Medica, Amsterdam.

Stenius-Aarniala B, Piirila P and Teramo K (1988) Asthma and pregnancy: a prospective study of 198 pregnancies. *Thorax* **43**, 12–18.

Stern L, Ramos A and Leduc J (1968) Urinary catecholamine excretion in infants of diabetic mothers. *Pediatrics* **42**, 598–605.

Streissguth AP, Barr HM and Sampson PD (1990) Moderate prenatal alcohol exposure: effects on child IQ and learning problems at age 7½ years. *Alcohol. Clin. Exp. Res.* **14**, 662–669.

Tappin DM, Ford RP and Schluter PJ (1997) Smoking during pregnancy measured by population cotinine testing. *NZ Med. J.* **110**, 311–314.

To WW and Tang MH (1999) The association between maternal smoking and fetal hydrancephaly. *J. Obstet. Gynaecol. Res.* **25**, 39–42.

Tomoda S, Tamura T, Sudo Y and Ogita S (1996) Effects of obesity on pregnant women: maternal hemodynamic change. *Am. J. Perinatol.* **13**, 73–78.

Tsang RC, Kleinman LI, Sutherland JM and Light IJ (1972) Hypocalcemia in infants of diabetic mothers. Studies in calcium, phosphorus, and magnesium metabolism and parathormone responsiveness. *J. Pediat.* **80**, 384–395.

Vigil-de Gracia PE, Tenorio-Maranon FR, Cejudo-Carranza E, Helguera-Martinez A and Garcia-Caceres E (1996) Difference between preeclampsia, HELLP syndrome and eclampsia, maternal evaluation. *Ginecol. Obstet. Mexico* **64**, 377–382.

Waller DK, Mills JL, Simpson JL, Cunningham GC, Conley MR, Lassman MR and Rhoads GG (1994) Are obese women at higher risk for producing malformed offspring? *Am. J. Obstet. Gynecol.* **170**, 541–548.

Warner JO, Jones CA, Kilburn SA (2000) Pre-natal sensitisation in humans. *Pediatr. Allergy Immunol.* **13**(Suppl.), 6–8.

Watkins ML, Scanlon KS, Mulinare J and Khoury MJ (1996) Is maternal obesity a risk factor for anencephaly and spina bifida? *Epidemiology* **7**, 507–512.

Wechsler B, Le Thi Huong D and Piette JC (1999) Pregnancy and systemic lupus crythcmatosus. *Ann. Med. Interne (Paris)*, **150**, 408–418.

West JR, Perrotta DM and Erickson CK (1998) Fetal alcohol syndrome: a review for Texas physicians. *Texas Med.* **94**, 61–67.

Whitelaw AG (1976) Influence of maternal obesity on subcutaneous fat in the newborn. *Br. Med. J.* **1**, 985–986.

Widness JA, Susa JB, Garcia JF, Singer DB, Sehgal P, Oh W, Schwartz R and Schwartz HC Increased erythropoiesis and elevated erythropoietin in infants born to diabetic mothers and in hyper-insulinemic rhesus fetuses. *J. Clin. Invest.* **67**, 637–642.

Willatts P, Forsyth JS, DiModugno MK, Varma S and Colvin M (1998) Effect of long-chain polyunsaturated fatty acids in infant formula on problem solving at 10 months of age. *Lancet* **352**, 688–691.

Wilson AC, Stewart Forsyth J, Greene SA, Irvine L, Hau C and Howie P (1998) Relation of infant diet to childhood health: seven year follow up of a cohort of children in Dundee infant feeding study. *Br. J. Med.* **316**, 21–25.

Yip R (2000) Significance of an abnormally low or high hemoglobin concentration during pregnancy: special consideration of iron nutrition. *Am. J. Clin. Nutr.* **72**, 272S–279S.

Zeiger RS and Heller S (1995) The development and prediction of atopy in high-risk children: follow-up at age seven years in a prospective randomised study of combined maternal and infant food allergen avoidance. *J. Allergy Clin. Immunol.* **95**, 1179–1190.

Zhang LM and Ding H (1994) Analysis of national maternal death surveillance: 1989–1991. *Zhonghua Fu Chan Ke Za Zhi* **29**, 514–517, 572.

6

THE FETUS AT BIRTH: MATERNAL AND FETAL PREPARATIONS FOR POSTNATAL DEVELOPMENT

Mary McNabb

LEARNING OUTCOMES

- Identify changes in the pattern of secretion and physiological functions of insulin and glucagon during fetal and neonatal development.

- Consider the nutritional implications of developmental changes in pancreatic β-cells during fetal and neonatal phases of development.

- Consider the neonatal significance of changes in maternal metabolism from late pregnancy to birth.

- Consider the changing metabolic effects of maternal oxytocin during labour and lactation.

Introduction

To understand the influences of maternal metabolic adaptations on the transition from fetal to neonatal metabolism, it is necessary to examine the changes in gastro-intestinal and metabolic functions during pregnancy and labour, in relation to nutritional and hormonal regulation of fetal growth. This involves the maturation of pancreatic, hepatic and gastro-intestinal organs during the perinatal period and the transition from carbohydrate to lipid metabolism immediately after birth (Uvnas-Moberg, 1989; Girard *et al.*, 1992; Pegorier *et al.*, 1998; Kassem *et al.*, 2000).

The relationship between pancreatic β-cell development and adult diabetes has been explored by examining the effects of restricted growth during a critical or sensitive period in fetal or early neonatal life on long-term changes in a number of regulatory systems, including sympathoadrenal and glucocorticoid activity, leading to glucose intolerance and cardiovascular disease in adult life. While considerable empirical evidence has accumulated in support of this paradigm, the molecular mechanisms affecting developmental changes in β-cell activity during fetal and neonatal life have not been conclusively identified (Petry and Hales, 2000). A research model on rats has focused on the effects of introducing a high-carbohydrate milk formula during the period of suckling on diabetes and obesity in later life (Aalinkeel *et al.*, 1999). This nutritional modification induces profound alterations in pancreatic function with the immediate onset of hyperinsulinaemia which persists into adulthood. The findings suggest that disruption of the early neonatal phase of pancreatic development with a low-fat, high-carbohydrate milk formula stimulates hyperinsulinaemia in the neonate and thus impairs insulin sensitivity and glucose tolerance, leading to obesity in later life (Aalinkeel *et al.*, 1999). Material in Chapters 1, 3, 4 and 7 should be read in relation to this chapter.

Transition from Fetal to Neonatal Metabolism

In small and large for gestation human neonates, a negative correlation has been found between the volume of formula milk supplementation of breast-feeds and peak blood ketone body concentrations, around 48 h following birth (De Rooy and Hawdon,

2000). If confirmed, this result is very significant, given the peculiar dependence of neonatal metabolism on the oxidation of fatty acids and ketogenesis (Persson, 1974; Cunnane *et al.*, 1999; Van der Lee *et al.*, 2000). Throughout the suckling period, ketone bodies are generated in the liver and small intestine, mainly from dietary lipids. In rats, the total ketone body concentration in blood is six times higher than in adult fed rats and the concentration of free fatty acids (FFAs) is three to four times higher (Page *et al.*, 1971). Ketone bodies provide the main circulating energy fuels for the brain, heart and peripheral tissues and precursors for essential myelination of the neonatal brain, which continues linear growth following birth (Van der Lee *et al.*, 2000).

The high capacity for fatty acid oxidation and ketogenesis that characterizes the period of suckling has opposing effects on the insulin–glucagon molar ratio (Menuelle and Plas, 1991). In humans, monkeys and sheep, plasma concentrations of glucagon at term are similar to maternal plasma values (Milner *et al.*, 1973). Following vaginal birth, glucagon undergoes a 3-fold increase to peak between 0 and 2 h postpartum and values remain significantly greater than at birth throughout the period of suckling (Luyck *et al.*, 1972; Girard *et al.*, 1992). Recent animal experiments suggest that in the presence of low concentrations of insulin, glucagon and long-chain fatty acids (LCFAs) have a key role in regulating the enzymes involved in lypolysis, glycogenolysis, gluconeogenesis and ketogenesis, throughout the suckling period (Pegorier *et al.*, 1998).

In contrast to glucagon, basal and stimulated insulin secretion appears to decline immediately following birth in a variety of species, including humans. In rats, insulin secretion remains low throughout the period of suckling (Sperling, 1994; Aalinkeel *et al.*, 1999). At the same time, hepatic responsiveness to insulin is reduced and glucose-stimulated insulin secretion remains low (Tozzo *et al.*,

1995; Aalinkeel *et al.*, 1999). Lipid oxidation does not seem to augment insulin secretion and administration of insulin to suckling rats decreases blood ketone body concentration through a direct anti-ketogenic effect on the liver (Yeh and Zee, 1976).

This developmental period of low insulin secretion coincides with significant structural modifications in the endocrine pancreas. In humans, this extends from the third trimester of pregnancy to the first 6 months postpartum (Kassem *et al.*, 2000). Within the Islets of Langerhans, β-cell proliferation steadily declines in the human fetus from 32 weeks gestation, while the frequency of apoptosis (cell death) peaks at birth and then declines over the next 2 months. By 6 months after birth, both proliferation and apoptosis have reached very low levels and β-cell distribution approaches that in adults (Kassem *et al.*, 2000).

Digestion and Metabolism in Human Pregnancy

Maternal digestion and absorption are enhanced during human pregnancy and lactation by decreased gastro-intestinal motility and enlargement of the duodenal villi. Transit time in the small intestine increases as pregnancy advances and there is enhanced absorption of a number of nutrients including glucose, lipids, amino acids, iron and calcium throughout pregnancy and lactation (Lawson *et al.*, 1985; Barrett *et al.*, 1994; Kovacs and Kronenberg, 1997; Kalhan, 2000). Many of these changes are regulated by rising levels of insulin, prolactin, growth hormone (GH) placental lactogen (PL), oestrogen, progesterone and an increased parasympathetic tone that characterizes both pregnancy and lactation (Uvnas-Moberg, 1989).

Increased glucose-induced insulin secretion in early pregnancy appears to stimulate maternal anabolism with increased accretion of nitrogen and fatty acids, while progesterone, prolactin and GH act centrally to increase maternal appetite (Fraser, 1991; Byatt *et al.*, 1993; Kalhan, 2000). At the same time, chorionic gonadotrophin, oestrogen and progesterone stimulate the adipose–brain hormone leptin, to reset hypothalamic control of energy balance in such a way as to stimulate an increase and subsequent decline in maternal adipose tissue stores with a characteristic distribution peculiar to pregnancy and lactation (Schubring *et al.*, 1998). In the periphery, progesterone reduces gastro-intestinal motility and may operate with cholecystokinin and somatostatin, to increase gastric emptying time and also with prolactin and PL, to enhance glucose-stimulated insulin secretion and fat deposition (Brelje *et al.*, 1993; Freemark *et al.*, 2001).

Maternal, placental and foetal metabolism

For mother and fetus, the latter half of pregnancy marks a very distinct period of metabolic transition. Maternal weight gain slows down, while that of the fetus accelerates. Fetal growth velocity increases between 18 and 34 weeks of gestation and then continues at a considerably slower rate towards term (Moore and Persaud, 1993). From 26 to 40 weeks of gestation, fetal weight increases more than 4-fold and, by term, fat accumulation accounts for over 90 per cent of energy consumed by the fetus (Feldman *et al.*, 1998). While overall fetal weight gain increases more slowly from around 34 weeks of gestation, the rate of fat accretion is approximately linear between 36 and 40 weeks, and the brain also exhibits a linear growth pattern during the last trimester and continues growing at a slower rate, until 18–24 months (Dobbing and Sands, 1973; Van Aerde *et al.*, 1998).

From around 35 weeks of pregnancy, the earlier maternal tendency to accumulate adipose tissue and retain nitrogen diminishes while nitrogen loss and branch-chained amino acid transamination is reduced to favour increased fetal nitrogen accretion. As a result of a reduction in the number of insulin receptors on adipocytes during late pregnancy and early lactation, lipogenesis declines and maternal lipid stores begin to fall, as enhanced adipose tissue lipolysis becomes a characteristic feature of both fed and fasted states (Herrera *et al.*, 1987). The altered pattern of fetal growth during the last trimester is accompanied by a rapid rise in the transplacental supply of glucose, amino acids, fatty acids and ketone bodies, increased deposition of glycogen in a number of organs, including the liver, skeletal muscle and subcutaneous adipose tissue, increased accretion of long- and short-chain fatty acids in adipose, hepatic and brain tissue, and a decline in the weight-specific consumption of glucose (Jones, 1976; Haggarty *et al.*, 1997).

Considerable demands are made on maternal energy during the second half of pregnancy because of the need to support the metabolic requirements of the accumulated increase in maternal, placental and fetal tissues (Butte *et al.*, 1999). In addition to meeting the increased glucose, amino and fatty acid requirements of the rapidly growing feto-placental unit, maternal fuels are also used to sustain daily glucose consumption of the enlarged maternal red cell mass and the glucose and fatty acid consumption of skeletal and uterine muscle, metabolically active mammary gland and the greatly expanded cardio-respiratory system (Butte *et al.*, 1999). Evidence from animal and human studies suggests that maternal, placental and fetal nutrient requirements during late pregnancy are met by increased and more frequent intakes of food and by significant metabolic modifications in both the fed and fasted states (Lopez-Luna *et al.*, 1994; Butte *et al.*, 1999).

Maternal glucose and lipid metabolism

In the second half of pregnancy, longitudinal glucose tolerance tests on women living in Westernized societies reveal a greater and more prolonged hyperglycaemia in the fed state compared with non-pregnant and early pregnant values. This metabolic shift is accompanied by a large increase in glucose-stimulated insulin secretion (Fraser, 1991). In relation to lipid metabolism, the latter half of pregnancy is characterized by increased intestinal absorption of triacylglycerol (TG) and hepatic esterification of FFAs, along with diminished rate of lipogenesis and enhanced mobilization of adipose tissue stores, which accelerates during lactation (Knopp *et al.*, 1981; Schubring *et al.*, 1998).

In the fasted state, plasma glucose concentrations decline progressively as pregnancy advances because of increased secretion of glucagon, and there is an accelerated activation of lipolysis significantly above that observed in the fed state (Knopp *et al.*, 1981; Daniel *et al.*, 1974; Herrera *et al.*, 1990; Fraser, 1991). Overall, less maternal glucose is converted to fatty acids, while more glycerol is converted to glucose and additional lipids are made available by increased absorption, hepatic synthesis and adipose tissue lipolysis. In both fed and fasted states, the second half of pregnancy is characterized by a physiological hyperlipidaemia and in humans this reflects maternal fatty acid intake, before and during pregnancy (Herrera *et al.*, 1988; Dutta-Roy, 1997).

The increased glucose and lipids that become available as a result of these changes are utilized through specific alterations in the metabolic capacities of the liver, placenta and mammary gland in both fed and fasted states. During the second half of pregnancy, the placenta progressively increases uptake of glucose and fatty acids, while the mammary gland and liver demonstrate a complementary pattern of increased uptake of fatty acids during both fed and fasted states (Lopez-Luna *et al.*, 1994).

Placental metabolism of glucose

Current evidence suggests that the increased placental and fetal requirements for glucose during the second half of pregnancy are met by a rise in overall placental transport capacity and an increase in transplacental glucose concentration gradient which is thought to be due to a greater fall in fetal relative to maternal plasma glucose concentrations (Hay, 1995). Serial studies on human infants have found that the maternal–fetal concentration gradient increases from mid-gestation to term (Bozzetti *et al.*, 1988). This seems to result from increased glucose clearance, secondary to increased fetal insulin secretion and insulin sensitivity, because of an increased number of receptors, particularly in the rapidly growing mass of adipose and muscle tissues (Kaplan, 1981; Hill and Milner, 1985).

Placental metabolism of lipids

During the latter half of pregnancy, the placenta has a growing capacity to remove TG from the maternal circulation and selectively removes particular groups of essential fatty acids, through its unique population of plasma membrane fatty acid binding proteins (Dutta-Roy, 1997). Results from studies on rats suggest that the removal of TG is due to the increased expression of lipoprotein lipase, which hydrolyses the TG component of circulating lipoproteins, to provide FFAs and glycerol for placental uptake and regulated transfer to the fetus (Herrera *et al.*, 1988). Research on placental delivery of essential fatty acids (EFAs) suggests that a number of hormonal mechanisms are involved in a complicated process that selectively provides docosahexaenoic acid (*n*-3) and arachidonic acid (*n*-6) for the distinct requirements of placental metabolism and central nervous system (CNS) development of the fetus during the third trimester (Dhutta-Roy, 1997; Cunnane *et al.*, 1999).

Interrelationship between the liver and mammary gland

The mammary gland and liver demonstrate a growing capacity to remove TG from the maternal circulation during the last trimester. Experimental evidence from rats has demonstrated increased hepatic expression of a fatty acid binding protein in late pregnancy and lipoprotein lipase activity has been found to increase rapidly in the mammary gland in the fed state during the last trimester. Further increases have also been found just prior to parturition (Ramirez *et al.*, 1983; Lopez-Luna *et al.*, 1994). This means that the diminished lipid accumulation and enhanced mobilization of adipose tissue stores that occur during the fed state are accompanied by enhanced lipid accumulation in the mammary gland which redirects high circulating levels of TG away from adipose tissue and into the gland for milk synthesis, in preparation for the next phase of lactation (Knopp *et al.*, 1981; Herrera *et al.*, 1988; Lopez-Luna *et al.*, 1994). Lipoprotein lipase activity in the mammary gland is stimulated by heightened insulin secretion and rising serum prolactin that particularly characterizes the latter part of pregnancy (Ramos and Herrera, 1996). Pregnancy-induced changes in plasma concentrations of prolactin and stimulated insulin secretion are shown in Figures 6.1 and 6.2. Under the influence of placental oestrogen, maternal serum prolactin begins to rise in the first trimester and increases progressively to 10 times the concentration of non-pregnant women at term.

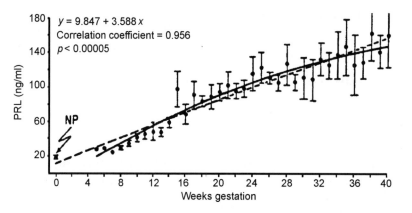

Figure 6.1   Mean ± SEM serum prolactin concentrations as a function of duration of pregnancy. [Reproduced from Rigg *et al.* (1977) *Am. J. Obstet. Gynecol.* **129**, 455 with permission of Mosby Inc.]

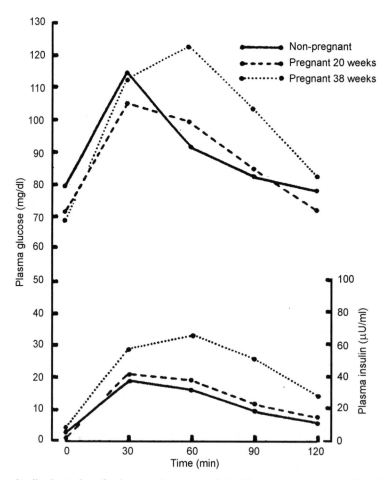

Figure 6.2   Longitudinal study of plasma glucose and insulin response to a 50 g load in 19 healthy primigravidae at 2 and 38 weeks of gestation and 10–12 weeks postpartum. [Reproduced from Fraser (1991) *Clinical Physiology in Obstetrics*, p. 206 by permission of Blackwell Science]

During the fasted state, most longitudinal studies in women show a progressive fall in plasma glucose that begins during the first trimester and reaches around 4 mmol/l during the last trimester (Fraser, 1991; Mills *et al.*, 1998). In rats, the simultaneous decline in glucose and insulin during the fasted state is accompanied by maximal stimulation of adipose tissue lipolysis and a fall in lipid uptake by the mammary gland (Lopez-Luna *et al.*, 1994). The rapid increase in circulating levels of non-esterified fatty acids (NEFA) in the fasted state in late pregnancy is thought to stimulate a slight, but significant, increase in plasma glucagon, which has also been noted in women and a rise in lipoprotein lipase activity in the liver (Daniel *et al.*, 1974; Lopez-Luna *et al.*, 1994). From being an exporter of a variety of lipoprotein fractions during the fed state, the liver becomes a temporary acceptor of TG and these are used as substrates for free fatty acid and ketone body synthesis, which then become available in preference to glucose as the metabolic fuel for a variety of maternal and fetal tissues (Daniel *et al.*, 1974; Herrera *et al.*, 1988; Lopez-Luna *et al.*, 1994).

Placental Transport of Ketones

The complete permeability of the human placenta to ketone bodies provides the fetus with additional substrates that may be used as energetic fuels and lipogenic substrates, during maternal fasting (Felig and Lynch, 1970). Concentrations of ketone bodies in the maternal circulation increase during the third trimester and reach similar levels in the fetal plasma (Sabata *et al.*, 1968; Persson, 1974; Herrera *et al.*, 1990). While the fetus has a very low capacity for ketogenesis, a number of tissues, notably the brain, heart, liver, kidneys and brown adipose tissue, express the enzymes required to utilize ketone bodies, and studies

on rats indicate that their activity increases during periods of maternal fasting or when the mother is fed a diet high in lipids (Dahlquist *et al.*, 1972; Herrera *et al.*, 1992). As a result of these changes in maternal metabolism in late pregnancy, the placenta receives and selectively transports increasing supplies of EFAs and ketones and maintains a fairly constant supply of glucose for the foetus across the fed–fasted state (Sangild, 1999).

Fetal Metabolism – Glycogenesis and Lipogenesis

From as early as the ninth week of gestation, glycogen is deposited in fetal tissues and increases significantly in placental and fetal tissues during the third trimester (Shelley and Bassett, 1975). While the largest store of glycogen is found in the liver, where it reaches two to three times the normal adult concentration after 24 weeks of gestation, smaller amounts of glycogen are also deposited in a number of tissues, including subcutaneous adipose tissue, skeletal and cardiac muscle, brain tissues, lungs and intestines (Shelley, 1961; Persson, 1974; Sperling, 1994). By term, the well-grown fetus has two-and-a-half times more glycogen in adipose tissue during the first 4 h of life than older infants; it has two to three times more glycogen in skeletal muscle and 10 times more in cardiac muscle, compared with the adult (Novak and Monkus, 1972).

Fat accretion in the human fetus is greater than in all other land-based mammals but, in contrast to many other species, brown fat makes up only 3–6 per cent of total adipose tissue in humans (Battaglia, 1978; Marcus *et al.*, 1988). Between 26 and 30 weeks of gestation, non-fat and fat energy contribute equally to the energy content of the fetus. Beyond that point, fat accumulation far exceeds the non-fat components and by term fat deposition accounts for more than 90 per cent of energy accumulated (Van Aerde *et al.*, 1998). The main lipogenic substrates are maternally derived glucose and fatty acids. The fetus displays an increasing capacity for lipid synthesis from glucose with advancing gestation and converts approximately 70 per cent of glucose uptake to fat (Persson, 1974; Van Aerde *et al.*, 1998).

Studies on rats indicate that the increasing fetal capacity for glycogenesis and lipogenesis seems to be largely regulated by rising levels of insulin, prolactin, hPL and cortisol in the fetal circulation (Freemark, 1999b). As well as the increased expression of insulin receptors, prolactin receptors increase in a variety of organs, including the liver, pancreas and adipose tissue, and have been shown to function as high-affinity binding proteins for hPL, prolactin and growth hormone in a variety of organ systems (Freemark, 1999a; Fleenor *et al.*, 2000). Insulin stimulates hepatic lipogenesis, while insulin and cortisol induce the expression of enzymes required for glycogenesis (Freemark, 1999a). PL and insulin stimulate placental glycogenesis, and prolactin and PL have a direct lipogenic effect on adipose cells (Freemark, 1999b).

Feto-placental Regulation of Metabolism

The fetus is essentially a parenterally nourished organism receiving a fairly constant supply of simple nutrients from the maternal circulation across the feto-placental barrier. During this period of enhanced anabolic metabolism, the maternal circulation selectively provides large amounts of glucose and amino acids and relatively small amounts of non-essential fatty acids (Girard *et al.*, 1992). While suckling and swallowing reflexes are present during the third trimester, the intake of luminal nutrients from amniotic fluid remains very small compared with that transferred across the placenta. Consequently, the enzymatic, hormonal and physiological capacities of the fetal gut and exocrine pancreas remain relatively under-developed and significant maturational changes occur in both organs during birth and the period of suckling (Bird *et al.*, 1996; Sangild, 1999; Zangen *et al.*, 2001). In addition, there is no requirement for endocrine pancreatic cells to regulate pre- and post-feeding cycles, as the feto-placental unit organizes maternal metabolism to supply glucose, amino acids and EFAs across the fed–fasted cycle (Nolan and Proietto, 1994).

Developmental Changes in the Fetal Pancreas

Experiments on mice suggest that ectodermal and endodermal layers of the embryo give rise to the endocrine and exocrine pancreas (Portha, 1990). In a variety of species, including humans, pancreatic primordial cells evaginate from foregut endoderm in early fetal life and a developmental process of differentiation, proliferation, apoptosis and maturation occurs in exocrine and endocrine cells during fetal and neonatal development (Jaffe *et al.*, 1982; Sangild, 1999). The initial formation of the pancreatic diverticulum is followed by cell differentiation. In humans, this process commences at around 8 weeks of gestation, with rapid, interrelated differentiation of endocrine α-glucagon-secreting cells and exocrine acini cells, followed by the appearance of smaller numbers of insulin-producing β-cells, somatostatin-producing δ-cells and pancreatic polypeptide (PP)-producing cells (Clark and Grant, 1983; Portha, 1990). At this stage of development, some β-cells are found alongside α-cells and most endocrine cells are either dispersed in the exocrine parenchyma or situated in small buds originating from the epithelium of minute ducts (Sperling, 1994).

By term, endocrine cells predominate in the central portion of the distinct lobules that characterize pancreatic formation as only minimal acinar development occurs until the intake of luminal nutrients begins after birth (Jaffe *et al.*, 1982). In humans, synthesis of proteases matures during fetal life while amylase and lipase secretion does not increase until the period of suckling (Lebenthal and Lee, 1980a). The exocrine pancreatic response to secretagogues (stimulators of secretion) is immature in term infants and this is thought to protect the immature microvillus membrane from proteolytic enzymes. It allows prolonged activity of essential brush border enzymes and prevents physiologically active non-nutritive milk proteins from being digested (Lebenthal and Lee, 1980b).

In contrast to the pancreas, evidence from pigs and humans suggests that, during the last 4–6 weeks of gestation, rapid growth and maturational changes begin to occur in the intestinal mucosa, in preparation for the shift from parenteral to enteral feeding (Lebenthal and Lee, 1980a; Menard *et al.*, 1999; Sangild, 1999). During human pregnancy, insulin stimulates intestinal growth and maturation before and during labour; fetal cortisol accelerates differentiation of gastric epithelial cells, stimulates gastrin and gastric acid secretion and regulates the processing of lipoproteins in the small intestine, which facilitates digestion and uptake of milk lipids from the mammary gland (Menard *et al.*, 1999).

Morphological development of pancreatic β-cells

In humans, insulin is present in the pancreas from 8–9 weeks gestation and increases 8–10-fold between 17 and 32 weeks of gestation

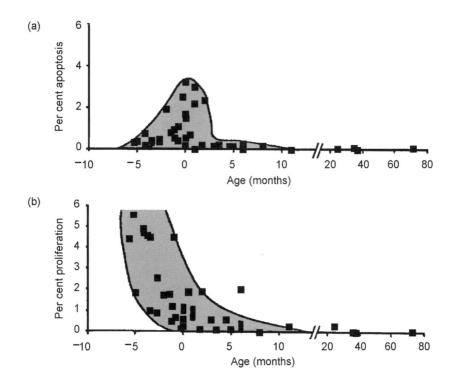

Figure 6.3 Percentage β-cell proliferation and apoptosis during fetal and neonatal life. [Adapted from Kassem *et al.* (2000) *Diabetes* **49**, 1329–1330. Copyright © 2000 American Diabetes Association. Reprinted with permission from the American Diabetes Association]

(Van Assche *et al.*, 1984). As illustrated in Figure 6.3 β-cell proliferation progressively declines from around 20 weeks to very low levels at 6 months postpartum, while apoptosis begins at a very low level around 20 weeks, peaks around the time of birth and declines over the first 6 months postpartum (Kassem *et al.*, 2000). During this process of developmental apoptosis, β-cell proliferation declines and the small poorly formed islets and dispersed cells that stain positive for insulin gradually give way to well-formed islets that characterize the adult gland, by around 6 months postpartum. These changes coincide with the suckling weaning transition and have a key role in regulating functional maturation of the glucoregulatory role of insulin secretion (Girard *et al.*, 1992; Kassem *et al.*, 2000).

The pattern of cell proliferation is shown to decline from around 5 per cent at 20 weeks gestation to very low levels from around 6 months following birth, while apoptosis rises from low levels at 20 weeks and peaks around the time of birth before declining to low levels around 6 months following birth (Figure 6.3).

During fetal life, proliferation of pancreatic β-cells is stimulated by glucose, amino acids, PL, prolactin, GH and insulin-like growth factors (IGF), and evidence from rats and humans suggests that this is particularly sensitive to poor maternal nutrition and low energy intake during pregnancy (Petry and Hales, 2000). In a variety of studies during fetal and neonatal life, physiological concentrations of glucose and amino acids stimulate β-cell growth and replication while *in vitro* experiments on human fetal pancreatic tissue have found that GH, IGFs, prolactin and PL induce β-cell growth and replication and promote the formation of islet-like cell clusters (Fleenor *et al.*, 2000). In cultured human pancreas at 12–21 weeks of gestation, hPL and GH stimulate a 50 per cent increase in insulin content and release in the presence of glucose (Freemark, 1999b). This evidence suggests that fetal β-cell growth and development is regulated by IGFs, lactogenic and somatogenic hormones coupled with the metabolism of glucose and amino acids (Fleenor *et al.*, 2000).

Insulin and Glucagon During Fetal and Early Neonatal Development

Evidence from a variety of studies suggests that insulin and glucagon have a number of unique developmental features that change significantly immediately following birth and again at weaning, when both hormones take on an adult pattern of secretion (Fowden, 1989; Girard *et al.*, 1992; Sperling, 1994; Aalinkeel *et al.*, 1999). In the human fetus, circulating insulin levels rise sharply in late pregnancy and insulin concentrations in the fetus at term are much higher than in the adult (Ktorza *et al.*, 1985). In addition, the number and/or affinity of insulin receptors in a variety of tissues is higher in the fetus and neonate than corresponding levels in the adult, and insulin receptors seem to be largely upregulated in response to hyperinsulinaemia, while those in the adult are down-regulated (Thorsson and Hintz, 1977; Kaplan, 1981; Ktorza *et al.*, 1985). This means that the anabolic effects of insulin on fetal glucose, amino acid and fatty acid metabolism are enhanced by raised insulin secretion which in turn is regulated by basal maternal insulin and glucose concentrations (Caruso *et al.*, 1998; Soltani-K *et al.*, 1999).

In adult life insulin is the major glucoregulatory hormone. Pulsatile β-cell secretion of insulin is stimulated primarily in response to raised plasma glucose and follows a well-characterized biphasic pattern, with cessation of secretion when blood glucose levels fall below 3 mmol/l. Glucose-stimulated insulin secretion affects homeostatic control by suppressing gluconeogenesis and proteolysis and accelerating peripheral utilization of glucose (Howell, 1991). A variety of experimental studies in humans and other animals have shown that, during late fetal and early neonatal development, critical components of this homeostatic system are absent or partially functional, while others are highly developed, compared with the adult (Lagercrantz and Slotkin, 1986; Cowett, 1988; Slotkin *et al.*, 1990; Widmaier, 1990).

Evidence from a variety of species including humans suggests that, during fetal and early neonatal development, glucose metabolism is not regulated by insulin and glucagon in the way that occurs in adults (Sperling, 1994). *In vitro* studies on fetal rats have shown that glucose-stimulated insulin secretion is present from mid-pregnancy onwards but to a much smaller extent than in adult β-cells (Aoyagi *et al.*, 1997; Bergsten *et al.*, 1998). Female rats made slightly or highly hyperglycaemic by a continuous glucose infusion during the last week of pregnancy have slightly hyperglycaemic fetuses that show marked hyperinsulinaemia, while highly hyperglycaemic fetuses show no change in insulin secretion compared with controls (Bihoreau *et al.*, 1986). In human studies at term, a maternal intravenous glucose load administered either before or during labour induces a marked rise in maternal glucose and serum insulin concentrations and a fall in FFA levels. However, despite a rapid rise in fetal glucose concentrations, fetal serum insulin levels show highly variable responses, including diminished, delayed and absent secretion (Coltart *et al.*, 1969; Tobin *et al.*, 1969).

In term and to a lesser extent in preterm human infants, a sustained, nearly complete suppression of glucose production occurs in response to an intravenous infusion of glucose at moderate levels of glycaemia and substantially lower insulin concentrations than in the adult (Denne *et al.*, 1995; Farrag *et al.*, 1997). At higher rates of intravenous insulin, glucose utilization rates far exceeded the maximal adult response, indicating enhanced peripheral insulin sensitivity, but proteolysis is not suppressed, although this response occurs in adults, when insulin is raised only slightly above basal concentrations (Denne *et al.*, 1995; Farrag *et al.*, 1997). Combined with findings on the morphological changes in pancreatic β-cells during fetal and neonatal development, the high number and affinity of insulin receptors in the newborn and the low level of glucose-stimulated insulin secretion during suckling, the evidence suggests that β-cell function undergoes developmental changes during the perinatal period and does not show evidence of mature regulatory responses until the infant receives a high carbohydrate–low fat diet at weaning (Girard *et al.*, 1992; Aalinkeel *et al.*, 1999).

Developmental characteristics of glucagon

During fetal and early neonatal life, glucagon does not seem to function as a physiological antagonist of insulin. This is in marked contrast to the adult, where glucagon has a key role in regulating glucose metabolism, by stimulating glycogenolysis, gluconeogenesis and ketogenesis, in response to hypoglycaemia (Devaskar *et al.*, 1984; Ktorza *et al.*, 1985). While glucagon is present in fetal plasma at concentrations similar to maternal values at term, in a variety of species, including humans, these high levels do not inhibit glycogen storage. In addition, glucagon secretion is not noticeably modified by acute changes in glucose, and hyperglycaemia, which suppresses glucagon in the adult, does not suppress fetal glucagon secreton in rats, lambs or monkeys (Ktorza *et al.*, 1985; Menuelle and Plas, 1991; Sperling, 1994).

In experimental studies on sheep, physiological doses of glucagon in late gestation produce no alteration or very modest increases in plasma glucose (Lawrence *et al.*, 1989). *In vitro* studies on the human fetal pancreas gave similar results (Schaeffer *et al.*, 1973; Sperling, 1994). At pharmacological doses in fetal sheep, glucagon stimulates an acute rise in circulating glucose but has no effect on hepatic fatty acid oxidation, as it does in the adult (Philipps *et al.*, 1983). In marked contrast to insulin, fetal glucagon receptors in a variety of species are fewer in number than in the adult and are poorly connected to the membrane receptor (Ktorza *et al.*, 1985). Taken together, these findings suggest that the fetal liver seems to have a physiological resistance to glucagon, which would allow the anabolic effects of insulin to remain unopposed during this phase of development (Sperling, 1994).

Following birth, a dramatic fall in insulin and an acute rise in glucagon reverses the high plasma insulin/glucagon molar ratio of fetal life, suggesting that the low plasma insulin/ glucagon molar ratio following birth has a key role in regulating the dramatic rise in fatty acid oxidation and ketogenesis that begins soon after birth (Pegorier *et al.*, 1998). While glucagon concentrations show a 3–5-fold increase from fetal levels soon after birth, in a variety of species, including humans, the regulation of secretion and the metabolic functions of glucagon are not the same as in the adult. In contrast to adults, the acute rise in glucagon following birth in rats does not seem to be regulated by neonatal glucose concentrations. Studies on suckling rats have found that, in direct contrast to the adult, glucagon levels rise during feeding and fall during fasting, and studies on lambs have found that admnistration of glucagon during experimentally induced hyperinsulinaemia results in a persistent decline in plasma glucose, without a significant change in endogenous glucose production (Beaudry *et al.*, 1977; Cowett *et al.*, 1999).

In all mammals, including humans, these hormonal changes mark the transition from internal to external gestation, when the mammary gland replaces the placenta and mammary secretions begin to supply neuro- hormonal and immunological regulators, trophic, appetite and digestive factors, and a high fat–low carbohydrate diet, specifically designed to meet the final phase of dependent growth and development, which ends at spontaneous weaning (Peaker, 1998; Lyle *et al.*, 2001). From late pregnancy onwards changes in maternal prolactin, GH and oxytocin are particularly involved in regulating maternal appetite and metabolism in preparation for suckling and lactation.

Hormonal Regulation of Maternal Nutrient Metabolism during Pregnancy and Labour

Recent findings from a number of species suggest that PL, prolactin and GH are selectively involved in regulating islet β-cell proliferation, insulin secretion, accumulation of adipose tissue stores, glucose intolerance, lipolysis and growth and uptake of nutrients in the mammary gland during pregnancy and lactation (Goodman *et al.*, 1991; Brelje *et al.*, 1993; Ramos *et al.*, 1999; Freemark *et al.*, 2001).

In direct contrast to prolactin, pituitary GH is markedly suppressed during pregnancy. During the first trimester, GH is detectable in plasma but is unresponsive to many physiological stimuli and declines progressively as pregnancy advances (Eriksson *et al.*, 1989). As illustrated in Figure 6.4(A), from 15 weeks to term, pituitary GH is gradually replaced by GH-V, a placental variant that becomes the major form of circulating GH in the maternal circulation (Frankenne *et al.*, 1988; Alsat *et al.*, 1997). GH-V differs from GH by 13 amino acid substitutions and has major sequence homology with PL and prolactin, evolving from a common precursor gene (Alsat *et al.*, 1997). Up to 20 weeks of gestation relaxinstimulated growth hormone from the pituitary is the main form present in the maternal circulation. From 15 to 20 weeks this is largely

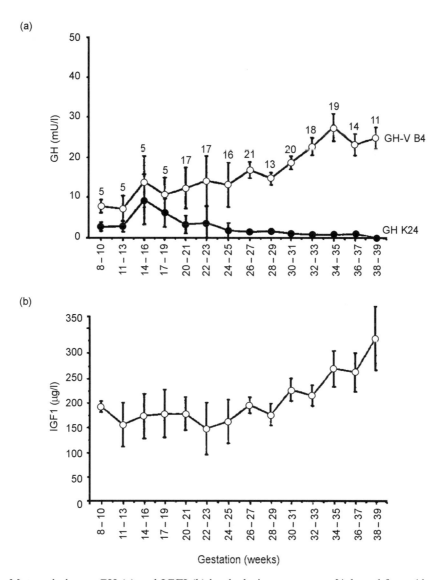

Figure 6.4   Maternal plasma GH (a) and IGFI (b) levels during pregnancy. [Adapted from Alsat *et al.* (1997) *Am. J. Obstet. Gynecol.* **177**, 1529 with permission]

replaced by GH-V, which is secreted only into the maternal circulation and appears to regulate maternal IGF1.

Because of these structural similarities, GH-V is thought to have similar influences on food intake, carbohydrate and lipid metabolism (Byatt *et al.*, 1993). *In vitro* evidence suggests that acute administration of GH and GH-V accelerates carbohydrate utilization, while

chronic administration decreases glucose uptake, stimulates insulin resistance and enhances lipolysis (Goodman *et al.*, 1991). Recent findings suggest that GH-V may play a key role in reorganizing maternal metabolism to sustain feto-placental growth and development during the latter half of pregnancy (Patel *et al.*, 1995; Zumkeller, 2000). In contrast to PL and prolactin, release of GH-V is stimulated by hypoglycaemia and exerts its metabolic effects alongside the progressive increase in fasting plasma glucagon during the third trimester (Daniel *et al.*, 1974). During the fasted state, both hormones inhibit maternal uptake of glucose and enhance adipose tissue lipolysis, generating FFAs and glycerol as alternative sources of fuel for maternal tissues and as a source of ketones and gluconeogenic precursors in the liver, to supply glucose and ketones for the fetus (Nolan and Proietto, 1994).

As happens in the non-pregnant state, an acute release of human prolactin occurs in synchrony with food ingestion throughout pregnancy in humans, and central prolactin is known to stimulate appetite in female rats in a dose-dependent manner (Quigley *et al.*, 1982; Noel and Woodside, 1993). Systemic and central infusions of prolactin stimulate increased food intake, fat deposition and weight gain in both rats and humans (McGarry and Beck 1962; Noel and Woodside, 1993). Chronic hyperprolactinaemia, as occurs in the second half of human pregnancy, stimulates islet β-cell proliferation, decreases the glucose stimulation threshold for insulin secretion, modulates lipid metabolism in the liver, and operates along with insulin to stimulate uptake of lipids by the mammary gland (Quigley *et al.*, 1982; Ramos and Herrera, 1996; Weinhaus *et al.*, 1996; Ramos *et al.*, 1999). Taken together, this evidence suggests that rising levels of prolactin during human pregnancy have a key role in regulating maternal appetite, insulin secretion and lipid metabolism in the liver, adipose tissue and mammary gland.

Current evidence suggests that the progressive rise in prolactin, GH-V and PL directly stimulates a gradual increase in the number and responsiveness of maternal pancreatic islet β-cells until the end of pregnancy, when the process is reversed by the combined effects of high concentrations of progesterone, oestrogen and glucocorticoids (Frankenne *et al.*, 1990; Philippe and Missotten, 1990; Lambillotte *et al.*, 1997). *In vitro* evidence suggests that

placental steroids, particularly progesterone, inhibit islet β-cell proliferation while glucocorticoids inhibit insulin release and stimulate apoptosis (Brelje *et al.*, 1993; Weinhaus *et al.*, 1996, 2000; Lambillotte *et al.*, 1997).

These changes allow a progressive rise in glucose-stimulated insulin secretion during pregnancy, followed by a sharp decline during late pregnancy and labour. Following the period of enhanced maternal anabolism and insulin sensitivity during the first half of pregnancy, chronically elevated levels of GH-V, oestrogen and glucocorticoids during the second half seem to induce mild glucose intolerance, increased insulin resistance and rising plasma concentrations of FFAs (Goodman *et al.*, 1991).

In vitro evidence suggests that the insulin-stimulating actions of prolactin and PL and the lipolytic actions of GH-V and glucocorticoids are counteracted during the latter stages of pregnancy by the more rapid rise in progesterone (Williams and Coultard, 1978; Weinhaus *et al.*, 2000). In human studies, circulating TG concentrations decline between 40 weeks of gestation and 2 weeks postpartum, and the degree of decline is predictably more pronounced in women who are lactating (Darmady and Postle, 1982). Experimental studies on rats suggest that, during late pregnancy and labour, insulin secretion falls and circulating TGs begin to decline (Martin-Hidalgo *et al.*, 1994). In rats, high maternal concentrations of TGs begin to decline during late pregnancy and labour, associated with a progressive rise in lipoprotein lipase activity in the mammary gland, which is thought to be induced by high circulating levels of prolactin and local increases in insulin (Flint *et al.*, 1979; Ramirez *et al.*, 1983; Ramos *et al.*, 1999).

Maternal oxytocin from pregnancy to lactation

In all mammals, including humans, oxytocin is recognized for its regulatory role of reproductive functions, including sexual activity, ovulation, uterine contractions, the initiation of maternal behaviour and lactation (Johnston and Amico, 1986; Fuchs *et al.*, 1991; Modney and Hatton, 1994). These and other regulatory activities are mediated by highly dynamic, central and peripheral systems, where oxytocin operates as an intranuclear peptide regulator and neurotransmitter, peripheral circulating hormone and local paracrine/autocrine factor within the uterus (Cunningham and Sawchenko, 1991; Neumann *et al.*, 1996; Jiang and Wakerley, 1995; Mitchell and Schmid, 2001).

Anatomical studies on rats have identified distinct groups of oxytocin-containing neurons in the cerebral diencephalon which forms the core of the forebrain. Situated beneath and between the cerebral hemispheres, the diencephalon is composed of the thalamus, hypothalamus and epithalamus. Oxytocin neurons that make up the neuroendocrine system have large (magnocellular) neurosecretory cells mainly grouped within the bilateral supraoptic (SON) and paraventricular (PVN) nuclei, while additional collections are found in smaller accessory groups in the medial and lateral hypothalamus. Each magnocellular neuron sends a single axon to the neurohypophysis which gives rise to 2000–10 000 neurosecretory endings packed with secretory granules, where oxytocin is stored prior to its release into the general circulation in response to a variety of stimuli, including vaginal stretching, uterine contractions, maternal–infant sensory contact and suckling (Johnston and Amico, 1986; Fuchs *et al.*, 1991; Leng and Brown, 1997; Mattheisen *et al.*, 2001). Afferent imputs to the magnocellular neurosecretory system have been demonstrated from a number of forebrain, brain stem and spinal regions, associated with a large number of autonomic reflexes and behavioural responses (Cunningham and Sawchenko, 1991). In addition to the magnocellular system, oxytocin has also been found in several other groups of small (parvocellular)

neurons, particularly in the PVN, and these send axons to a number of central locations, including the forebrain brain stem and spinal cord. Here they regulate a variety of autonomic reflexes and behavioural responses, including food ingestion, gastric activity, pain threshold and anxiety (Cunningham and Sawchenko, 1991; Uvnas-Moberg, 1998).

Indirect studies in women and direct experiments in rats suggest that, from mid-pregnancy until the end of lactation, oxytocinergic systems in the brain undergo a number of morphological and biochemical reorganizations under the stimulatory influence of placental steroids, uterine contractions and suckling that are reversed again at weaning (Johnston and Amico, 1986; Modney and Hatton, 1994; Jiang and Wakerley, 1995). Under the stimulatory influence of oestrogen, central and peripheral sensitivity to oxytocin is increased during pregnancy and labour by a parallel rise in oxytocin receptor mRNA in a number of brain regions and in the uterus. Increases in brain receptor mRNA levels have been demonstrated in rats during pregnancy and lactation, while in humans there is a > 300-fold increase in oxytocin receptor mRNA in the myometrium at term, compared with non-pregnant values, and these display a gradient expression with highest and lowest concentrations in the fundus and cervix, respectively (Kimura *et al.*, 1996).

Studies in rats during the latter half of pregnancy and labour have also found increases in oxytocin mRNA in the SON, PVN and in accessory cell groups in the forebrain and brain stem, indicating increased synthesis of the peptide (Luckman, 1995). In the rat, increased oxytocin synthesis outstrips secretion because of enhanced restraint at neurosecretory terminals. This allows the pituitary content of oxytocin to increase by around 50 per cent during pregnancy, in preparation for increased secretion during labour and lactation (Johnston and Amico, 1986; Leng and Brown, 1997). At mid-pregnancy in the rat, endogenous opioid restraint on oxytocin secretion is strong and in late pregnancy activated histaminergic neurons increase oxytocin synthesis while histaminergic and opioid neurons inhibit its premature release from the neurohypophysis (Leng and Brown, 1997; Luckman and Larsen, 1997).

During the last week or so of pregnancy, κ-opioid receptors in the neurohypophysis are down-regulated and desensitized while, close to term, the neural imputs that drive the activity of central oxytocin neurons are restrained by opioid neuronal circuits, within the SON and PVN (Leng and Brown, 1997). Alongside these modulating influences on oxytocin neurons, direct experiments on rats and indirect studies on women suggest that the peptide is simultaneously released from magnocellular dendrites in the SON and PVN during late pregnancy, labour and lactation, and this intranuclear release is not subject to endogenous opioid restraint (Neumann et al., 1996). While endogenous opioids have a negative feedback effect on the pulsatile activation of oxytocin neurons, intranuclear release of oxytocin seems to generate a synchronous bursting activity of oxytocin neurons (Jiang and Wakerley, 1995). Indirect evidence on women and direct experiments in rats suggest that the sensitivity of these neurons is low in late pregnancy, high during lactation and low again at weaning (Johnston and Amico, 1986; Fuchs et al., 1991; Jiang and Wakerley, 1995; Matthiesen et al., 2001).

The next section will examine how these changes in central and peripheral oxytocin systems during late pregnancy and labour influence maternal appetite and metabolism during labour in relation to the transition from fetal to neonatal metabolism immediately after birth.

Prolactin, GH-V and oxytocin – maternal appetite and metabolism in labour

Towards the end of pregnancy in the rat, oxytocin from the median eminence released into the anterior pituitary may indirectly increase maternal appetite, through its stimulatory action on prolactin (Noel and Woodside, 1993). In humans, indirect evidence suggests that the stimulatory effect of oxytocin on prolactin secretion may operate during the last week of pregnancy and the first 5 h of labour, when food appetite seems to increase (Crawford, 1956). Recent studies on rats suggest that oxytocin receptors on prolactin-releasing cells increase dramatically at the end of pregnancy, allowing oxytocin to exert its full potential as a prolactin releasing factor before and after birth, as the stimulus for prolactin secretion switches from placenta to mother and neonate (Brenton et al., 1995).

In early human labour GH-V levels decline followed by an equally sharp fall in prolactin around 2 h prior to birth (see Figure 6.5; Rigg and Yen, 1977; Mirlesse et al., 1993). This is followed by a dramatic surge during the first 2 h after birth, when sucking reflexes are activated. Taken together, these changes can be expected to dramatically enhance glucose tolerance and reduce insulin secretion as labour progresses. At the same time, continuing high levels of placental oestrogen, progesterone and adrenal cortisol during labour can be expected to maintain their combined inhibition of islet β-cell proliferation and insulin secretion (Golde et al., 1982; Jovanovic and Peterson, 1983; Lambillotte et al., 1997; Weinhaus et al., 2000).

The progressive decline in circulating lipids from the end of pregnancy seems to be initiated by the more rapid rise in progesterone relative to GH-V and glucocorticoids and by the increased uptake of fatty acids by the mammary gland in response to rising levels of insulin and prolactin (Flint et al., 1979; Ramos et al., 1999). From early labour, this trend is sustained by the sharp fall in GH-V coupled with the lipogenic actions of progesterone and the insulin-like actions of oxytocin on maternal adipose tissue (Rigg and Yen, 1977; Muchmore et al., 1981; Mirlesse et al.,

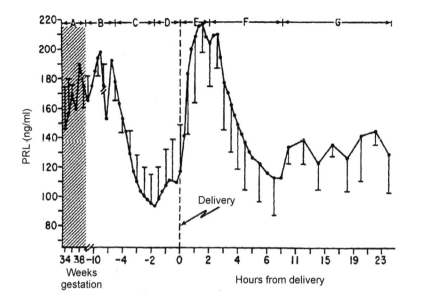

Figure 6.5 Plasma prolactin concentrations before, during and following birth (Reproduced from Rigg and Yen, 1977 with permission of Mosby Inc.)

1993; Martin-Hildago *et al.*, 1994). These combined hormonal changes can be expected to induce a further fall in circulating lipids and a decline in basal maternal glucose levels during active labour with a correspondingly greater fall in glucose concentrations in the fetus (Bozzetti *et al.*, 1988).

Oxytocin, food intake and gastro-intestinal function

As labour progresses, cervical stretching and myometrial contractions stimulate uterine afferent nerve pathways to the hypothalamus that stimulate both central and peripheral release of oxytocin (Antonijevic *et al.*, 1995). In a number of experimental studies on fasted rats, central administration of oxytocin inhibits food and salt ingestion in a dose-related manner (Verbalis *et al.*, 1995). In both fed and fasted states, similar treatment

reversibly suppresses oral intake of glucose in a dose-related manner (Lokrantz *et al.*, 1997).

Other experimental models have also demonstrated that central administration of oxytocin specifically decreases the stimulatory effects of a_2 adrenoreceptors on feeding rhythms across the diurnal cycle (Morien *et al.*, 1999; Diaz-Cabiale *et al.*, 2000). An infusion of oxytocin into the vagal complex in the medulla reduces intestinal mobility and stimulates the release of some gastro-intestinal and pancreatic hormones via cholinergic vagal efferent pathways, while central administration of oxytocin reduces gastric acid secretion (McCann and Rogers, 1990; Asad *et al.*, 2001). These findings suggest that, during periods of stimulation, as occur during labour and suckling, oxytocin operates via central and peripheral mechanisms to inhibit food intake and gastro-intestinal activity. On the basis of current findings on the activation of oxytocin during established labour, maternal food appetite can be expected to fall to non-existent levels as labour progresses.

Oxytocin, glucose homeostasis and adipose tissue metabolism

Current evidence from rats and humans suggests that the changing patterns of peripheral oxytocin release during labour and lactation have opposing effects on glucose homeostasis and adipose tissue metabolism (Muchmore et al., 1981; Widmaier et al., 1991; Eriksson et al., 1994). In women during labour, basal plasma concentrations of oxytocin remain at $\sim 0.17\,\mu U/ml$, while pulse amplitude increases moderately from 0.92 to $1.4\,\mu U/ml$ as labour progresses and pulse frequency increases from 1.2/30 min at term, to 6.7/30 min during the second and third stages of labour (Fuchs et al., 1991). Immediately after birth, opioid restraint on oxytocin neurons is removed. Basal levels of oxytocin rise significantly and sensory stimulation and suckling increase pulse frequency and amplitude of oxytocin release compared with

labour and birth (Mattheisen et al., 2001). As illustrated in Figures 6.6 and 6.7 basal concentrations of oxytocin increase in women immediately following birth and decline during the first 12 weeks of lactation, while suckling-induced concentrations increase progressively in exclusive breast-feeding women, as lactation continues (Johnston and Amico, 1986; Uvnas-Moberg et al., 1990).

Experiments on male rats suggest that doses of oxytocin introduced into the peripheral circulation similar to those found in labour have no significant regulatory influence on plasma glucose or glucagon, while elevated levels of oxytocin, as seen in response to suckling, stimulate a rise in glucagon and glucose that is blocked by the oxytocin antagonist (Widmaier et al., 1991; Bjorkstrand et al., 1996). Opposing effects of the increased intranuclear release of oxytocin on pancreatic function during labour and lactation have been suggested by findings of a dual central effect of physiological doses of oxytocin on insulin secretion in male rats. A microinjection of oxytocin into the cerebral ventricles has a

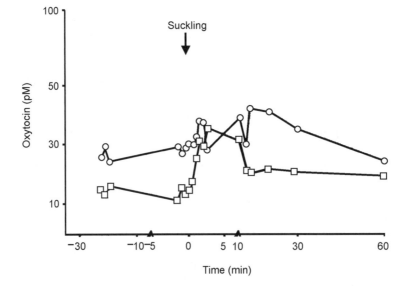

Figure 6.6 Oxytocin levels in relation to suckling on day 4 and at 3–4 months postpartum. [Reproduced from Uvnas-Moberg et al. (1990) Acta Obstet. Scand. **69**, 301–306 with permission from Blackwell Publishing Ltd]

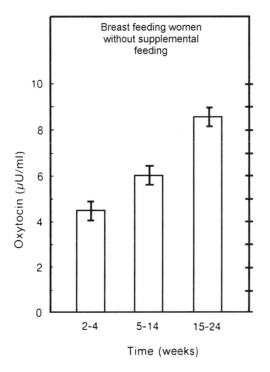

Figure 6.7 Mean ± stimulated plasma oxytocin levels in four exclusively breast-feeding women between 2 and 24 weeks following birth. (Reproduced with permission from Johnston and Amico, 1986)

stimulatory influence on insulin secretion while a similar dose administered into the brain stem induces a vagally mediated decline (Siaud *et al.*, 1991; Bjorkstrand *et al.*, 1996). Clinical studies on women suggest that reflex myometrial stimulation of brain-stem feedback on oxytocin neurons may inhibit insulin secretion during labour, while the sensory-suckling reflex may augment glucose-induced insulin secretion during episodes of suckling (Eriksson *et al.*, 1994; Bjorkstrand *et al.*, 1996).

In women, fasting plasma insulin levels are low between late pregnancy and birth and progressively increase in response to suckling (Widstrom *et al.*, 1984; Eriksson *et al.*, 1994; Chen *et al.*, 1998). During labour, a sharp decline has also been found in insulin required by well-controlled diabetics undergoing induc-

tion of labour with synthetic oxytocin (Golde *et al.*, 1982; Jovanovic and Peterson, 1983). In the first of these studies, 48 per cent of women did not need insulin in labour despite large requirements during pregnancy. Taken together, these findings suggest that the combined inhibitory effects of placental steroids and glucocorticoids on insulin secretion are maintained during labour and may be enhanced by intranuclear oxytocin release, while the insulin-like actions of low concentrations of oxytocin on adipose tissue, along with the lipogenic effects of progesterone and the sharp decline in GH-V, may explain the reduced insulin requirements observed in clinical studies on well-controlled diabetics (Golde *et al.*, 1982; Jovanovic and Peterson, 1983; Weinhaus *et al.*, 2000).

In relation to changes in adipose tissue metabolism between labour and lactation, experiments on isolated adipocytes suggest that doses of oxytocin similar to those found during labour stimulate increased glucose transport and oxidation, glycogen synthesis and lipogenesis and inhibit catecholamine-stimulated lipolysis. On the other hand, high concentrations of oxytocin, comparable to those found following birth and during suckling, activate glycogenolysis and adipose tissue lypolysis (Muchmore *et al.*, 1981; Augert and Exton, 1988). Increased lipolysis and either glycogenolysis or gluconeogenesis have been demonstrated in women following intravenous injections of high concentrations of oxytocin, while increased glycogenolysis has been found during episodes of suckling in the fasted state (Burt *et al.*, 1964; Tigas *et al.*, 2002). In women following childbirth, doses of oxytocin between 10 and 400 mu/kg body weight induce consistent increases in plasma concentrations of NEFA in association with delayed hypoglycaemia. However, episodes of suckling during the fasted state between 6 weeks and 3 months postpartum result in a significant rise in glucose production by increased rates of glycogenolysis, even though gluconeogenesis,

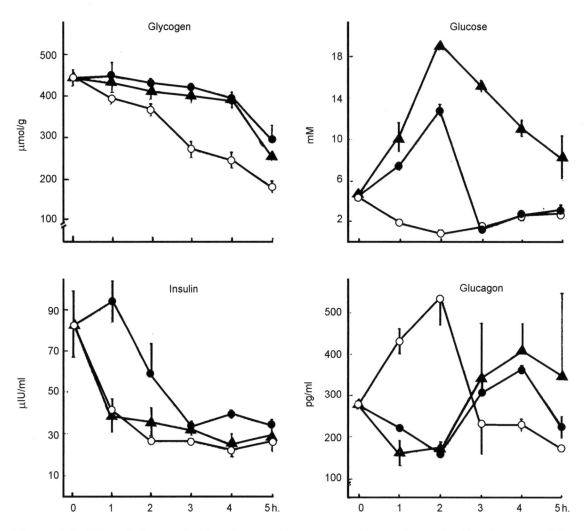

Figure 6.8 Effect of glucose administration in newborn rats, on plasma glucose, insulin, glucagon and liver glycogen over the first 5 h of extrauterine life. Immediately following birth, rats were injected intraperitoneally with NaCl (○), glucose (●) or glucose plus mannoheptulose (▲). [Reprinted from Martin *et al.* (1981) *Biochem. Biophys. Acta* **672**, 264, copyright by permission of Elsevier Science]

lypolysis and ketogenesis remained unchanged (Burt *et al.*, 1964; Tigas *et al.*, 2002). Taken together, this evidence suggests that elevated secretion of oxytocin during episodes of suckling may stimulate lypolysis, glycogenolysis or gluconeogenesis to maintain glucose homeostasis and regulate nutrient uptake by the mammary gland during the fed–fasted cycle.

The contrasting effects of low and high concentrations of oxytocin on maternal metabolism complement the changing maternal energy requirements associated with labour and lactation. In contrast to the need for rapid utilization of glucose for milk lactose secretion during lactation, myometrial contractions during labour impose no additional demand on maternal energy stores (Steingrimsdottir *et al.*, 1993; Tigas *et al.*, 2002). Like all smooth muscle, the myometrium has a low energy requirement and an increased capacity for glycogen storage, which increases up to 10-fold during pregnancy, peaks at term and is used as a predominant source of energy for contractions during and after labour (Steingrimsdottir et al., 1993). At the same time, skeletal muscle activity is characteristically reduced and it has been suggested that maternal neocortical or higher brain requirements for glucose may also decline during labour, as women tend to withdraw and become remote from verbal communications around them (Odent, 1992).

Maternal and neonatal glucose

Current evidence from animal experiments suggests that the physiological fall in maternal glucose from the end of pregnancy may have important regulatory influences on maternal, foetal and early neonatal metabolism. Effects of experimentally induced hyperglycaemia have been studied in adequately nourished pregnant rats and underfed ewes during the last 3–7 days of pregnancy as well as in newborn rats immediately following birth (Ktorza et al., 1981; Martin et al., 1981; Bihoreau et al., 1986; Clarke et al., 1996). The effects of maternal glucose infusions include a significant increase in fetal insulin secretion following mild but not high maternal hyperglycaemia with decreased foetal glucagon secretion and expression of key regulatory enzymes of gluconeogenesis. In newborn rats, an intraperitoneal injection of glucose inhibits the simultaneous fall in insulin and rise in glucagon secretion and the decline in liver glycogen that normally occur immediately following birth (Figure 6.8, Martin et al., 1981).

Fetal Neurohormonal Responses to Labour and Birth

During adult life, the sympatho-adrenal system functions to maintain homeostasis, in response to a wide variety of stressful stimuli, through activation of sympathetic nerve pathways and adrenomedullary secretions. These responses are largely controlled by the central nervous system through stimulation of splanchnic nerves that synapse with prevertebral ganglia in the spinal cord (Slotkin, 1990). In a number of species, including humans, chromaffin cells in the adrenal medulla and abdominal aorta function independently of sympathetic innervation throughout gestation, which gives them a unique capacity to respond directly to specific stressful stimuli like haemorrhage or hypoxia (Phillippe, 1983; Slotkin, 1990). In the human fetus this developmental capacity begins to change a few days following birth, when the highly active extra-adrenal islets of chromaffin cells start to degenerate and the adrenal medulla begins to acquire sympathetic innervation from the splanchnic nerves; the adrenal medulla retains its ability to respond directly to stressful stimuli for some weeks after birth (Lagercrantz and Slotkin, 1986).

The dominance of non-neurogenic catecholamine release in response to labour and birth seems to be part of a phased maturation of the 'stress axis'. Before and after birth, this selective response induces maturational changes in particular organ systems, in preparation for extrauterine life, while other well-defined stressors like low oxygen tension and hypoglycaemia do not evoke any adrenomedullary secretion. In newborn lambs, a decreased rate of glucose production has been demonstrated in response to adrenaline compared with the adult (Cowett, 1988; Slotkin, 1990). As illustrated in Figure 6.9, catecholamine levels rise in the human fetus throughout labour, to reach 20 times adult resting values immediately following birth. Current evidence suggests that the intermittent squeezing of the fetal head during human labour triggers the rapid surge in catecholamine release (Lagercrantz and Slotkin, 1986). At the same time, free cortisol levels double in association with labour and rise further in the

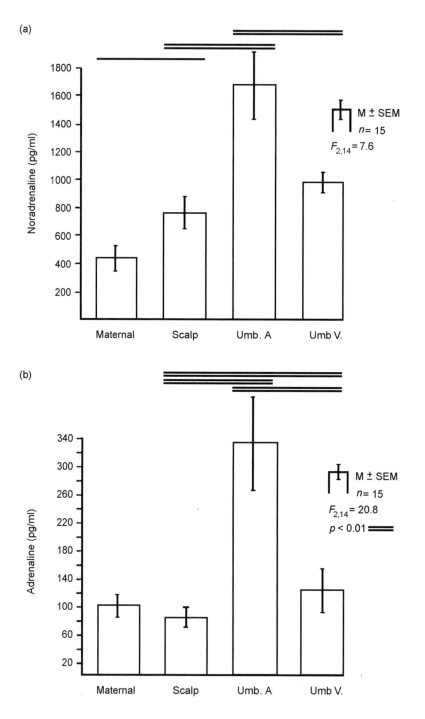

Figure 6.9 Comparison of maternal noradrenaline (a) and adrenaline (b) to fetal scalp, umbilical artery and vein. This result indicates that fetal catecholamines, particularly noradrenaline, rise dramatically during labour and are 3–5-fold higher than those in the maternal circulation following birth. (Reproduced with permission from Artal, 1980)

first hour or two following birth, while a dramatic surge in thyroid-stimulating hormone (TSH) at birth stimulates striking increases in thyroid hormones during the first 24 h of neonatal life (Pearson Murphy and Branchaud, 1994; Girard et al., 1992).

These hormonal responses to labour regulate fetal cardio-respiratory and metabolic adaptations to extrauterine life. Thyroid hormones are essential for activating gluconeogenesis in fetal sheep during late gestation, and immediately following birth TSH is the prime activator of lipolysis in white adipose tissue in human neonates, while catecholamines stimulate a sharp rise in plasma glucagon and a corresponding fall in plasma insulin (Lagercrantz and Slotkin, 1986; Marcus et al., 1988; Fowden et al., 2001). In the presence of low concentrations of insulin and glucose, glucagon and adrenaline stimulate glycogenolysis while glucagon and LCFAs stimulate gene transcription of key enzymes that initiate gluconeogenesis and ketogenesis (Pegorier et al., 1998). As a result of these changes, the neonate is stimulated to actively utilize its prenatally stored reserves of carbohydrate and adipose tissue immediately after birth. As carbohydrate stores decline, FFAs formed by lipolysis of triglycerides are supplied as fuels primarily to liver, muscle and brain tissues and form a major substrate for gluoconeogenesis, which underlies the role of fat provision in the regulation of glucose homeostasis following birth (Girard et al., 1992).

Hormonal regulation of suckling metabolism

When catecholamine levels decline a few hours after birth, glucagon is released in high concentrations in response to suckling and declines with fasting. While longitudinal studies have not been done on suckling human neonates,

experiments on rats suggest that this pattern continues until spontaneous weaning onto a high-carbohydrate diet, when glucagon markedly declines and secretion becomes responsive to hypoglycaemia, as it does in the adult (Girard et al., 1992). Throughout the period of suckling, insulin concentrations remain low and hepatic insulin resistance has been demonstrated during the suckling period in rats and dogs (Issad et al., 1987; Cowett et al., 1999). In a variety of animal studies, these hormonal patterns persist throughout the suckling period in response to the high fat–low carbohydrate composition of maternal milk and reflect their opposing regulatory functions on lipid metabolism during this period of development (Figure 6.10; Girard et al., 1992).

In suckling human neonates, plasma levels of ketone bodies increase a few hours after birth and maximum levels are reached by the second to third day, and this increase has been shown to parallel increased fatty acid oxidation (Persson, 1974; Hawdon et al., 1992; De Rooy and Hawdon, 2000). Throughout the suckling period, hepatic and intestinal ketogenesis synthesizes ketone bodies from dietary lipids and these provide the main circulating energy fuels for the brain, heart and peripheral tissues and precursors for essential myelination of the neonatal brain (Cunnane et al., 1999). This high capacity for oxidation of lipids does not seem to augment insulin secretion and administration of insulin to suckling rats has been shown to decrease blood ketone body concentration through a direct anti-ketogenic effect on the liver (Yeh and Zee, 1976).

Following birth, the infant's capacity to metabolize lactose is 5–10 times more rapid than glucose (Kliegman and Sparks, 1985). Following birth human infants demonstrate glucose intolerance in response to exogenous glucose, while a galactose infusion results in a lower insulin response and a smaller rise in plasma glucose (Persson, 1974; Kliegman et al.,

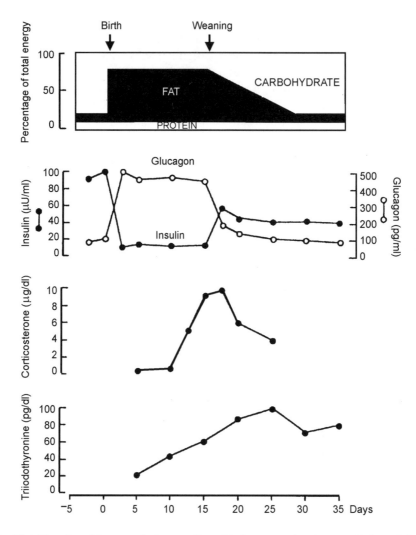

Figure 6.10 Nutritional and hormonal changes from birth to weaning in rats. [Adapted from Girard *et al.* (1992) *Physiol. Rev.* **72**, 507–562; reproduced by permission of The American Physiological Society]

1983). In conjunction with the low insulin requirements during suckling, the significance of these findings for the long-term health of β-cell function has recently been demonstrated in a series of nutritional experiments on rats. Feeding a high-carbohydrate milk formula during this critical period of pancreatic development stimulates the immediate onset of hyperinsulinaemia followed by enhanced glucose-stimulated insulin secretion during adult life (Aalinkeel *et al.*, 1999).

Maternal hypothalamic–pituitary–adrenocortical axis and Oxytocin – Influences on Neonatal Metabolic Adaptations

Distinct changes occur in maternal food appetite and metabolism during active labour that regulate the transplacental supply of glucose, ketones and fatty acids until the moment of birth. Existing evidence suggests that the transition from carbohydrate to lipid metabolism in the neonate following birth is stimulated by transplacental supplies of ketones and fatty acids and inhibited by increased supplies of glucose during labour (Ktorza *et al.*, 1981; Martin *et al.*, 1981; Girard *et al.*, 1992; Chen *et al.*, 1998). In humans, glucocorticoids and oxytocin may influence this transition through their opposing effects on maternal metabolism during active labour.

In humans and other primates, basal levels of glucocorticoids show a raised profile from approximately 25 weeks, in conjunction with adaptations in the hypothalamic–pituitary–adrenocortical (HPA) axis that seem to be stimulated by rising levels of oestrogen and a progressive decline in fasting glucose concentrations during the second half of pregnancy (Nolten *et al.*, 1981; Allolio *et al.*, 1990). Oestrogen enhances the production of a corticosteroid-binding globulin (CBG) that increases 3-fold in the maternal circulation during pregnancy (Vamvakopoulos and Chrousos, 1993). While this increase in CBG could be expected to inactivate the higher levels of cortisol by increasing its binding capacity, a number of studies have demonstrated that unbound, biologically active cortisol levels also rise during the third trimester (Allolio *et al.*, 1990; Reis *et al.*, 1999). This trend is influenced by the progressive increase in progesterone that competes with circulating cortisol for CBG binding sites. This action is confirmed by findings that progesterone displays circadian variations that are inversely related to cortisol during the second half of pregnancy. In contrast to cortisol, the lowest levels of progesterone have been found at 08:00 h and the highest levels between 16:00 and 20:00 h (Allolio *et al.*, 1990).

Placental corticotrophin-releasing hormone

In humans and other primates, placental corticotrophin-releasing hormone (CRH) operates as part of the maternal and fetal HPA axis and is regulated by a positive feedback mechanism within the placenta (Reis *et al.*, 1999). Longitudinal studies on women suggest that, from around 15 weeks of gestation, placenta CRH is released into the circulation and progressively increases throughout pregnancy to reach levels equivalent to those found in hypothalamic portal blood in response to stress (Reiss *et al.*, 1999). According to some but not all research findings, CRH activity is buffered by the presence of higher concentrations of CRH-binding protein (CRH-BP) until the last 3 weeks of pregnancy, when a rapid rise in plasma CRH is accompanied by a 50 per cent fall in CRH-BP (Reiss *et al.*, 1999).

Hyporesponsiveness of the maternal HPA axis during pregnancy and labour

In humans and other primates, the progressive rise in placental CRH is accompanied by suppression of hypothalamic CRH neurons and reduced anterior pituitary corticotrophin responses to CRH. Despite highly elevated levels of circulating CRH during the second half of pregnancy, adrenocorticotrophic hormone (ACTH) remains within the normal range and no increase has been found in plasma ACTH in response to exogenous CRH during the third trimester (Reiss *et al.*, 1999). However, in humans, evidence of an enhanced HPA axis has been found during labour, with significant increases in maternal ACTH and cortisol during late pregnancy, labour and birth (Fajardo *et al.*, 1994; Chen *et al.*, 1998).

In humans, emotional stress and heightened sensitivity to pain seem to be associated with greater increases in maternal cortisol and glucose between late pregnancy and birth and higher concentrations of cortisol and glucose in cord blood immediately following birth (Chen *et al.*, 1998). Hormonal profiles on a small sample of women before and after labour have demonstrated increased levels of cortisol, low concentrations of insulin and maternal serum glucose levels of around 6.8 mmol/l soon after birth (Chen *et al.*, 1998). In this study, mean cord glucose concentrations were 5.9 mmol/l and this blood value emerged as the most predictive of delayed lactogenesis.

These findings suggest that emotional stress and heightened sensitivity to pain during labour are associated with increased HPA activity and cortisol-induced hyperglycaemia, which has been shown to counteract the shift from carbohydrate to lipid metabolism in the neonate immediately following birth (Martin *et al.*, 1981; Chen *et al.*, 1998). Direct evidence from rats suggests that, from late pregnancy onwards, the activation of oxytocin neurons may counter this effect, through its capacity to ameliorate anxiety (Douglas *et al.*, 1998; Neumann *et al.*, 1999). During active labour and birth, central oxytocin may also reduce maternal glucose levels by inhibiting appetite, while the relatively low pulsatile release of oxytocin in the peripheral circulation may reduce glucose concentrations by stimulating glucose transport, oxidation and lipogenesis and by inhibiting catecholamine stimulated lipolysis in adipose tissue (Muchmore *et al.*, 1981).

Conclusion

At present, the factors responsible for the shift from glucose to fat metabolism in the human neonate are not completely understood. Insulin and glucagon have a number of unique developmental features during fetal and early neonatal life and neither hormone has the full metabolic capacities or the secretory patterns of the adult until the onset of weaning. Indirect studies on humans and direct evidence from rats suggest that suckling is characterized by a developmental period of low insulin secretion which coincides with significant structural modifications in the endocrine pancreas. In humans this extends from the third trimester of pregnancy to the first 6 months postpartum (Kassem *et al.*, 2000). Since recent experiments on rats suggest that disruption of this critical phase of development stimulates neonatal hyperinsulinaemia and impairs insulin sensitivity in later life, it is essential to gain a greater understanding of the changes in maternal metabolism during labour to identify their possible influences on the transition from glucose to lipid metabolism in the neonate immediately following birth.

References

Aalinkeel R, Srinivasan M, Kalhan SC, Laychock SG and Patel MS (1999) A dietary intervention (high carbohydrate) during the neonatal period causes islet dysfunction in rats. *Am. J. Physiol.* **277**(40), E1061–E1069.

Allolio B, Hoffmann J, Linton EA, Winkelman W, Kusche M and Schulte HM (1990) Diurnal salivary cortisol patterns during pregnancy and after delivery: relationship to plasma corticotrophin-releasing-hormone. *Clin. Endocrinol.* **33**, 279–289.

Alsat E, Guibourdenche J, Lutton D, Frankenne F and Evian-Brion D (1997) Human placental growth hormone. *Am. J. Obstet. Gynecol.* **177**(6), 1526–1534.

Antonijevic IA, Leng G, Luckman SM, Douglas AJ, Bicknell RJ and Russell JA (1995) Induction of uterine activity with oxytocin in late pregnant rats replicates the expression of *c-fos* in neuroendocrine and brain stem neurones as seen during parturition. *Endocrinology* **136**(1), 154–163.

Aoyagi K, Bergstern P, Eriksson UJ, Ebendal T and Hellestrom C (1997) In vitro regulation of insulin release and biosynthesis of fetal rat pancreatic cells explanted on pregnancy day 16. *Biol. Neonate* **71**, 60–68.

Artal R (1980) Fetal adrenal medulla. *Clin. Obstet. Gynaecol.* **23**(3), 825–836.

Asad M, Shewade DG, Koumaravelou K, Abraham BK, Vasu S and Ramaswamy S (2001) Effect of centrally administered oxytocin on gastric and duodenal ulcers in rats. *Acta Pharmac. Sin.* **22**(6), 488–492.

Augert G and Exton JH (1988) Insulin and oxytocin effects on phosphoinsitide metabolism. *J. Biol. Chem.* **263**(8), 3600–3609.

Barrett JFR, Whittaker PG, Williams JG and Lind T (1994) Absorption of non-haem iron from food during normal pregnancy. *Br. Med. J.* **309**, 79–82.

Battaglia FC (1978) Commonality and diversity in fetal development: bridging the interspecies gap. *Pediatr. Res.* **12**, 736–742.

Beaudry M-A, Chiasson J-L and Exton J-H (1977) Gluconeogenesis in the suckling rat. *Am. J. Physiol.* **233**(3), E175–E180.

Bergsten P, Aoyagi K, Persson E, Eriksson UJ and Hellestrom C (1998) Appearance of glucose-induced insulin release in fetal rat B-cells. *J. Endocrinol.* **158**, 115–120.

Bihoreau MT, Ktorza A, Kervran A and Picon L (1986) Effect of gestational hyperglycemia on insulin secretion in vivo and in vitro by fetal rat pancreas. *Am. J. Physiol.* **251**(14), E86–E91.

Bird JA, Spence JAD, Mould T and Symonds ME (1996) Endocrine and metabolic adaptation following caesarean section or vaginal delivery. *Arch. Dis. Child.* **74**, F132–F134.

Bjorkstrand E, Erksson M and Uvnas-Moberg K (1996) Evidence of a peripheral and a central effect of oxytocin on pancreatic hormone release in rats. *Neuroendocrinology* **63**, 377–383.

Bozzetti P, Ferrari MM, Marconi AM, Ferrazzi E, Pardi G, Makowski EL and Battaglia FC (1988) The relationship of maternal and fetal glucose concentration from mid-gestation until term. *Metabolism* **37**(4), 358–363.

Brelje CT, Scharp DW, Lacy PE, Ogren L, Talamantes F, Robertson M, Friesen HG and Sorenson RL (1993) Effect of homologous placental lactogens, prolactins, and growth hormones on islet B-cell division and insulin secretion in rat, mouse, and human islets: implications for placental lactogen regulation of islet function during pregnancy. *Endocrinogy* **132**(2), 879–887.

Brenton C, Pechoux C, Morel G and Zingg HH (1995) Oxytocin receptor messenger ribonucleic acid: characterisation, regulation, and cellular localization in the rat pituitary gland. *Endocrinology* **136**(7), 2928–2936.

Burt RL, Leake NH and Dannenburg WN (1964) Sex differences in metabolic effects of oxytocin. *Nature* **201**, 829–830.

Butte NF, Hopkinson JM, Mehta N, Moon JK,

O'Brien D and Smith E (1999) Adjustments in energy expenditure and substrate utilization during late pregnancy and lactation. *Am. J. Clin. Nutr.* **69**, 299–307.

Byatt JC, Staten NR, Salgiver WJ, Kostelc JG and Collier RJ (1993) Stimulation of food intake and weight gain in mature female rats by bovine prolactin and bovine growth hormone. *Am. J. Physiol.* **264**(27), E986–E992.

Caruso A, Paradisi G, Ferrazani Slucchese A, Moretti S and Fulghesu AM (1998) Effect of maternal carbohydrate metabolism on fetal growth. *Obstet. Gynaecol.* **92**(1), 8–12.

Chen DC, Nommsen-Rivers L, Dewey KG and Lonnerdal B (1998) Stress during labour and delivery and early lactation performance. *Am. J. Clin. Nutr* **68**, 335–344.

Clark A and Grant AM (1983) Quantitative morphology of endocrine cells in human fetal pancreas. *Diabetologia* **25**, 31–34.

Clarke L, Andrews DC, Lomax MA and Symonds ME (1996) Effect of maternal glucose infusion on brown adipose tissue and liver development in the neonatal lamb. *Reprod. Fertil. Devl.* **8**, 1045–1054.

Coltart TM, Beard RW, Turner RC and Oakley NW (1969) Blood glucose and insulin relationships in the human mother and fetus before onset of labour. *Br. Med. J.* **4**, 17–19.

Cowett RM (1988) Decreased response to catecholamines in the newborn: effect on glucose kinetics in the lamb. *Metabolism* **37**(8), 736–740.

Cowett RM, Rapoza RE and Gelardi NL (1999) Insulin counterregulatory hormones are ineffective in neonatal hyperinsulinemic hypoglycaemia. *Metabolism* **48**(5), 568–574.

Crawford JS (1956) Some aspects of obstetric anaesthesia. *Br. J. Anaesth.* **28**, 201–208.

Cunnane SC, Menard CR, Likhodii SS, Brenna JT and Crawford MA (1999) Carbon recycling into *de novo* lipogenesis is a major pathway in neonatal metabolism of linoleate and *ax*-linolenate. *Prostagland. Leukotrienes Essential Fatty Acids* **60**(5–6), 387–392.

Cunningham ET and Sawchenko PE (1991) Reflex control of magnocellular vasopressin and oxytocin secretion. *Trends Neurosci.* **14**(9), 406–411.

Dahlquist G, Persson U and Persson B (1972) The activity of D-B-hydroxybutyrate dehydrogenase in fetal, infant and adult rat brain and the influence of starvation. *Biol. Neonate* **20**, 40–50.

Daniel RR, Metzger BE, Frienkel N, Faloona GR, Unger RH and Nitzan M (1974) Carbohydrate metabolism in pregnancy XI. Response of plasma glucagon to overnight fast and oral glucose during normal pregnancy and in gestational diabetes. *Diabetes* **23**, 771–776.

Darmady J and Postle AD (1982) Lipid metabolism in pregnancy. *Br. J. Obstet. Gynaecol.* **89**, 211–215.

Denne SC, Karn CA, Wang J and Liechty EA (1995) Effect of intravenous glucose and lipid on proteolysis and glucose production in normal newborns. *Am. J. Physiol.* **269**(32), E361–E367.

De Rooy LJ and Hawdon JM (2000) The influence of breastfeeding and size for gestational age on neonatal metabolic adaptations. *Arch. Dis. Child.* **82**(Suppl 1), A1.

Devaskar SU, Ganguli S, Styer D, Devaskar UP and Sperling MA (1984) Glucagon and glucose dynamics in sheep: evidence for glucagon resistance in the fetus. *Am. J. Physiol.* **246**(9), E256–265.

Diaz-Cabiale Z, Narvaez JA, Petersson M, Uvnas-Mobers K and Fuxe K (2000) Oxytocin/alpha$_2$-adrenoceptor interactions in feeding responses. *Neuroendocrinology* **71**, 209–218.

Dobbing J and Sands J (1973) Quantitative growth and development of human brain. *Arch. Dis. Child.* **48**, 757–767.

Douglas AJ, Johnstone HA, Wigger A, Landgraf R, Russell JA and Neumann ID (1998) The role of endogenous opioids in neurohypophysial and hypothalamo–pituitary–adrenal axis hormone secretory responses to stress in pregnant rats. *J. Endocrinol.* **158**, 285–293.

Dutta-Roy AK (1997) Fatty acid transport and metabolism in the feto-placental unit and the role of the fatty acid-binding proteins. *Nutr. Biochem.* **8**, 548–557.

Eriksson L, Frankenne F, Eden S, Hennen G and Von Schoultz B (1989) Growth hormone 24h serum profile during pregnancy – lack of pulsatility for the secretion of the placental variant. *Br. J. Obstet. Gynaecol.* **96**, 949–953.

Eriksson M, Bjorkstrand E, Smedh U, Alster P, Matthiesen A-S and Uvnas-Moberg K (1994) Role of vagal nerve activity during suckling. Effects on plasma levels of oxytocin, prolactin, VIP, somatostatin, insulin, glucagon, glucose and milk secretion in lactating rats. *Acta Physiol. Scand.* **151**, 453–459.

Fajardo MC, Florido J, Villaverde C, Oltras CM, Gonzalez-Ramirez AR and Gonzalez-Gomez F (1994) Plasma levels of *B*-endorphin and ACTH during labour and immediate puerperium. *Eur. J. Obstet. Gynaecol. Reprod. Biol.* **55**, 105–108.

Farrag HM, Nawrath LM, Healey JE, Dorcus EJ, Rapozo RE, Oh W and Cowett R (1997) Persistent glucose production and greater peripheral sensitivity to insulin in the neonate vs. the adult. *Am. J. Physiol.* **272**(35), E86–E93.

Feldman M, Van Aerde JE and Clandinin MT (1998) Lipid accretion in the fetus and newborn. In: *Fetal and Neonatal Physiology*, ed. Polin RA and Fox WW, pp. 299–314. WB Saunders, Philadelphia, PA.

Felig P and Lynch V (1970) Starvation in human pregnancy: hypoglycaemia, hypoinsulinaemia and hyperketonemia. *Science* **170**, 990–992.

Fleenor D, Petryk A, Driscoll P and Freemark M (2000) Constitutive expression of placental lactogen in pancreatic beta cells: effects on cell morphology, growth and gene expression. *Pediat. Res.* **47**, 136–142.

Flint DJ, Sinnett-Smith PA, Clegg RA and Veronon RG (1979) Role of insulin receptors in the changing metabolism of adipose tissue during pregnancy and lactation in the rat. *Biochem. J.* **182**, 421–429.

Fowden AL (1989) The role of insulin in prenatal growth. *J. Devl. Physiol.* **12**, 173–182.

Fowden AL, Mapstone J and Forhead AJ (2001) Regulation of gluconeogenesis by thyroid hormones in foetal sheep during late gestation. *J. Endocrinol.* **170**, 461–469.

Frankenne F, Closset J, Gomez F, Scippo ML, Smal J and Hennen G (1988) The physiology of growth hormone (GHs) in pregnant women and partial characterisation of the placental GH variant. *J. Clin. Endocrinol. Metab.* **66**(6), 1171–1180.

Frankenne F, Scippo M-L, Beeumen JV, Igout A and Hennen G (1990) Identification of placental human growth hormone as the growth hormone-V gene expression product. *J. Clin. Endocrinol. Metab.* **71**(1), 15–18.

Fraser RB (1991) Carbohydrate metabolism. In: *Clinical Physiology in Obstetrics*, ed. Hytten F and Chamberlain G, pp. 204–212. Blackwell Scientific, Oxford.

Freemark M (1999a) Editorial: the fetal adrenal and the maturation of the growth hormone and prolactin axes. *Endocrinology* **140**(5), 1963–1965.

Freemark M (1999b) The role of growth hormone, prolactin, and placental lactogen in human fetal development. In: *Molecular and Cellular Pediatric Endocrinology*, ed. Handwerger S, pp. 57–83. Humana Press, Totwa, NJ.

Freemark M, Fleenor D, Driscoll P, Binark N and Kelly PA (2001) Body weight and fat deposition in prolactin receptor-deficient mice. *Endocrinology* **142**(2), 532–537.

Fuchs A-R, Romero R, Keefe D, Parra M, Oyarzun E and Behnke E (1991) Oxytocin secretion and human parturition: pulse frequency and duration increase during spontaneous labour. *Am. J. Obstet. Gynecol.* **165**(5), 1515–1523.

Girard J, Ferre P, Pegorier J-P and Duee P-H (1992) Adaptations of glucose and fatty acid metabolism during perinatal period and suckling–weaning transition. *Physiol. Rev.* **72**(2), 507–562.

Golde SH, Good-Anderson B, Montro M and Artal R (1982) Insulin requirements during labour: a reappraisal. *Am. J. Obstet. Gynecol.* **144**(5), 556–559.

Goodman MH, Tai L-R, Ray J, Cooke NE and Liebhaber SA (1991) Human growth hormone variant produces insulin-like and lipolytic responses in rat adipose tissue. *Endocrinology* **129**(4), 1779–1783.

Haggarty P, Page K, Abramovich DR, Ashton J and Brown D (1997) Long-chain polyunsaturated fatty acid transport across the perfused human placenta. *Placenta* **18**, 635–642.

Hawdon JM, Ward Platt MP and Aynsley-Green A (1992) Patterns of metabolic adaptation for preterm and term infants in the first neonatal week. *Arch. Dis. Child.* **67**, 357–365.

Hay WW (1995) Metabolic interrelationships of placenta and fetus. *Placenta* **16**, 19–30.

Herrera E, Gomez-Coronodo D and Lasuncion MA (1987) Lipid metabolism in pregnancy. *Biol. Neonate* **51**, 70–77.

Herrera E, Lasuncion MA, Gomez-Coronado D, Aranda P, Lopez-Luna P and Maier I (1988) Role of lipoprotein lipase activity on lipoprotein metabolism and the fate of circulating triglycerides in pregnancy. *Am. J. Obstet. Gynecol.* **158**(6), 1575–1583.

Herrera E, Lasuncion MA, Gomez-Coranado L, Martin A and Bonet B (1990) Lipid metabolic interactions in the mother during pregnancy and their fetal repercussions. In: *Endocrine and Biochemical Development of the Fetus and Neonate*, ed. Cuezva JM, Pascual-Leon AM and Patel MS, pp. 213–230. Plenum Press, New York.

Herrera E, Lasuncion MA and Asuncion M (1992) Placental transport of free fatty acids, glycerol, and ketone bodies. In: *Fetal and Neonatal Physiology*, ed. Polin RA and Fox WW, pp. 291–298. WB Saunders, Philadelphia.

Hill DJ and Milner RDG (1985) Insulin as a growth factor. *Pediatr. Res.* **19**(9), 879–886.

Howell SL (1991) Insulin biosynthesis and secretion. In: *Textbook of Diabetes*, Vol. 1, ed. Pickup J and Williams E, pp. 72–83. Oxford, Blackwell Scientific.

Issad T, Coupe C, Ferre P and Girard J (1987) Insulin resistance during suckling period in rats. *Am. J. Physiol.* **253**(16), E142–E148.

Jaffe R, Hashida Y and Yunis EJ (1982) The endocrine pancreas of the neonate and infant. *Perspect. Pediatr. Pathol.* **7**, 137–165.

Jiang QB and Wakerley JB (1995) Analysis of bursting responses of oxytocin neurons in the rat in late pregnancy, lactation and after weaning. *Am. J. Physiol.* **486**(1), 237–248.

Johnston JM and Amico JA (1986) A prospective longitudinal study of the release of oxytocin and prolactin in response to infant suckling in long term lactation. *J. Clin. Endocrinol. Metab.* **62**(4), 653–657.

Jones CT (1976) Lipid metabolism and mobilization in the guinea pig during pregnancy. *Biochem. J.* **156**, 357–365.

Jovanovic L and Perterson CM (1983) Insulin and glucose requirements during the first stage of labour in insulin-dependent diabetic women *Am. J. Med.* **75**, 607–612.

Kalhan SC (2000) Protein metabolism in pregnancy. *Am. J. Clin. Nutr.* **71**(Suppl), 1249S–1255S.

Kaplan SA (1981) The insulin receptor. *Pediatr. Res.* **15**, 1156–1162.

Kassem SA, Ariel L, Thornton PS, Scheimberg I and Glaser B (2000) B-cell proliferation in the developing normal human pancreas and in hyperinsulinism of infancy. *Diabetes* **49**, 1325–1333.

Kimura T, Takemura M, Nomura S, Nobunaga T, Kubota Y, Ionue T, Hashimoto K, Kumazawa I, Hashimoto K, Kumazawa I, Ito Y, Ohashi K, Koyama M, Azuma C, Kitamura Y and Saji F (1996) Expression of oxytocin receptor in human myometrium. *Endocrinology* **137**, 780–785.

Kliegman RM and Sparks JW (1985) Perinatal galactose metabolism. *J. Pediatr.* **107**(6), 831–841.

Kliegman RM, Miettinen EL and Morton S (1983) Potential role of galactokinase in neonatal carbohydrate assimilation. *Science* **220**, 302–304.

Knopp RH, Montes A, Childs M, Job R and Mabuchi H (1981) Metabolic adjustments in normal and diabetic pregnancy. *Clin. Obstet. Gynaecol.* **24**(1), 21–49.

Kovacs CS and Kronenberg HM (1997) Maternal–foetal calcium and bone metabolism during pregnancy, puerperium, and lactation. *Endocr. Rev.* **18**(6), 832–872.

Ktorza A, Girard J, Kinebanyan MF and Picon L (1981) Hyperglycaemia induced by glucose infusion in unrestrained pregnant rat during the last 3 days of gestation: metabolic and hormonal changes in the mother and the fetus. *Diabetologia* **21**, 569–574.

Ktorza A, Bihoreau M-T, Nurjhan N, Picon L and Girard J (1985) Insulin and glucagon during the perinatal period: secretion and metabolic effects on the liver. *Biol. Neonate* **48**, 204–220.

Lagercrantz H and Slotkin TA (1986) The "stress" of being born. *Sci. Am.* **254**, 920–102.

Lambillotte C, Gilon P and Henquin J-C (1997) Direct glucocorticoid inhibition of insulin secretion. *J. Clin. Invest.* **9**(3), 414–423.

Lawrence A, Wallin C, Fawcett P and Rosenfeld CR (1989) Oxytocin stimulates glucagon and insulin secretion in fetal and neonatal sheep. *Endocrinology* **125**(5), 2289–2296.

Lawson M, Kern F and Everson GT (1985) Gastrointestinal transit time in human pregnancy: prolongation in the second and third trimesters followed by postpartum normalization. *Gastroenterology* **89**, 996–1000.

Lebenthal E and Lee PC (1980a) The development of the small intestinal function in the perinatal period. *Proceedings of Symposium on Breastfeeding*, Tel Aviv, Israel, pp. 85–89.

Lebenthal E and Lee PC (1980b) The development of the exocrine pancreatic function in the perinatal period. *Proceedings of Symposium on Breastfeeding*, Tel Aviv, Israel, pp. 90–95.

Leng G and Brown D (1997) The origins and significance of pulsatility in hormone secretion from the pituitary. *J. Neuroendocrinol.* **9**, 493–513.

Lokrantz C-M, Uvnas-Moberg K and Kaplan JM (1997) Effect of central oxytocin administration on intraoral intake of glucose in deprived and non-deprived rats. *Physiol. Behav.* **62**(2), 347–352.

Lopez-Luna P, Olea J and Herrera E (1994) Effect of starvation on lipoprotein lipase activity in different tissues during gestation in the rat. *Biochim. Biophys. Acta* **1215**, 275–279.

Luckman SM (1995) Fos expression within regions of the prefrontal area, hypothalamus and brainstem during pregnancy and parturition. *Brain Res.* **669**, 115–124.

Luckman SM and Larsen PJ (1997) Evidence for the involvement of histaminergic neurones in the regulation of the rat oxytocinergic system during pregnancy and lactation. *J. Physiol.* **501**(3), 649–655.

Luyck A, Massi-Benedetti F, Farloni A and Lefevre PJ (1972) Presence of pancreatic glucagon in the portal plasma of human neonates. Differences in the insulin and glucagon response to glucose between normal infants and infants from diabetic mothers. *Diabetologia* **8**, 230–296.

Lyle RE, Kincaid SC, Bryant JC, Prince AM and McGehee ER Jr (2001) Human milk contains detectable levels of immunoreactive leptin. In: *Bioactive Components of Human Milk*, ed. Newburg E, pp. 87–92. Kluwer Academic/Plenum, New York.

Marcus C, Ehren H, Bolme P and Arner P (1988) Regulation of lipolysis during the neonatal period. *J. Clin. Invest.* **82**, 1793–1797.

Martin AT, Benito CM and Medina JM (1981) Regulation of glycogenolysis in the liver of the newborn rat in vivo, inhibitory effect of glucose. *Biochim. Biophys. Acta* **672**, 262–267.

Martin-Hidalgo A, Holm C, Belfrage P, Schotz MC and Herrera E (1994) Lipoprotein lipase and hormone-sensitive lipase activity and mRNA in rat adipose tissue during pregnancy. *Am. J. Physiol.* **266**(29), E930–935.

Matthiesen A-S, Ransjo-Arvidson A-BR, Nissen E and Uvnas-Moberg K (2001) Postpartum maternal oxytocin release by newborns: effects of infant hand massage and suckling. *Birth* **28**(1), 13–19.

McCann MJ and Rogers RC (1990) Oxytocin excites gastric-related neurons in rat dorsal vagal complex. *J. Physiol.* **428**, 95–108.

McGarry EE and Beck JC (1962) Some metabolic effects of ovine prolactin in man. *Lancet* **ii**, 915–916.

Menard D, Corriveau L and Becaulieu J-F (1999) Insulin modulates cellular proliferation in developing human jejunum and colon. *Biol. Neonate* **75**, 143–151.

Menuelle P and Plas C (1991) Variation in the antagonistic effects of insulin and glucagons on glycogen metabolism in cultured foetal hepatocytes. *Biochem. J.* **277**, 111–117.

Mills JL, Jovanovic L, Knopp R, Aarons J, Conley M, Park E, *et al.* (1998) Physiological reduction in fasting plasma glucose concentration in the first trimester of normal pregnancy: the Diabetes in Early Pregnancy Study. *Metabolism* **47**(9), 1140–1144.

Milner RDG, Chauskey SK, Mickleson KNP and Assan P (1973) Plasma pancreatic glucagon and insulin:glucagon ratio at birth. *Arch. Dis. Child.* **48**, 241–242.

Mirlesse V, Frankenne F, Alsat E, Poncelet M, Hennen G and Evain-Brion D (1993) Placenta growth hormone levels in normal pregnancy and in pregnancies with intrauterine growth retardation. *Pediatr. Res.* **34**(4), 439–442.

Mitchell BF and Schmid B (2001) Oxytocin and its receptor in the process of parturition. *J. Soc. Gynaecol. Invest.* **8**(3), 122–133.

Modney BK and Hatton GI (1994) Maternal behaviours: evidence that they feed back to alter brain morphology and function. *Acta Paediatr. Suppl.* **397**, 29–32.

Moore KL and Persaud TVN (1993) *The Developing Human*, p. 98. WB Saunders, Philadelphia, PA.

Morien A, Cassone VM and Wellman PJ (1999) Diurnal changes in paraventricular hypothalamic ax_1 and ax_2-adrenoreceptors and food intake in rats. *Pharmacol. Biochem. Behav.* **63**(1), 33–38.

Muchmore DB, Little SA and deHaens C (1981) A dual mechanism of action of oxytocin in rat epididymal fat cells. *J. Biol. Chem.* **256**(1), 365–372.

Neumann I, Douglas AJ, Pittman QJ, Russell JA and Landraf R (1996) Oxytocin released within the supraoptic nucleus of the rat brain by positive feedback action is involved in parturition-related events. *J. Neuroendocrinol.* **8**, 227–233.

Neumann ID, Torner L and Wigger A (1999) Brain oxytocin differential inhibition of neuroendocrine stress-responses and anxiety-related behaviour in virgin, pregnant and lactating rats. *Neuroscience* **95**(2), 567–575.

Noel M and Woodside B (1993) Effect of systemic and central prolactin injections on food intake, weight gain and estrous cyclicity in female rats. *Physiol. Behav.* **54**, 151–154.

Nolan CJ and Proietto J (1994) The feto-placental glucose steal phenomenon is a major cause of maternal metabolic adaptation during late pregnancy in the rat. *Diabetologia* **37**, 976–998.

Nolten WE, Holt LH and Rueck PA (1981) Deoxycorticosterone in normal pregnancy: III. Evidence of a foetal source of deoxycorticosterone. *Am. J. Obstet. Gynecol.* **139**(4), 477–482.

Novak M and Monkus E (1972) Metabolism of subcutaneous adipose tissue in the immediate postnatal period of human newborns. 1. Developmental changes in lipolysis and glycogen content. *Pediatr. Res.* **6**, 73–80.

Odent M (1992) *The Nature of Birth and Breastfeeding*, pp. 61–62. Bergin and Garvey, Westport, CT.

Page MA, Krebs HA and Williamson DH (1971) Activities of enzymes of ketone-body utilization in brain and other tissues of suckling rats. *Biochem. J.* **121**, 49–53.

Patel N, Alsat E, Igout A, Baron F, Hennen G, Porquet D and Evian-Brion D (1995) Glucose inhibits human placental GH secretion, in vitro. *J. Clin. Endocrinol. Metab.* **80**(5), 1743–1746.

Peaker M (1998) Milk: integrative signalling between mother and off-spring. *Biochem. Soc. Trans.* **26**, 103–107.

Pearson Murphy BE and Branchaud CL (1994) The fetal adrenal. In: *Maternal–Fetal Endocrinology*, ed. Tulchinsky D and Little AB, pp. 275–295. WB Saunders, Philadelphia, PA.

Pegorier J-P, Chatelain F, Thumelin S and Girard J (1998) Role of long-chain fatty acids in postnatal induction of genes coding for liver mitochondrial B-oxidative enzymes. *Biochem. Soc. Trans.* **26**, 113–130.

Persson B (1974) Carbohydrate and lipid metabolism in the newborn infant. *Acta Anaesthes. Scand. Suppl.* **55**, 50–57.

Petry CJ and Hales NC (2000) Long-term effects on offspring of intrauterine exposure to deficits in nutrition. *Hum. Reprod. Update* **6**(6), 578–586.

Philippe J and Missotten M (1990) Dexamethasone inhibits insulin biosynthesis by destabilizing insulin messenger ribonucleic acid in hamster insulinoma cells. *Endocrinology* **127** (4), 1640–1645.

Phillippe M (1983) Fetal catecholamines. *Am. J. Obstet. Gynecol.* **146**(7), 840–855.

Philipps AF, Dubin JW, Matty PJ and Raye JR (1983) Influence of exogenous glucagon on fetal glucose metabolism and ketone production. *Pediatr. Res.* **17**, 51–56.

Portha B (1990) Development of the pancreatic B-cells: growth pattern and functional maturation. In: *Endocrine and Biochemical Development of the Fetus and Neonate*, ed. Cuezva JM, Pascual-Leone AM, Patel MS, pp. 33–43. Plenum Press, New York.

Quigley ME, Ishizuka B, Ropert JF and Yen SSC (1982) The food-entrained prolactin and cortisol release in late pregnancy and prolactinoma patients. *J. Clin. Endocrinol. Metab.* **54**(6), 1109–1112.

Ramirez I, Llobera M and Herrera E (1983) Circulating triacyglycerols, lipoproteins, and tissue lipoprotein lipase activities in rat mothers and offspring during the perinatal period: effect of postmaturity. *Metabolism* **32**, 333–341.

Ramos P and Herrera E (1996) Comparative

responsiveness to prolonged hyperinsulinemia between adipose-tissue and mammary-gland lipoprotein lipase activities in pregnant rats. *Early Pregnancy: Biol. Med.* **2**, 29–35.

Ramos P, Martin-Hidalgo A and Herrera E (1999) Insulin-induced up-regulation of lipoprotein lipase messenger ribonucleic acid and activity in mammary gland. *Endocrinology* **140**(3), 1089–1093.

Reis FM, Fadalti M, Florio P and Petraglia F (1999) Putative role of placental corticotrophin-releasing factor in the mechanism of human parturition. *J. Soc. Gynaecol. Invest.* **6**(3), 109–119.

Rigg LA and Yen SSC (1977) Multiphasic prolactin secretion during parturition in human subjects. *Am. J. Obstet. Gynecol.* **128**(2), 215–218.

Rigg LA, Lein A and Yen SSC (1977) Pattern of increase in circulating prolactin levels during human pregnancy. *Am. J. Obstet. Gynecol.* **129**(4), 454–456.

Sabata V, Wolf H and Lausmann S (1968) The role of free fatty acids, glycerol, ketone bodies and glucose in the energy metabolism of mother and foetus during delivery. *Biol. Neonate* **13**, 7–17.

Sangild PT (1999) Biology of the pancreas before birth. In: *Biology of the Pancreas in Growing Animals*, ed. Pierzynowski SG and Zabielski, pp. 1–13. Elsevier Science, Amsterdam.

Schaeffer LD, Wilder ML and Williams RH (1973) Secretion and content of insulin and glucagon in human fetal pancreas slices in vitro. *Proc. Soc. Exp. Biol. Med.* **143**, 314–319.

Schubring C, Engloaro P, Siebler T, Blum WF, Demirakca T, Kratzsch J and Kiess W (1998) Longitudinal analysis of maternal serum leptin levels during pregnancy, at birth and up to six weeks after birth: relation to body mass index, skinfolds, sex steroids and umbilical cord blood leptin levels. *Horm. Res.* **50**, 276–283.

Shelley HJ (1961) Glycogen reserves and their changes at birth and in anoxia. *Br. Med. Bull.* **17**(2), 137–143.

Shelley HJ and Bassett JM (1975) Control of carbohydrate metabolism in the fetus and newborn. *Br. Med. Bull.* **31**(1), 37–43.

Siaud P, Puech R, Assenmacher I and Alonso G (1991) Microinjection of oxytocin into the dorsal vagal complex decreases pancreatic insulin secretion. *Brain Res.* **546**, 190–194.

Slotkin TA (1990) Development of the sympathoadrenal axis. In: *Neuroendocrine Perspectives*, ed. Muller EE and MacLeod RM, pp. 69–96. Springer, New York.

Slotkin TA, Kudlacz EM, Hou Q-C and Seidler FJ (1990) Maturation of the sympathetic nervous system: role of neonatal physiological adaptations and in cellular development of perinatal tissues. In: *Endocrine and Biochemical Development of the Fetus and Neonate*, ed. Cuezva JM, Pascula L and Patel MS, pp. 67–75. Plenum Press, New York.

Soltani-K H, Bruce C and Fraser RB (1999) Observational study of maternal anthropometry and fetal insulin. *Arch. Dis. Child.* **81**, F122–F124.

Sperling MA (1994) Carbohydrate metabolism: insulin and glucagon. In: *Maternal and Fetal Endocrinology*, ed. Tulchinsky D and Little AB, pp. 379–400. WB Saunders, Philadelphia, PA.

Steingrimsdottir T, Ronquist G and Ulmsten U (1993) Energy economy in the pregnant human uterus at term: studies on arteriovenous differences in metabolites of carbohydrate, fat and nucleotides. *Eur. J. Obstet. Gynaecol. Reprod. Biol.* **51**, 209–215.

Thorsson AV and Hintz RL (1977) Insulin receptors in the newborn: increase in receptor affinity and number. *New Engl. J. Med.* **297**, 908–912.

Tigas S, Sunehag A and Haymond MW (2002) Metabolic adaptation to feeding and fasting during lactation in humans. *J. Clin. Endocrinol. Metab.* **87**(1), 302–307.

Tobin JD, Roux JF and Soeldner JS (1969) Human foetal insulin response after acute maternal glucose administration during labour. *Pediatrics* **44**(5), 668–671.

Tozzo E, Tessier F and Desbuquis B (1995) Expression of the hepatic insulin receptor gene in the rat during postnatal development. *Horm. Metab. Res.* **27**, 163–168.

Uvnas-Moberg K (1989a) The gastrointestinal tract in growth and reproduction. *Sci. Am.* **July**, 60–65.

Uvnas-Moberg K (1998) Antistress pattern induced by oxytocin. *News Physiol. Sci.* **13**, 22–26.

Uvnas-Moberg K, Widstrom A-M, Werner S, Mattheisen A-S and Winberg J (1990) Oxytocin and prolactin levels in breast-feeding women. *Acta Obstet. Scand.* **69**, 301–306.

Vamvakopoulos N and Chrousos GP (1993) Evidence of direct estrogen regulation of human corticotrophin-releasing hormone gene expression. *J. Clin. Invest.* **92**, 1896–1902.

Van Aerde JE, Feldman M and Clandinin MT (1998) Accretion of lipid in the fetus and newborn. In: *Fetal and Neonatal Physiology*, ed Polin RA and Fox WW, pp. 458–477. Marcel Dekker, New York.

Van Assche FA, Hoet JJ and Jack PMB (1984) Endocrine pancreas of the pregnant mother, fetus and newborn. In: *Fetal Physiology and Medicine*, pp. 127–152. Marcel Dekker, New York.

Van der Lee KAJM, Vork MM, De Vries JE, Willemsen PHM, Glatz JFC, Reneman RS, *et al.* (2000) Long-chain fatty acid-induced changes in gene expression in neonatal cardiac myocytes. *J. Lipid Res.* **41**, 41–47.

Verbalis JG, Blackburn RE, Hoffman GE and Stricker EM (1995) Establishing behavioral and physiological functions of central oxytocin: insights from studies of oxytocin and ingestive behaviours. In: *Oxytocin*, ed. Ivell R and Russell J, pp. 209–225. Plenum Press, New York.

Weinhaus AJ, Stout LE and Sorenson RL (1996) Glucokinase, hexokinase, glucose transporter 2, and glucose metabolism in islets during pregnancy and prolactin-treated islets *in vitro*: mechanisms for long-term up-regulation of islets. *Endocrinology* **127**(5), 1640–1649.

Weinhaus AJ, Bhagroo NV, Brelje CT and Sorenson RL (2000) Dexamethasone counteracts the effects of prolactin on islet function: implications for islet regulation in late pregnancy. *Endocrinology* **141**(4), 1384–1393.

Widmaier EP (1990) Glucose homeostasis and hypothalamic-pituitary-adrenocortical axis during development in rats. *Am. J. Physiol.* **259**(22), E601–E613.

Widmaier EP, Shah PR and Lee G (1991) Interactions between oxytocin, glucagon and glucose in normal and streptozotocin-induced diabetic rats. *Regulat. Pept.* **34**, 235–249.

Widstrom AM, Winberg J, Werner S, Hamberger B, Eneroth P and Uvnas-Moberg K (1984) Suckling in lactating women stimulates the secretion of insulin and prolactin without concomitant effects on gastrin, growth hormone, calcitonin, vasopressin or catecholamines. *Early Hum. Devl.* **10**, 115–122.

Williams C and Coultard TM (1978) Adipose tissue metabolism in pregnancy: the lipolytic effect of human placental lactogen. *Br. J. Obstet. Gynaecol.* **85**, 43–46.

Yeh Y and Zee P (1976) Insulin: a possible regulator of ketosis in newborn and suckling rats. *Pediatr. Res.* **10**, 192–197.

Zangen S, Lorenzo CD, Zangen T, Mertz H, Schwankovsky L and Hyman P (2001) Rapid maturation of gastric relaxation in newborn infants. *Pediatr. Res.* **50**(5), 620–632.

Zumkeller W (2000) The role of growth hormone and insulin-like growth factors for placental growth and development. *Placenta* **21**, 451–467.

7

FETAL, INFANT AND CHILDHOOD GROWTH AND ADULT HEALTH

Keith M. Godfrey and David J.P. Barker

LEARNING OUTCOMES

- Understand what programming is and the basis of the fetal origins of adult disease hypothesis.

- Understand how this could be related to the development of coronary heart disease, diabetes mellitus and hypertension.

- Understand how the concept of programming could inform public health policies.

- Understand why optimal maternal nutrition is important in breaking the cycle of socio-economic deprivation and high disease risk in later life.

Introduction

Programming and the 'Fetal Origins' Hypothesis

The 'fetal origins' hypothesis proposes that alterations in fetal nutrition and endocrine status result in developmental adaptations that permanently change structure, physiology and metabolism, thereby predisposing to cardiovascular, metabolic and endocrine disease in adult life (Barker, 1998). For example, it is thought that coronary heart disease may be a consequence of fetal adaptations to undernutrition that are beneficial for short-term survival, even though they are detrimental to health in postreproductive life (Barker, 1998).

In fetal life the tissues and organs of the body go through what are called 'critical' periods of development. These may coincide with periods of rapid cell division. In common with other living creatures, human beings are 'plastic' in their early life, and are moulded by the environment. Although the growth of a fetus is influenced by its genes, studies in humans and animals suggest that it is usually limited by the environment, in particular the nutrients and oxygen received from the mother (Harding, 2001; McCance and Widdowson, 1974). There are many possible evolutionary advantages in the body remaining plastic during development, rather than having its development driven only by genetic instructions acquired at conception.

'Programming' is sometimes used to describe the process whereby a stimulus or insult during a critical period of development has lasting or lifelong effects (Harding, 2001). Experimental studies in animals have documented many examples of fetal programming, with recent studies showing that alterations in maternal nutrition can have long-term effects on the offspring that are of relevance to human cardiovascular disease. For example, feeding pregnant rats a low-protein diet results in life-long elevation of blood pressure in the offspring (Langley-Evans and Jackson, 1994). Rats whose mothers had been fed a diet with a low ratio of protein to energy during pregnancy exhibited a permanently altered balance between hepatic glucose production and utilization; control rats fed the same diet during postnatal life had no alterations in hepatic glucose metabolism (Desai et al., 1995). Other notable long-term effects of alterations in maternal nutrition include changes in cholesterol metabolism, insulin secretion and renal development (Barker, 1998).

Although some effects of nutrition may be direct consequences of alterations in substrate availability, a number are thought to be mediated by hormonal effects (Barker, 1998). These may alter the development of specific fetal tissues during critical periods, or lead to long-lasting changes in hormone secretion or tissue hormone sensitivity. Experimental studies have implicated the fetal hypothalamus as a key site that can be programmed by transient changes in prenatal endocrine status (Barker, 1998). Material in Chapters 1, 3, 6 and 9 should be read in relation to this chapter.

Fetal Growth and Cardiovascular Disease

At the start of this century the incidence of coronary heart disease rose steeply in Western countries so that it became the most common cause of death. In many of these countries the steep rise has been followed by a fall over recent decades that cannot be accounted for by changes in adult lifestyle. The incidence of coronary heart disease is now rising in other parts of the world to which Western influences are extending, including China, India and Eastern Europe.

An important clue suggesting that coronary heart disease might originate during fetal development came from studies of death rates among babies in Britain during the early 1900s (Barker, 1998). The usual certified cause of death in newborn babies at that time was low birth-weight. Death rates in the newborn differed considerably between one part of the country and another, being highest in some of the northern industrial towns and the poorer rural areas in the north and west. This geographical pattern in death rates was shown to closely resemble today's large variations in death rates from coronary heart disease (Barker, 1998), variations that form one aspect of the continuing north–south divide in health in Britain. One possible conclusion suggested by this observation was that low rates of growth before birth are in some way linked to the development of

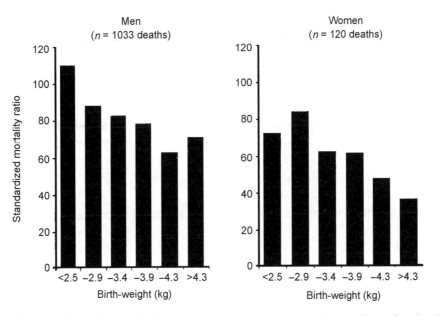

Figure 7.1 Coronary heart disease death rates, expressed as standardized mortality ratios, in 10 141 men and 5585 women born in Hertfordshire, UK according to birth-weight. Derived from Osmond *et al.* (1993).

coronary heart disease in adult life. Although it has been suggested that events in childhood influence the pathogenesis of coronary heart disease, a focus on intrauterine life offered a new point of departure for research.

More direct evidence that an adverse intrauterine environment might have long-term consequences came from follow-up studies of men and women in middle and late life whose body measurements at birth had been recorded. A study of people born in Hertfordshire, UK, showed for the first time that those who had had low birth-weights had increased death rates from coronary heart disease in adult life (Barker, 1998; Osmond *et al.*, 1993). Thus, among 15 726 people born during 1911–1930, death rates from coronary heart disease fell progressively with increasing birth-weight in both men and women (Figure 7.1). A small rise at the highest birth-weights in men could relate to the macrosomic infants of women with gestational diabetes. Another study, of 1586 men born in Sheffield during 1907–1925, showed that it was particularly people who

were small at birth as a result of growth retardation, rather than those born prematurely, who were at increased risk of the disease (Barker *et al.*, 1993a).

Replication of the UK findings has led to wide acceptance that low rates of fetal growth are associated with coronary heart disease in later life. For example, confirmation of a link between low birth-weight and adult coronary heart disease has come from studies of 1200 men in Caerphilly, South Wales (Frankel *et al.*, 1996) and of 70 297 nurses in the USA (Rich-Edwards *et al.*, 1997). The latter study found a two-fold fall in the relative risk of non-fatal coronary heart disease across the range of birth-weight (Rich-Edwards *et al.*, 1997). Similarly, among 517 men and women in Mysore, South India, the prevalence of coronary heart disease in men and women aged 45 years or older fell from 15 per cent in those who weighed 2.5 kg or less at birth, to 4 per cent in those who weighed 3.2 kg or more (Stein *et al.*, 1996).

The Hertfordshire records and the Nurses and Caerphilly studies did not include

measurements of body size at birth other than
weight. The weight of a newborn baby without
a measure of its length is a crude summary of
its physique. The addition of birth length
allows derivation of ponderal index (birth-
weight/length³) as a measure of thinness, but
cannot adequately distinguish variations in fat
and lean mass. With the addition of head
circumference the baby whose body and trunk
is small in relation to its head, as a result of
'brain-sparing', can also be distinguished.
Thinness, shortness and a small trunk are
thought to reflect differing fetal adaptations to
undernutrition, hypoxia and other influences
(Barker, 1998).

Follow-up studies of men and women born
in Sheffield and Helsinki suggest different long-
term consequences for particular patterns of
body proportions at birth. Patterns which
predict death from coronary heart disease
may be summarized as a small head circumference, shortness or thinness, which reflect
retarded fetal growth, and either low placental
weight or an altered ratio of placental weight
to birth-weight (Barker, 1998; Barker et al.,
1993a; Forsen et al., 1997; Eriksson et al.,
1999, 2001; Martyn et al., 1996). The pattern
for stroke is different. Whereas stroke was
similarly associated with low birth-weight, it
was not associated with thinness or shortness.
Instead there were increased rates among men
who had a low ratio of birth-weight to head
circumference (Martyn et al., 1996a; Eriksson
et al., 2000a). One interpretation of these
associations is that normal head growth has
been sustained at the cost of interrupted
growth of the body in late gestation.

Infant and Child Growth and Coronary Heart Disease

Figure 7.2 shows the growth of 357 boys who
in later life were either admitted to hospital
with coronary heart disease or died from it.
They belong to a cohort of 4630 men who were

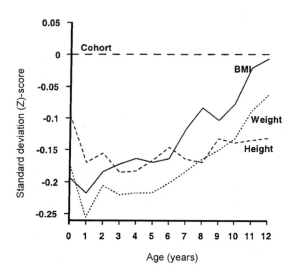

Figure 7.2 Growth of 357 boys who later
developed coronary heart disease in a cohort of 4630
boys born in Helsinki

born in Helsinki (Eriksson et al., 2001), and
their growth is expressed as Z-scores (see p 301
for definition). The Z-score for the cohort is set
at zero, and a boy maintaining a steady
position as large or small in relation to other

Table 7.1 Hazard ratios for coronary heart disease
according to body size at birth

	Hazard ratio (95% CI)	Number of cases/ number of men
Birth-weight (g)		
≤2500	3.63 (2.02–6.51)	24/160
2501–3000	1.83 (1.09–3.07)	45/599
3001–3500	1.99 (1.26–3.15)	144/1775
3501–4000	2.08 (1.31–3.31)	123/1558
>4000	1.00	21/538
p for trend	0.006	
Ponderal index (kg/m³)		
≤25	1.66 (1.11–2.48)	104/1093
25.1–27	1.44 (0.97–2.13)	135/1643
27.1–29	1.18 (0.78–1.78)	84/1260
>29	1.00	31/578
p for trend	0.0006	

Table 7.2 Hazard ratios for coronary heart disease according to body size at 1 year

	Hazard ratio (95% CI)	Number of cases/ number of men
Weight (kg)		
⩽9	1.82 (1.25–2.64)	96/781
9.1–10	1.17 (0.80–1.71)	85/1126
10.1–11	1.12 (0.77–1.64)	89/1243
11.1–12	0.94 (0.62–1.44)	49/852
>12	1.00	38/619
p for trend	<0.0001	
Height (cm)		
⩽73	1.55 (1.11–2.18)	79/636
73.1–75	0.90 (0.63–1.27)	68/962
75.1–77	0.94 (0.68–1.31)	87/1210
77.1–79	0.83 (0.58–1.18)	64/1011
>79	1.00	59/802
p for trend	0.007	
Body mass index (kg/m²)		
⩽16	1.83 (1.28–2.60)	72/654
16.1–17	1.61 (1.15–2.25)	89/936
17.1–18	1.29 (0.91–1.81)	83/1136
18.1–19	1.12 (0.77–1.62)	59/941
>19	1.00	54/954
p for trend	0.0004	

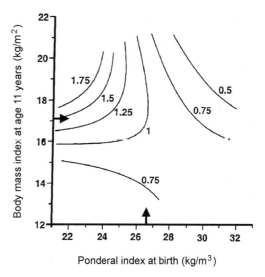

Figure 7.3 Hazard ratios for coronary heart disease according to ponderal index at birth and body mass index at 11 years. Arrows indicate average values: lines join points with the same hazard ratios

boys would follow a horizontal path on the figure. Boys who later developed coronary heart disease, however, were small at birth, remained small in infancy but had accelerated gain in weight and body mass index thereafter. In contrast, their heights remained below average (Eriksson *et al.*, 2001). Table 7.1 shows hazard ratios for coronary heart disease according to size at birth. The hazard ratios fall with increasing birth-weight and, more strongly, with increasing ponderal index (birth-weight/length³), a measure of thinness at birth. These trends were found in babies born at term or prematurely and therefore reflect slow intrauterine growth. Table 7.2 shows that the hazard ratios also fell with increasing weight, height and body mass index at age one year (Eriksson *et al.*, 2001). Small size at this age

predicts coronary heart disease independently of size at birth. In a simultaneous analysis with birth-weight the hazard ratio associated with each unit decrease in Z-score for weight between birth and 1 year was 1.21 (1.08–1.36, *p*=0.001).

This association with poor weight gain in infancy was first shown in Hertfordshire (Osmond *et al.*, 1993): the strength of the association is similar in the Hertfordshire and Helsinki studies. The association with rapid childhood weight gain was first shown in a study of an older cohort of men born in Helsinki (Ericksson *et al.*, 1999), while the association with low rates of height growth is consistent with the known association between the disease and short adult stature in men (Marmot *et al.*, 1984).

Figure 7.3, based on the same data as used in Figure 7.2, shows the combined effects of ponderal index at birth and body mass index in childhood in the Helsinki cohort (Eriksson *et al.*, 2001). The figure uses body mass indexes at age 11 years, but body mass indexes at ages around this give similar results. The lines on the figure join points with the same hazard

Table 7.3 Prevalence of non-insulin-dependent diabetes (NIDDM, 2 h glucose $\geqslant 11.1$ mmol/l) and impaired glucose tolerance (2 h glucose 7.8–11.0 mmol/l) in 370 men aged 59–70 years

Birth-weight in pounds (kg)	Number of men	Percentage with 2 h plasma glucose $\geqslant 11.1$ mmol/l	Percentage with 2 h plasma glucose $\geqslant 7.8$ mmol/l	Odds ratio (95% CI)[a] of NIDDM or impaired glucose tolerance
$\leqslant 5.5$ (<2.54)	20	10	40	6.6 (1.5–28)
5.6–6.5 (2.55–2.95)	47	13	34	4.8 (1.3–17)
6.6–7.5 (2.96–3.41)	104	6	31	4.6 (1.4–16)
6.7–8.5 (3.42–3.86)	117	7	22	2.6 (0.8–8.9)
8.6–9.5 (3.87–4.31)	54	9	13	1.4 (0.3–5.6)
>9.5 (>4.31)	28	0	14	1.0
All	370	7	25	

[a]Adjusted for current body mass index.
Derived from Hales *et al.* (1991).

ratios. For example, the line for the highest ratio, 1.75, is associated with low ponderal index at birth, but above-average body mass index in childhood. Boys who had a low ponderal index at birth increased their risk of coronary heart disease if they attained even average body mass index in childhood. In contrast, among boys with a high ponderal index no increased risk was associated with a high childhood body mass index. The interaction between ponderal index at birth and body mass index in childhood is strongly statistically significant ($p<0.001$). Findings among girls are similar, and again the risk of coronary heart disease is determined more by the tempo of weight gain than the body size attained (Forsen *et al.*, 1999).

Confounding variables

These findings suggest that influences linked to fetal and placental growth have an important effect on the risk of coronary heart disease and stroke. It has been argued, however, that people whose growth was impaired *in utero* may continue to be exposed to an adverse environment in childhood and adult life, and it is this later environment that produces the effects attributed to programming. There is strong evidence that this argument cannot be sustained. In four of the studies which have replicated the association between birth-weight and coronary heart disease, data on adult lifestyle factors including smoking, employment, diet, alcohol consumption and exercise were collected (Frankel *et al.*, 1996; Rich-Edwards *et al.*, 1997; Barker *et al.*, 2001; Leon *et al.*, 1997). Allowance for them had little effect on the association between birth-weight and coronary heart disease.

In studies exploring the mechanisms underlying these associations, the trends in coronary heart disease with birth-weight are paralleled by similar trends in two of its major risk factors – hypertension and non-insulin-dependent diabetes mellitus (Barker *et al.*, 1989; Eriksson *et al.*, 2000b; Hales *et al.*, 1991; Huxley *et al.*, 2000; Law *et al.*, 2001). Table 7.3 illustrates the size of these trends, the prevalence of non-insulin-dependent diabetes mellitus and impaired glucose tolerance falling 3-fold between men who weighed 5.5 lb (2.5 kg) at birth and those who weighed 9.5 lb (4.3 mg); (Hales *et al.*, 1991). These associations with small size at birth were again independent of social class, cigarette smoking and alcohol consumption. Influences in adult life, however, add to the effects of the intrauterine environment. For example, the prevalence of impaired glucose tolerance is highest in people who had low birth-weight but became obese as adults.

Hypertension

Associations between low birth-weight and raised blood pressure in childhood and adult life have been extensively demonstrated around the world. A systematic review of published papers described the associations between birth-weight and blood pressure (Huxley *et al.*, 2000) in 80 studies of people of all ages in many countries. These associations were not confounded by socio-economic conditions at the time of birth or in adult life. The difference in systolic pressure associated with a 1 kg difference in birth-weight was around 2.0 mmHg. In clinical practice this would be a small difference but this is a large difference between the mean values of populations and may correspond to a substantial proportion of total attributable mortality.

The association between low birth-weight and raised blood pressure depends on babies who were born small for dates after reduced fetal growth, rather than on babies born pre-term (Barker, 1998). Although in these studies alcohol consumption and higher body mass were also associated with raised blood pressure, the associations between birth-weight and blood pressure were independent of them. Nevertheless, body mass remains an important influence on blood pressure and, in humans and animals, the highest pressures are found in those who were small at birth but become overweight as adults (Eriksson *et al.*, 2000b).

As already discussed, birth-weight is a crude measure of fetal growth that does not distinguish thinness or short length, differences in head size, or variations in the balance of fetal and placental size. Analyses of babies born in Preston, UK, defined two groups who developed raised adult blood pressures (Barker *et al.*, 1992). The first group had below-average placental weight and were thin with a low ponderal index and a below-average head circumference. The second had above-average placental weight and a short crown–heel length in relation to their head circumference; such short babies tend to be fat and may have above-average birth-weight. In contrast to the associations between birth size and coronary heart disease, those between birth-weight and blood pressure are generally as strong as those between thinness, shortness and blood pressure. Associations between blood pressure and thinness and shortness have been found in some studies but not in others (Barker, 1998). In a longitudinal study of young people in Adelaide, associations between blood pressure and thinness and shortness were not apparent at age 8 years, but emerged at age 20 (Moore *et al.*, 1999).

Placental size and blood pressure

Table 7.4 shows the systolic pressure of a group of men and women who were born at term in Preston, UK, 50 years ago (Barker *et al.*, 1992). Subjects are grouped according to their birth-weights and placental weights. As in other studies, systolic pressure falls between subjects with low and high birth-weight. In addition, however, there is an increase in blood pressure with increasing placental weight. Subjects with a mean systolic pressure of 150 mmHg or more, a level sometimes used to define hypertension in clinical practice, comprise a group who as babies were relatively small in relation to the size of their placentas. There are similar trends with diastolic pressure. A rise in blood pressure with increasing placental weight and a higher ratio of placental weight to birth-weight was also found in 4-year-old children in Salisbury, UK, and among young adults in Adelaide, Australia

Table 7.4 Mean systolic blood pressure (mmHg) of men and women aged 50, born after 38 completed weeks of gestation, according to placental weight and birth-weight

Birth-weight, lb (kg)	≤1.0 (454)	1.1–1.25 (455–568)	1.3–1.5 (569–681)	>1.5 (>681)	All
		Placental weight, lb (g)			
≤6.5 (2.9)	149 (24)	152 (46)	151 (18)	167 (6)	152 (94)
6.6–7.5 (3.0–3.4)	139 (16)	148 (63)	146 (35)	159 (23)	148 (137)
>7.5 (>3.4)	131 (3)	143 (23)	148 (30)	153 (40)	149 (96)
All	144 (43)	148 (132)	148 (83)	156 (69)	149[a] (327)

[a]sd=20.4.
Figures in parentheses are numbers of subjects.

(Law *et al.*, 1991; Moore *et al.*, 1999). In studies of children and adults the association between placental enlargement and raised blood pressure has, however, been inconsistent. For example, in a study of men and women born in Aberdeen, Scotland, after World War II, at a time when food was still rationed, raised blood pressure was associated with small placental size (Campbell *et al.*, 1996). As referred to later, animal studies offer a possible explanation of this inconsistency. In sheep the placenta enlarges in response to moderate undernutrition in mid-pregnancy (Robinson *et al.*, 1994). This effect, thought to be an adaptive response to extract more nutrients from the mother, is however only seen in ewes that were well nourished before pregnancy.

Mother's blood pressure

In some studies the blood pressures of the mothers during and after pregnancy have been recorded. They correlate with the offspring's blood pressure. However, the associations between body size and proportions at birth and later blood pressure are independent of the mothers' blood pressures (Barker, 1998; Law *et al.*, 1991; Martyn *et al.*, 1995).

Childhood growth

There are a number of possible mechanisms by which restricted intrauterine growth could either initiate raised blood pressure or lead to accentuated amplification of blood pressure in later life. Studies in the USA, the UK and Holland have shown that blood pressure in childhood predicts the likelihood of developing hypertension in adult life. These predictions are strongest after adolescence. In children the rise of blood pressure with age is closely related to growth and is accelerated by the adolescent growth spurt. These observations have led Lever and Harrap to propose that essential hypertension is a disorder of growth (Lever and Harrap, 1992). The hypothesis that hypertension is a disorder of accelerated childhood growth can be reconciled with the association with low birth-weight by postulating that rapid postnatal compensatory growth plays an important role in amplifying changes established *in utero*.

Renin-angiotensin system

If the materno-placental supply of nutrients does not match fetal requirements in the last trimester of pregnancy the fetus diverts blood and nutrients to maintain brain metabolism at the expense of the trunk and limbs. This adaptation reduces blood flow to the fetal kidneys and may underlie activation of the fetal renin–angiotensin system in intrauterine growth retardation. This raises the possibility that changes in the system that may underlie the programming of hypertension. A follow-up study of men and women born in Sheffield, UK found, however, that those who had been small at birth had *lower* plasma concentrations of inactive and active renin (Martyn *et al.*, 1996b). Causes of raised blood pressure that are not mediated by increased renin release tend to result in low concentrations of renin; these findings therefore suggest that the association between impaired fetal growth and raised blood pressure involves mechanisms other than the renin–angiotensin system. Low concentrations of renin in adult life do not, however, exclude the possibility of an earlier but lasting influence of the renin–angiotensin system.

Renal structure

An alternative explanation for the low plasma renin concentrations of people who were small at birth is that they reflect a relative deficit of nephrons. Brenner suggested that retarded fetal growth leads to reduced numbers of nephrons, increasing pressure in the glomerular capillaries and leading to glomerular sclerosis (Mackenzie and Brenner, 1995). This sclerosis results in further loss of nephrons and a self-perpetuating cycle of hypertension and progressive glomerular injury. The numbers of nephrons in the normal population varies widely, from 300 000 to 1 100 000 or more (Mackenzie and Brenner, 1995). Fetal ultrasound has shown that babies that are small for gestational age have reduced renal growth during a critical period between 26 and 34 weeks of gestation. This reduces the antero-posterior size of the kidney but does not diminish kidney length (Konje *et al.*, 1996).

Endocrine

Animal studies have led to the hypothesis that impaired fetal growth alters the fetus's hypothalamic–pituitary–adrenal axis which in turn re-sets homeostatic mechanisms controlling blood pressure (Edwards *et al.*, 1993). Studies of men and women in Hertfordshire, Preston and Adelaide have shown that those who had been small at birth had increased fasting plasma cortisol concentrations (Phillips *et al.*, 2000), preliminary evidence that the hypothalamic–pituitary–adrenal axis can be programmed in humans.

Vascular structure

The content and arrangement of elastin in the aorta and large conduit arteries play an important part in minimizing the rise of blood pressure in systole and maintaining blood pressure in diastole. Elastin is only synthesized in early life and the gradual loss or fracture of elastin fibres is thought to contribute to the rise in systolic and pulse pressure with ageing. These considerations have led to the hypothesis that impaired fetal development may be associated with a relative deficiency in elastin synthesis, resulting in stiffer arteries and raised blood pressure in postnatal life (Martyn and Greenwald, 1997). This hypothesis is supported by a study of 50-year-old men and women showing that those who had a small abdominal circumference at birth tended to have a higher pulse wave velocity and decreased arterial elasticity in adult life (Martyn *et al.*, 1995).

In the growth-retarded fetus there are changes in blood flow in several vascular beds, including the descending aorta and cerebral vasculature (Al-Ghazali *et al.*, 1989). If sustained they may lead to reduced growth of the abdominal viscera and shortness at birth. Elastin deposition in fetal blood vessels is related to blood flow and 'brain-sparing' reflexes that reduce flow in the large arteries of the trunk and legs may diminish elastin deposition, leading to less compliant arteries and consequent hypertension.

Further studies suggest that, in addition to its associations with compliance, low birth-weight is also associated with persisting alterations in vascular structure and function. Hertfordshire men who had had low birth-weight had narrow bifurcation angles in their retinal blood vessels (Barker, 1998). People with hypertension have similar changes in retinal vascular geometry. In a study of children, those of low birth-weight had reduced flow-mediated dilatation in the brachial artery after the artery had been occluded and released. Flow-mediated dilatation depends on the endothelium. These findings suggest, therefore, a link between low birth-weight and endothelial dysfunction (Leeson *et al.*, 1997).

Nervous system

People with high blood pressure tend to have a high resting pulse rate. This is associated with high cardiac output, a hyperdynamic circulation and features of increased sympathetic nervous system activity. Among men and women in Preston, those who had low birth-weight had a higher resting pulse rate (Phillips and Barker, 1997). This is consistent with the hypothesis that retarded growth *in utero* establishes increased sympathetic nervous activity and leads to raised blood pressure in later life.

Non-insulin-dependent Diabetes

Insulin has a central role in fetal growth, and disorders of glucose and insulin metabolism are therefore an obvious possible link between early growth and cardiovascular disease. Although obesity and a sedentary lifestyle are known to be important in the development of non-insulin-dependent diabetes, they seem to lead to the disease only in predisposed individuals. Family and twin studies have suggested that the predisposition is familial, but the nature of this predisposition is unknown. The disease tends to be transmitted through the maternal rather than the paternal side of the family.

Size at birth and non-insulin dependent diabetes

A number of studies have confirmed the association between birth-weight and impaired glucose tolerance and non-insulin-dependent diabetes first reported in Hertfordshire (Table 7.3; Barker, 1998; Hales *et al.*, 1991; Lithell *et al.*, 1996; Curhan *et al.*, 1996; McCance *et al.*, 1994; Barker *et al.*, 1993b). In the Health Professionals Study, USA, the odds ratio for diabetes, after adjusting for current body mass, was 1.9 among men whose birth-weight was less than 5.5 lb (2.5 kg) compared with those who weighed 7.0–8.5 lb (3.2–3.9 kg; Curhan *et al.*, 1996). Among the Pima Indians, USA, the odds ratio for diabetes was 3.8 in men and women who weighed less than 5.5 lb (2.5 kg; McCance *et al.*, 1994). In Preston it was the thin babies who developed impaired glucose tolerance and diabetes. Lithell *et al.* (1996) confirmed the association with thinness in Uppsala, Sweden (Table 7.5); the prevalence of diabetes was three times higher among men in the lowest fifth of ponderal index at birth. Among the Pima Indians diabetes in pregnancy is unusually common and the association between birth-weight and non-insulin-dependent diabetes is U-shaped, with an increased prevalence in young people with birth-weights over 9.9 lb (>4.5 kg; McCance *et al.*, 1994). The increased risk of diabetes among those of high birth-weight was associated with maternal diabetes in pregnancy.

Table 7.5 Prevalence of non-insulin-dependent diabetes by ponderal index at birth among 60-year-old men in Uppsala, Sweden

Ponderal index at birth (kg/m^3)	Number of men	Prevalence (%) of diabetes
≤24.2	193	11.9
24.3–25.8	193	5.2
25.9–27.3	196	3.6
27.4–29.3	188	4.3
≥29.4	201	3.5
All	971	5.7
p value for trend		0.001

Insulin resistance

Both deficiency in insulin production and insulin resistance are thought to be important in the pathogenesis of non-insulin dependent diabetes. There is evidence that both may be determined in fetal life. Men and women with low birth-weight have a high prevalence of the 'insulin resistance syndrome' (Barker *et al.*, 1993b), in which impaired glucose tolerance, hypertension and raised serum triglyceride concentrations occur in the same patient; Table 7.6 shows results for a sample of 407 men in Hertfordshire. Phillips *et al.* (1994a) carried out insulin tolerance tests on 103 men and women in Preston. At each body mass, insulin resistance was greater in people who had had a low ponderal index at birth.

Conversely, at each ponderal index, resistance was greater in those with high body mass. The greatest insulin resistance was therefore in those with low ponderal index at birth but high current body mass.

A study in San Antonio, Texas, USA, confirmed the association between low birth-weight and the insulin resistance syndrome in 30-year-old Mexican-Americans and non-Hispanic white people (Valdez *et al.*, 1994). Among men and women in the lowest third of the birth-weight distribution and the highest third of current body mass 25 per cent had the syndrome. By contrast none of those in the highest third of birth-weight and lowest third of current body mass had it. A study of young adults in France showed that those who had had intrauterine growth retardation had raised plasma insulin concentrations when fasting and after a glucose challenge (Leger *et al.*, 1997). They did not show any of the other abnormalities that occur in the insulin resistance syndrome. This suggests that insulin resistance may be a primary abnormality to which other changes are secondary. A follow-up study of men and women who were *in utero* during the Dutch famine provides direct evidence that maternal undernutrition can programme insulin resistance and non-insulin-dependent diabetes (Ravelli *et al.*, 1998). Those exposed to famine *in utero* had higher 2 h plasma glucose and insulin concentrations than those born before or conceived after the famine.

Table 7.6 Prevalence of the insulin resistance syndrome in men aged 59–70 years according to birth-weight

Birth-weight, lb (kg)	Number of men	Percentage with insulin resistance syndrome	Odds ratio adjusted for body mass index (95% confidence interval)
≤5.5 (≤2.50)	20	30	18 (2.6–118)
5.6–6.5 (2.51–2.95)	54	19	8.4 (1.5–49)
6.6–7.5 (2.96–3.41)	114	17	8.5 (1.5–46)
7.6–8.5 (3.42–3.86)	123	12	4.9 (0.9–27)
8.6–9.5 (3.87–4.31)	64	6	2.2 (0.3–14)
>9.5 (4.31)	32	6	1.0
All	407	14	

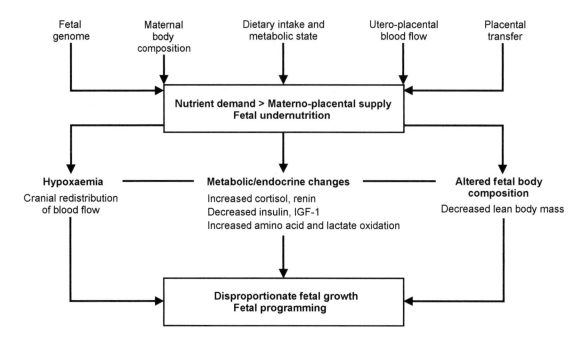

Figure 7.4   Framework for understanding the maternal regulation of fetal development and programming

Law *et al.* (1995) reported associations between thinness at birth and raised 30 min plasma glucose concentrations in 7-year-old children in Salisbury, UK. In a group of older children, Whincup *et al.* (1997) found that those who had lower birth-weight had raised plasma insulin concentrations, both fasting and after oral glucose, suggesting insulin resistance. Among these children, however, those who had low birth-weight had normal plasma glucose concentrations, which implies that, despite being insulin-resistant, they were currently able to maintain glucose homeostasis. These findings in children support an intrauterine origin for non-insulin-dependent diabetes and suggest that the seeds of diabetes in the next generation have already been sown and are apparent in today's children.

Mechanisms

The processes that link thinness at birth with insulin resistance in adult life are not known.

Babies born at term with a low ponderal index have a reduced mid-arm circumference and low muscle bulk. It is possible that thinness at birth is associated with abnormalities in muscle structure and function which originate in mid-gestation and have long-term consequences that interfere with insulin's ability to promote glucose uptake in skeletal muscle. Magnetic resonance spectroscopy studies show that people who were thin at birth have lower rates of glycolysis and glycolytic ATP production during exercise (Taylor *et al.*, 1995). In response to undernutrition a fetus may reduce its metabolic dependence on glucose and increase oxidation of other substrates, including amino acids and lactate (Figure 7.4). This has led to the hypothesis that a glucose-sparing metabolism persists into adult life, and that insulin resistance arises as a consequence of similar processes, possibly because of reduced rates of glucose oxidation in insulin-sensitive peripheral tissues.

When the availability of nutrients to the fetus is restricted concentrations of anabolic hormones, including insulin and insulin-like growth factor I, fall, while catabolic hormones, including glucocorticoids, rise (Figure 7.4). Persisting hormonal changes could underlie the development of insulin resistance. Bjorntorp (1995) has postulated that glucocorticoids, growth hormone and sex steroids may play major roles in the evolution of the metabolic syndrome.

Insulin deficiency

Infants who are small for dates have fewer pancreatic β-cells and there is evidence that nutritional and other factors determining fetal and infant growth influence the size and function of the adult β-cell complement (Hales and Barker, 1992). Whether and when non-insulin-dependent diabetes supervenes will be determined by the rate of attrition of β-cells with ageing, and by the development of insulin resistance, of which obesity is an important determinant.

While studies of adults in Preston (Phillips et al., 1994b) and Stockholm (Alvarsson et al., 1994) have found no association between birth-weight and insulin responses to infused glucose, it is possible that insulin resistance in adult life changes insulin secretion and obscures associations with fetal growth. Studies of younger people may resolve this. A study of men aged 21 years showed that those with lower birth-weight had reduced plasma insulin concentrations 30 min after a glucose challenge (Robinson et al., 1992). Another study of men of similar age showed that a low insulin response to glucose was associated with high placental weight and a high ratio of placental weight to birth-weight (Wills et al., 1996). In contrast, a study of young Pima Indians showed that those with low birth-weight had evidence of insulin resistance but no defect in insulin secretion (Dabelea et al., 1999).

In Mysore, South India, men and women with non-insulin-dependent diabetes showed

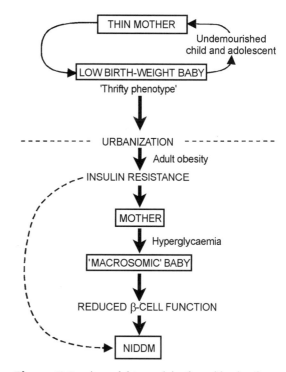

Figure 7.5 A model to explain the epidemic of non-insulin-dependent diabetes in urban India

signs of both insulin resistance and deficiency (Fall et al., 1998). As in people from South India living in Britain, there was a high prevalence of insulin resistance and central adiposity in this population. Those in Mysore who had non-insulin-dependent diabetes, however, also had a low insulin increment after a glucose challenge, indicating insulin deficiency as well as resistance. Whereas, however, insulin resistance was associated with low birth-weight, non-insulin-dependent diabetes was associated with shortness at birth in relation to birth-weight, that is a high ponderal index, and with maternal adiposity (Fall et al., 1998).

These findings led to a novel hypothesis to account for the epidemic of non-insulin-dependent diabetes in urban and migrant Indian populations (Fall et al., 1998; Figure 7.5). Widespread fetal undernutrition predisposes the Indian population to insulin resistance. On moving to cities, people's levels of physical activity diminish. Young women, no longer required to do agricultural work or walk long distances to fetch water and firewood, become fatter and therefore more insulin-resistant. They are therefore unable to maintain glucose homeostasis during pregnancy, even at relatively low levels of obesity, and become hyperglycaemic, although not necessarily diabetic. It is known that high plasma glucose concentrations within the normal range influence fetal growth and lead to macrosomia (Farmer *et al.*, 1988).

Serum cholesterol and blood clotting

Studies in Sheffield, UK, show that the neonate that has a short body and low birthweight in relation to the size of its head has persisting disturbances of cholesterol metabolism and blood coagulation (Barker, 1998). Disproportion in body length relative to head size is thought to result from cranial redistribution of blood flow associated with hypoxaemia and undernutrition in late gestation. The fetus diverts oxygenated blood away from the trunk to sustain the brain. This affects the growth of the liver, two of whose functions, regulation of cholesterol and of blood clotting, seem to be permanently perturbed. Disturbance of cholesterol metabolism and blood clotting are both important features of coronary heart disease.

The Sheffield records included abdominal circumference at birth, as well as length, and it was specifically reduction in this birth measurement that predicted raised serum low-density-lipoprotein cholesterol and plasma fibrinogen concentrations in adult life (Barker, 1998). The differences in concentrations across the range of abdominal circumference were large, statistically equivalent to 30 per cent differences in mortality from coronary heart disease. Findings for plasma fibrinogen con-

centrations, a measure of blood coagulability, were of similar size. One interpretation is that reduced abdominal circumference at birth reflects impaired liver growth and consequent re-programming of liver metabolism. Further understanding of liver programming came from experiments on rats showing that undernutrition *in utero* can permanently alter the balance of two liver enzymes, phosphoenolpyruvate carboxykinase and glucokinase, involved respectively in the synthesis and breakdown of glucose (Desai *et al.*, 1995). A low-protein diet during gestation permanently changes the balance of enzyme activity in the offspring in favour of synthesis. This is thought to reflect enhanced cell replication in the area around the portal vein, carrying blood from the gut to the liver, at the expense of the cells around the hepatic vein. These experiments are of particular interest because undernutrition after birth had no effect, and because the two enzymes are not normally synthesized until after birth, suggesting that their production can be regulated before the genes encoding them are transcribed.

Fetal Nutrition

The demonstration that normal variations in fetal size and proportions at birth have implications for health throughout life has prompted a re-evaluation of the regulation of fetal growth and development. Although the fetal genome determines *growth potential in utero*, the weight of evidence suggests that it plays a subordinate role in determining the growth that is actually achieved (Snow, 1989). Rather, it seems that the dominant determinant of fetal growth is the nutritional and hormonal milieu in which the fetus develops, and in particular the nutrient and oxygen supply.

Support for the importance of the intrauterine environment comes from animal cross-breeding experiments and from studies of half-siblings related either through the mother or the father (Morton, 1955). For example, among half-siblings, those with the same mother have similar birth-weights (correlation coefficient 0.58); birth-weights of half-siblings with the same father are dissimilar (correlation coefficient 0.1; Morton, 1955). A study of babies born after ovum donation illustrates how birth size is essentially controlled by the mother's body and the nutritional environment it affords (Brooks et al., 1995). The birth-weights of the babies were unrelated to the weights of the women who donated the eggs but strongly related to the weight of the recipient mother, heavier mothers having larger babies. While maternal cigarette smoking is known to restrict fetal growth, follow-up studies have generally shown that it is not related to levels of cardiovascular risk factors in the offspring (Law et al., 1991).

Animal experiments suggest that fetal undernutrition in early gestation produces small but normally proportioned offspring, whereas undernutrition in late gestation may alter body proportions but have less effect on birth-weight (Barker, 1998). The varying critical periods during which organs and systems mature indicate that an adverse intrauterine environment at different developmental stages is likely to have differing short- and long-term effects. For example, there is a critical period for gonadal development early in gestation, as compared with one for renal development later in gestation between 26 and 34 weeks of pregnancy. The observation that babies that were symmetrically small, short or thin at birth are predisposed to different disorders in adult life (Barker, 1998) may in part reflect an adverse intrauterine environment at different developmental stages.

With respect to timing, effects manifest late in pregnancy may commonly originate much earlier in gestation. For example, studies of the Dutch famine of 1944–1945 led to the dogma that thinness at birth results from exposure in the last trimester of pregnancy (Stein et al.,

1975). Outside the setting of famine, animal and human studies indicate that fetal under-nutrition in late pregnancy is, however, generally a consequence of an inadequate materno-placental supply capacity set up earlier in gestation (Godfrey et al., 1997). Thus, while the short- and long-term effects of an acute severe famine are of great scientific importance, we must be aware that they could result in erroneous conclusions about timing in the non-famine situation.

Maternal Influences on Fetal Nutrition

Size at birth reflects the product of the fetus's trajectory of growth, set at an early stage in development, and the materno-placental capacity to supply sufficient nutrients to maintain that trajectory. Failure of the materno-placental supply line to satisfy fetal nutrient requirements results in a range of fetal adaptations and developmental changes (Figure 7.4). It is thought that these may lead to permanent alterations in the body's structure and metabolism, and thereby to cardiovascular and metabolic disease in adult life. In Western communities, randomized controlled trials of maternal macronutrient supplementation have had relatively small effects on birth-weight (Kramer, 1993). These have led to the view that regulatory mechanisms in the maternal and placental systems act to ensure that human fetal growth and development is little influenced by normal variations in maternal nutrient intake, and that there is a simple relationship between a woman's body composition and the growth of her fetus. Recent experimental studies in animals and observational data in humans challenge these concepts (Barker, 1998). These suggest that a mother's own fetal growth and her dietary intakes and body composition can exert major effects on the balance between the fetal demand for nutrients and the materno-placental capacity to meet that demand.

Quite apart from any long-term effects on health in adult life, specific issues that have not been adequately addressed in previous studies of maternal nutrition include: (a) effects on the trajectory of fetal growth; (b) intergenerational effects; (c) paradoxical effects on placental growth; (d) effects on fetal proportions and specific tissues; and (e) the importance of the balance of macronutrients in the mother's diet and of her body composition.

The fetal growth trajectory

A rapid trajectory of growth increases the fetus's demand for nutrients. This reflects effects on both maintenance requirements, greater in fetuses that have achieved a larger size as a result of a faster growth trajectory, and on requirements for future growth. Although the fetal demand for nutrients is greatest late in pregnancy, the magnitude of this demand is thought to be primarily deter-mined by genetic and environmental effects on the trajectory of fetal growth set at an early stage in development. Experimental studies of pregnant ewes have shown that, although a fast growth trajectory is generally associated with larger fetal size and improved neonatal survival, it does render the fetus more vulner-able to a reduced materno-placental supply of nutrients in late gestation. Thus, maternal undernutrition during the last trimester adversely affected the development of rapidly growing fetuses with high requirements, while having little effect on those growing more slowly (Harding *et al.*, 1992). Rapidly growing fetuses were found to make a series of adapta-tions in order to survive, including fetal wasting and placental oxidation of fetal amino acids to maintain lactate output to the fetus (Harding *et al.*, 1992).

Although the identity of the major genes determining growth potential and the fetal growth trajectory is unknown, animal studies indicate that insulin-like growth factors and their receptors may be important. Experiments in animals have shown that periconceptional alterations in maternal diet and plasma progesterone concentrations can alter gene expression in the pre-implantation embryo to change the fetal growth trajectory (Walker *et al.*, 1996). Environmental effects have been demonstrated on both embryonic growth rates and on cell allocation in the pre-implantation embryo. New data from rats fed a 9 per cent casein low-protein diet in the periconceptional period found that this was not only associated with reduced trophectoderm and inner cell mass cell numbers at the expanding blastocyst stage, but also with permanently raised blood pressure in the offspring during adult life (Kwong *et al.*, 2000). Maternal progesterone treatment can also permanently alter the trajectory of fetal growth by changing the allocation of cells between the inner cell mass that develops into the fetus and the outer trophectoderm that becomes the placenta (Walker *et al.*, 1996). The trajectory of fetal growth is thought to increase with improve-ments in periconceptional nutrition, and is faster in male fetuses. The greater vulnerability of such fetuses on a fast growth trajectory may contribute to the rise in coronary heart disease with Westernization and the higher death rates in men.

Intergenerational effects

Experimental studies in animals have shown that undernutrition over many generations can have cumulative effects on reproductive performance over several generations. Thus, feeding rats a protein-deficient diet over 12 generations resulted in progressively greater fetal growth retardation over the generations; following re-feeding with a normal diet it then took three generations to normalize growth and development (Stewart *et al.*, 1980).

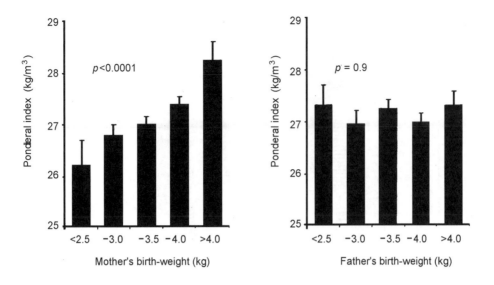

Figure 7.6   Ponderal index at birth in 492 term Southampton pregnancies according to the mother's and father's birth-weights. Values are means ($\pm$SE) adjusted for sex and gestation. Derived from Godfrey *et al*. (1997)

Strong evidence for major intergenerational effects in humans has come from studies showing that a woman's birth-weight influences the birth-weight of her offspring (Emanuel *et al*., 1992). We have, moreover, found that, whereas low-birth-weight mothers tend to have thin infants with a low ponderal index, the father's birth-weight is unrelated to ponderal index at birth (Figure 7.6); crown–heel length at birth is, however, more strongly related to the father's birth-weight than to the mother's (Godfrey *et al*., 1997). The effect of *maternal* birth-weight on thinness at birth is consistent with the hypothesis that the materno-placental supply line may be unable to satisfy fetal nutrient demand in low-birth-weight mothers. Potential mechanisms underlying this effect include alterations in the uterine or systemic vasculature, programmed changes in maternal metabolic status, and impaired placentation. The strong effect of *paternal* birth-weight on crown–heel length may reflect paternal imprinting of genes important for skeletal growth, such as those regulating the concentrations of insulin-like growth factors.

Placental size and transfer capabilities

Although the size of the placenta gives only an indirect measure of its capacity to transfer nutrients to the fetus, it is nonetheless strongly associated with fetal size at birth. Experiments in sheep have shown that maternal nutrition in early pregnancy can exert major effects on the growth of the placenta, and thereby alter fetal development (Robinson *et al*., 1994). As previously referred to, the effects produced depended on the nutritional status of the ewe in the peri-conceptional period. In ewes poorly nourished around the time of conception, high nutrient intakes in early pregnancy increased the size of the placenta. Conversely, in ewes well nourished around conception, high intakes in early pregnancy resulted in smaller placental size. Although this suppression appears paradoxical, in sheep farming it is common practice for ewes to be put on rich pasture prior to mating and then on poor pasture for a period in early pregnancy.

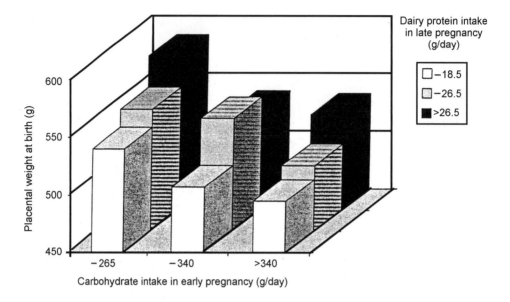

Figure 7.7   Diet in pregnancy and placental weight at birth in 538 term Southampton pregnancies. Values are adjusted for sex and the duration of gestation at delivery. *p*-Values for associations with placental weight: carbohydrate, *p*=0.002; dairy protein, *p*=0.005. Derived from Godfrey *et al.* (1996)

As part of a study designed to evaluate whether the normal variations in maternal diet found in Western communities could influence fetal growth and development, we have found evidence of a similar suppressive effect of high dietary intakes in early pregnancy on placental growth (Godfrey *et al.*, 1996). Thus, among 538 women who delivered at term, those with high dietary intakes in early pregnancy, especially of carbohydrate, had smaller placentas, particularly if combined with low intakes of dairy protein in late pregnancy (Figure 7.7; Godfrey *et al.*, 1996). These effects were independent of the mother's body size, social class and smoking, and resulted in alterations in the ratio of placental weight to birth-weight (placental ratio). Confirmation that maternal diet can alter placental growth has come from analyses of the Dutch famine, where famine exposure in early pregnancy increased placental weight (Lumey, 1998).

The U-shaped relation between the placental ratio and later coronary heart disease found in

men born earlier this century in Sheffield (Martyn *et al.*, 1996a) suggests that effects on placental growth could be of long-term importance. Babies with a disproportionately small placenta may suffer as a consequence of an impaired placental supply capacity; those with a disproportionately large placenta may experience fetal catabolism and wasting to supply amino acids for placental consumption (Robinson *et al.*, 1995). Consequent fetal adaptations may underlie the increased adult coronary heart death rates in those with both low and high placental ratios.

Effects on specific fetal tissues

Experimental studies in animals have shown that dietary manipulations during early development can have tissue-specific effects, leading to alterations in body proportions. For example, in pigs fed differing diets in the first year of life, those fed a protein-deficient diet had a disproportionately large head, ears and genitalia compared with those fed an energy-deficient diet (McCance and Widdowson, 1974). Experiments in guinea-pigs have shown that maternal undernutrition in pregnancy can result in offspring that have altered body proportions at birth and that exhibit profound elevation of serum cholesterol concentrations when fed a high-cholesterol diet in the post-weaning period (Kind et al., 1999).

In humans, few studies have examined the possibility of maternal nutrition during pregnancy having tissue-specific effects on the fetus, leading to greater alterations in neonatal proportions than in birth-weight. We have found that women with low dairy protein intakes in late pregnancy tended to have babies that were thinner at birth (Godfrey et al., 1997); maternal dairy protein intakes were not, however, related to birth-weight (Godfrey et al., 1996).

Maternal diet and body composition

Evidence supporting a long-term effect of *absolute* levels of maternal nutrient intake during pregnancy has come from a follow-up study of children whose mothers took part in a randomized controlled trial of calcium supplementation in pregnancy in Argentina (Belizan et al., 1997). This study found that maternal supplementation was associated with lowering of the offspring's blood pressure in childhood, even though supplementation was not associated with any change in birth-weight (Belizan et al., 1997). Follow-up studies following the Dutch famine of 1944–1945 found that severe maternal energy restriction at different stages of pregnancy was variously associated with obesity, dyslipidaemia and insulin resistance in the offspring, and there was preliminary evidence of an increased risk of coronary heart disease (Ravelli et al., 1998, 1999; Roseboom et al., 2000a,b).

Indications that the *balance* of macronutrients in the mother's diet can have important short- and long-term effects on the offspring has come from experimental studies in pregnant rats. These have found that maternal diets with a low ratio of protein to carbohydrate and fat alter fetal and placental growth, and result in lifelong elevation of blood pressure in the offspring (Langley-Evans and Jackson, 1994). In the Dutch studies, famine exposure *per se* was not associated with raised blood pressure in the offspring, but there was evidence for an effect of macronutrient balance; maternal rations with a low protein density were associated with raised blood pressure in the adult offspring (Roseboom et al., 2001). This adds to our studies from Aberdeen, UK, which found that maternal diets with either a low or a high ratio of animal protein to carbohydrate were associated with raised blood pressure in the offspring during adult life (Campbell et al., 1996). Maternal diets with a high protein density were also associated with insulin deficiency and impaired glucose tolerance in the offspring (Shiell et al., 2000).

While adverse effects of diets with a high protein density might appear counterintuitive, they are consistent with the results of controlled trials of dietary supplementation in pregnancy (Rush, 1989). Moreover, the Aberdeen findings have recently been replicated in a follow-up study of men and women in Motherwell, UK, whose mothers were advised to eat a high-meat-protein, low-carbohydrate diet during pregnancy (Shiell et al., 2001). The offspring's blood pressure was higher in those whose mothers reported greater intakes of meat and fish and lower intakes of carbohydrate in late pregnancy, particularly if the mother also had a low intake of green vegetables. One possibility is that the long-term effects may be consequences of the metabolic stress imposed on the mother by an unbalanced diet in which high intakes of essential amino acids are not accompanied by the other micronutrients required to utilize them (Shiell *et al.*, 2001).

With respect to maternal body composition, observations linking high maternal weight and adiposity with insulin deficiency, non-insulin-dependent diabetes and coronary heart disease in the offspring (Forsen *et al.*, 1997, 2000; Fall *et al.*, 1998) add to those of associations between gestational diabetes and adverse long-term outcomes (Silverman *et al.*, 1996). Of great importance is an increasing body of consistent evidence showing strong links between low weight and body mass index in the mother and insulin resistance and dyslipidaemia, but not raised blood pressure, in the adult offspring (Ravelli *et al.*, 1998; Shiell *et al.*, 2000; Mi *et al.*, 2000). In contrast, thin maternal skinfold thicknesses and low pregnancy weight gain have been consistently associated with raised blood pressure in the offspring (Margetts *et al.*, 1991; Godfrey *et al.*, 1994; Clark *et al.*, 1998; Adair *et al.*, 2001). For example, in studies of Jamaican children, we found strong associations between low pregnancy weight gain and thinner maternal triceps skinfold thickness in early pregnancy and raised blood pressure in the offspring, but no significant associations with maternal body mass index in early pregnancy (Godfrey *et al.*, 1994).

Responses to Adult Living Standards

Observations on animals show that the environment during development permanently changes not only the body's structure and function but also its responses to environmental influences encountered in later life (Bateson and Martin, 1999). Men who had low birthweight are more vulnerable to developing coronary heart disease and type 2 diabetes if they become overweight (Frankel *et al.*, 1996; Forsen *et al.*, 2000). Table 7.7 shows the effect of low income in adult life on coronary heart disease among men in Helsinki (Barker *et al.*, 2001). As expected, men who had a low taxable income had higher rates of the disease. There is no known explanation for this and it is a major component of the social inequalities in health in Western countries. The effect of low income, however, is confined to men who had slow fetal growth and were thin at birth, defined by a ponderal index less than $26 \, kg/m^3$. Men who were not thin at birth were resilient to the effects of low income on coronary heart disease, so that there was a statistically significant interaction between the effects of fetal growth and adult income (Barker *et al.*, 2001).

One explanation of these findings emphasizes the psychosocial consequences of a low

Table 7.7   Hazard ratios (95 per cent CI) for coronary heart disease according to ponderal index at birth (kg/m^3) at birth and taxable income in adult life

Household income×1000 marks (pounds sterling) per year	Ponderal index ≤26.0 ($n=1475$)	Ponderal index >26.0 ($n=2154$)
>140 (>15 700)	1.00	1.19 (0.65–2.19)
111–140 (12 401–15 700)	1.54 (0.83–2.87)	1.42 (0.78–2.57)
96–110 (10 701–12 400)	1.07 (0.51–2.22)	1.66 (0.90–3.07)
76–95 (8401–10 700)	2.07 (1.13–3.79)	1.44 (0.79–2.62)
≤75 (8400)	2.58 (1.45–4.60)	1.37 (0.75–2.51)
p for trend	<0.001	0.75

p for interaction between the effects of ponderal index at birth and income=0.005.

position in the social hierarchy, as indicated by low income and social class, and suggests that perceptions of low social status and lack of success lead to changes in neuroendocrine pathways and hence to disease (Marmot and Wilkinson, 2001). The findings in Helsinki seem consistent with this. People who are small at birth are known to have persisting alterations in responses to stress, including raised serum cortisol concentrations (Phillips *et al.*, 2000). Rapid childhood weight gain could exacerbate these effects.

Conclusion

The demonstration that normal variations in fetal size and thinness at birth have implications for health throughout life has prompted a re-evaluation of the regulation of fetal development. Impetus has been added to this re-evaluation by recent findings showing that a woman's diet and body composition in pregnancy are related to levels of cardiovascular risk factors and the prevalence of coronary heart disease in her offspring in adult life. These observations challenge the view that the fetus is little affected by changes in maternal nutrition, except in circumstances of famine.

The long time-scale over which the effects of an adverse intrauterine environment act dictate that we now need to progress beyond epidemiological associations to greater understanding of the cellular and molecular processes that underlie them. Szent-Gyorgi wrote that, 'for every complex problem, there is a simple, easy to understand, incorrect answer'; for fetal growth and development the complexities are such that currently available data form only a limited basis for changing dietary recommendations to pregnant women. Future work will need to identify the factors that set the trajectory of fetal growth, and the influences that limit the materno-placental delivery of nutrients and oxygen to the fetus. We also need to define how the fetus adapts to a limited nutrient supply, how these adaptations programme the structure and physiology of the body, and by what molecular mechanisms nutrients and hormones alter gene expression.

If, as we believe, a woman's own fetal growth, and her diet and body composition before and during pregnancy play a major role in programming the future health of her children, mothers will want to know what they can do to optimize the intrauterine environment they provide for their babies. A technical consultation organized by the United States Department of Agriculture, the World Bank and UNICEF concluded that a key area of focus to reduce the burden of low birthweight and its associated morbidities is to improve the nutritional status of adolescent girls and of pregnant women. Similarly, one of the two main recommendations of the Acheson Report on Inequalities in Health in the UK was that 'a high priority is given to policies aimed at improving health and reducing inequalities in women of childbearing age, expectant mothers and young children' (Independent Inquiry into Inequalities in Health, 1998). A strategy of interdependent clinical, animal and epidemiological research is required to identify specific recommendations for both whole populations and for vulnerable groups such as teenage pregnancies and single parents. Research is also required to identify the barriers to healthy eating among young women, whose diets are important both for their own health and the health of the next generation. Such an approach may allow us to reduce the prevalence of major chronic diseases and diminish social inequalities in health.

References

Adair LS, Kuzawa CW and Borja J (2001) Maternal energy stores and diet composition during pregnancy program adolescent blood pressure. *Circulation* **104**, 1034–1039.

Al-Ghazali W, Chita SK, Chapman MG and Allan LD (1989) Evidence of redistribution of cardiac output in asymmetrical growth retardation. *Br. J. Obstet. Gynaecol.* **96**, 697–704.

Alvarsson M, Efendic S and Grill VE (1994) Insulin responses to glucose in healthy males are associated with adult height but not with birth weight. *J. Intern. Med.* **236**, 275–279.

Barker DJP (1998) *Mothers, Babies and Health in Later Life*, 2nd edn. Churchill Livingstone, Edinburgh.

Barker DJP, Osmond C, Golding J, Kuh D and Wadsworth MEJ (1989) Growth *in utero*, blood pressure in childhood and adult life and mortality from cardiovascular disease. *Br. Med. J.* **298**, 564–567.

Barker DJP, Godfrey KM, Osmond C and Bull A (1992) The relation of fetal length, ponderal index and head circumference to blood pressure and the risk of hypertension in adult life. *Paediatr. Perinat. Epidemiol.* **6**, 35–44.

Barker DJP, Osmond C, Simmonds SJ and Wield GA (1993a) The relation of small head circumference and thinness at birth to death from cardiovascular disease in adult life. *Br. Med. J.* **306**, 422–426.

Barker DJP, Hales CN, Fall CHD, Osmond C, Phipps K and Clark PMS (1993b) Type 2 (non-insulin-dependent) diabetes mellitus, hypertension and hyperlipidaemia (syndrome X): relation to reduced fetal growth. *Diabetologia* **36**, 62–67.

Barker DJP, Forsen T, Uutela A, Osmond C and Eriksson JG (2001) Size at birth and resilience to the effects of poor living conditions in adult life: longitudinal study. *Br. Med. J.* **323**, 1273–1276.

Bateson P and Martin P (1999) *Design for a Life: how Behaviour Develops*. Jonathan Cape, London.

Belizan JM, Villar J, Bergel E, del Pino A, Di Fulvio S, Galliano SV and Kattan C (1997) Long term effect of calcium supplementation during pregnancy on the blood pressure of offspring: follow up of a randomised controlled trial. *Br. Med. J.* **315**, 281–285.

Bjorntorp P (1995) Insulin resistance: the consequence of a neuroendocrine disturbance? *Int. J. Obes. Relat. Metab. Disord.* **19**(Suppl. 1), S6–S10.

Brooks AA, Johnson MR, Steer PJ, Pawson ME and Abdalla HI (1995) Birth weight: nature or nurture? *Early Hum. Devl.* **42**, 29–35.

Campbell DM, Hall MH, Barker DJP, Cross J, Shiell AW and Godfrey KM (1996) Diet in pregnancy and the offspring's blood pressure 40 years later. *Br. J. Obstet. Gynaecol.* **103**, 273–280.

Clark PM, Atton C, Law CM, Shiell A, Godfrey K and Barker DJP (1998) Weight gain in pregnancy, triceps skinfold thickness and blood pressure in the offspring. *Obstet. Gynaecol.* **91**, 103–107.

Curhan GC, Willett WC, Rimm EB and Stampfer MJ (1996) Birth weight and adult hypertension and diabetes mellitus in US men. [Abstract] *Am. J. Hypertens.* **9**, 11A.

Dabelea D, Pettitt DJ, Hanson RL, Imperatore G, Bennett PH and Knowler WC (1999) Birth weight, type 2 diabetes, and insulin resistance in Pima Indian children and young adults. *Diabetes Care* **22**, 944–950.

Desai M, Crowther NJ, Ozanne SE, Lucas A and Hales CN (1995) Adult glucose and lipid metabolism may be programmed during fetal life. *Biochem. Soc. Trans.* **23**, 331–335.

Edwards CRW, Benediktsson R, Lindsay RS and Seckl JR (1993) Dysfunction of placental glucocorticoid barrier: link between foetal environment and adult hypertension? *Lancet* **341**, 355–357.

Emanuel I, Filakti H, Alberman E and Evans SJW (1992) Intergenerational studies of human birth-weight from the 1958 birth cohort. I. Evidence for a multigenerational effect. *Br. J. Obstet. Gynaecol.* **99**, 67–74.

Eriksson JG, Forsen T, Tuomilehto J, Winter PD, Osmond C and Barker DJP (1999) Catch-up growth in childhood and death from coronary heart disease: longitudinal study. *Br. Med. J.* **318**, 427–431.

Eriksson JG, Forsen T, Tuomilehto J, Osmond C and Barker DJP (2000a) Early growth, adult income and risk of stroke. *Stroke* **31**, 869–874.

Eriksson J, Forsen T, Tuomilehto J, Osmond C and Barker D (2000b) Fetal and childhood growth and hypertension in adult life. *Hypertension* **36**, 790–794.

Eriksson JG, Forsen T, Tuomilehto J, Osmond C and Barker DJP (2001) Early growth and coronary heart disease in later life: longitudinal study. *Br. Med. J.* **322**, 949–953.

Fall CHD, Stein CE, Kumaran K, Cox V, Osmond C, Barker DJP and Hales CN (1998) Size at birth, maternal weight, and type 2 diabetes in South India. *Diabet. Med.* **15**, 220–227.

Farmer G, Russell G, Hamilton-Nicol DR, Ogenbede HO, Ross IS, Pearson DWM, Thom H, Kerridge DF and Sutherland HW (1998) The influence of maternal glucose metabolism on fetal growth, development and morbidity in 917 singleton pregnancies in nondiabetic women. *Diabetologia* **31**, 134–141.

Forsen T, Eriksson JG, Tuomilehto J, Teramo K, Osmond C and Barker DJP (1997) Mother's weight in pregnancy and coronary heart disease in a cohort of Finnish men: follow up study. *Br. Med. J.* **315**, 837–840.

Forsen T, Eriksson JG, Tuomilehto J, Osmond C and Barker DJP (1999) Growth *in utero* and during childhood among women who develop coronary heart disease: longitudinal study. *Br. Med. J.* **319**, 1403–1407.

Forsen T, Eriksson J, Tuomilehto J, Reunanen A, Osmond C and Barker D (2000) The fetal and childhood growth of persons who develop type 2 diabetes. *Ann. Intern. Med.* **133**, 176–182.

Frankel S, Elwood P, Sweetnam P, Yarnell J and Davey Smith G (1996) Birthweight, body-mass index in middle age, and incident coronary heart disease. *Lancet* **348**, 1478–1480.

Godfrey KM, Forrester T, Barker DJP, Jackson AA, Landman JP, Hall JStE, Cox V and Osmond C (1994) Maternal nutritional status in pregnancy and blood pressure in childhood. *Br. J. Obstet. Gynaecol.* **101**, 398–403.

Godfrey K, Robinson S, Barker DJP, Osmond C and Cox V (1996) Maternal nutrition in early and late pregnancy in relation to placental and fetal growth. *Br. Med. J.* **312**, 410–414.

Godfrey KM, Barker DJP, Robinson S and Osmond C (1997) Maternal birthweight and diet in pregnancy in relation to the infant's thinness at birth. *Br. J. Obstet. Gynaecol.* **104**, 663–667.

Hales CN and Barker DJP (1992) Type 2 (non-insulin-dependent) diabetes mellitus: the thrifty phenotype hypothesis. *Diabetologia* **35**, 595–601.

Hales CN, Barker DJP, Clark PMS, Cox LJ, Fall C, Osmond C and Winter PD (1991) Fetal and infant growth and impaired glucose tolerance at age 64. *Br. Med. J.* **303**, 1019–1022.

Harding JE (2001) The nutritional basis of the fetal origins of adult disease. *Int. J. Epidemiol.* **30**,15–23.

Harding JE, Liu L, Evans P, Oliver M and Gluckman P (1992) Intrauterine feeding of the growth-retarded fetus: can we help? *Early Hum. Devl.* **29**, 193–197.

Huxley RR, Shiell AW and Law CM (2000) The role of size at birth and postnatal catch-up growth in determining systolic blood pressure: a systematic review of the literature. *J. Hypertens.* **18**, 815–831.

Independent Inquiry into Inequalities in Health (1998) *Report of the Independent Inquiry into Inequalities in Health.* The Stationery Office, London.

Kind KL, Clifton PM, Katsman AI, Tsiounis M, Robinson JS and Owens JA (1999) Restricted fetal growth and the response to dietary cholesterol in the guinea pig. *Am. J. Physiol.* **277**, R1675–1682.

Konje JC, Bell SC, Morton JJ, de Chazal R and Taylor DJ (1996) Human fetal kidney morphometry during gestation and the relationship between weight, kidney morphometry and plasma active renin concentration at birth. *Clin. Sci.* **91**, 169–175.

Kramer MS (1993) Effects of energy and protein intakes on pregnancy outcome: an overview of the research evidence from controlled clinical trials. *Am. J. Clin. Nutr.* **58**, 627–635.

Kwong WY, Wild AE, Roberts P, Willis AC and Fleming TP (2000) Maternal undernutrition during the preimplantation period of rat development causes blastocyst abnormalities and programming of postnatal hypertension. *Development* **127**, 4195–4202.

Langley-Evans SC and Jackson AA (1994) Increased systolic blood pressure in adult rats induced by fetal exposure to maternal low protein diets. *Clin. Sci.* **86**, 217–222.

Law CM, Barker DJP, Bull AR and Osmond C (1991) Maternal and fetal influences on blood pressure. *Arch. Dis. Child.* **66**, 1291–1295.

Law CM, Gordon GS, Shiell AW, Barker DJP and Hales CN (1995) Thinness at birth and glucose tolerance in seven year old children. *Diabet. Med.* **12**, 24–29.

Law CM, Egger P, Dada O, Delgado H, Kylberg E, Lavin P, Tang GH, von Hertzen H, Shiell AW and Barker DJ (2001) Body size at birth and blood pressure among children in developing countries. *Int. J. Epidemiol.* **30**, 52–57.

Leeson CPM, Whincup PH, Cook DG, Donald AE, Papacosta O, Lucas A and Deanfield JE (1997) Flow-mediated dilation in 9- to 11-year old children. The influence of intrauterine and childhood factors. *Circulation* **96**, 2233–2238.

Leger J, Levy-Marchal C, Bloch J, Pinet A, Chevenne D, Porquet D, Collin D and Czernichow P (1997) Reduced final height and indications for insulin resistance in 20 year olds born small for gestational age: regional cohort study. *Br. Med. J.* **315**, 341–347.

Leon DA, Lithell H, Vagero D, McKeigue P and Koupilova I (1997) Biological and social influences on mortality in a cohort of 15,000 Swedes followed from birth to old age. [Abstract]. *J. Epidemiol. Community Health* **51**, 594.

Lever AF and Harrap SB (1992) Essential hypertension: a disorder of growth with origins in childhood? *J. Hypertens.* **10**, 101–120.

Lithell HO, McKeigue PM, Berglund L, Mohsen R, Lithell UB and Leon DA (1996) Relation of size at birth to non-insulin dependent diabetes and insulin concentrations in men aged 50–60 years. *Br. Med. J.* **312**, 406–410.

Lumey LH (1998) Compensatory placental growth after restricted maternal nutrition in early pregnancy. *Placenta* **19**, 105–111.

McCance DR, Pettitt DJ, Hanson RL, Jacobsson LTH, Knowler WC and Bennett PH (1994) Birth weight and non-insulin dependent diabetes: thrifty genotype, thrifty phenotype, or surviving small baby genotype? *Br. Med. J.* **308**, 942–945.

McCance RA and Widdowson EM (1974) The determinants of growth and form. *Proc. R. Soc. Lond. B* **185**, 1–17.

Mackenzie HS and Brenner BM (1995) Fewer nephrons at birth: a missing link in the etiology of essential hypertension? *Am. J. Kidney Dis.* **26**, 91–98.

Margetts BM, Rowland MGM, Foord FA, Cruddas AM, Cole TJ and Barker DJP (1991) The relation of maternal weight to the blood pressures of Gambian children. *Int. J. Epidemiol.* **20**, 938–943.

Marmot MG, Shipley MJ and Rose G (1984) Inequalities in death – specific explanations of a general pattern? *Lancet* **i**, 1003–1006.

Marmot M and Wilkinson RG (2001) Psychosocial and material pathways in the relation between income and health: a response to Lynch *et al. Br. Med. J.* **322**, 1233–1236.

Martyn CN, Barker DJP, Jespersen S, Greenwald S, Osmond C and Berry C (1995) Growth *in utero*, adult blood pressure, and arterial compliance. *Br. Heart J.* **73**, 116–121.

Martyn CN, Barker DJP and Osmond C (1996a) Mothers' pelvic size, fetal growth, and death from stroke and coronary heart disease in men in the UK. *Lancet* **348**, 1264–1268.

Martyn CN, Lever AF and Morton JJ (1996b) Plasma concentrations of inactive renin in adult life are related to indicators of foetal growth. *J. Hypertens.* **14**, 881–886.

Martyn CN and Greenwald SE (1997) Impaired synthesis of elastin in walls of aorta and large conduit arteries during early development as an initiating event in pathogenesis of systemic hypertension. *Lancet* **350**, 953–955.

Mi J, Law C, Zhang K-L, Osmond C, Stein C and Barker D (2000) Effects of infant birthweight and maternal body mass index in pregnancy on components of the insulin resistance syndrome in China. *Ann. Intern. Med.* **132**, 253–260.

Moore VM, Cockington RA, Ryan P and Robinson JS (1999) The relationship between birth weight and blood pressure amplifies from childhood to adulthood. *J. Hypertens.* **17**, 883–888.

Morton NE (1955) The inheritance of human birth weight. *Ann. Hum. Genet.* **20**, 123–134.

Osmond C, Barker DJP, Winter PD, Fall CHD and Simmonds SJ (1993) Early growth and death from cardiovascular disease in women. *Br. Med. J.* **307**, 1519–1524.

Phillips DIW, Hirst S, Clark PMS, Hales CN and Osmond C (1994a) Fetal growth and insulin secretion in adult life. *Diabetologia* **37**, 592–596.

Phillips DIW, Barker DJP, Hales CN, Hirst S and Osmond C (1994b) Thinness at birth and insulin resistance in adult life. *Diabetologia* **37**, 150–154.

Phillips DIW and Barker DJP (1997) Association between low birth-weight and high resting pulse in adult life: is the sympathetic nervous system involved in programming the insulin resistance syndrome? *Diabet. Med.* **14**, 673–677.

Phillips DI, Walker BR, Reynolds RM, Flanagan DE, Wood PJ, Osmond C, Barker DJ and Whorwood CB (2000) Low birth weight predicts elevated plasma cortisol concentrations in adults from 3 populations. *Hypertension* **35**, 1301–1306.

Ravelli ACJ, van der Meulen JHP, Michels RPJ, Osmond C, Barker DJP, Hales CN and Bleker OP (1998) Glucose tolerance in adults after prenatal exposure to famine. *Lancet* **351**, 173–177.

Ravelli AC, van der Meulen JHP, Osmond C, Barker DJ and Bleker OP (1999) Obesity at the age of 50 y in men and women exposed to famine prenatally. *Am. J. Clin. Nutr.* **70**, 811–816.

Rich-Edwards JW, Stampfer MJ, Manson JE, Rosner B, Hankinson SE, Colditz GA, Willett WC and Hennekens CH (1997) Birth weight and risk of cardiovascular disease in a cohort of women followed up since 1976. *Br. Med. J.* **315**, 396–400.

Robinson S, Walton RJ, Clark PM, Barker DJP, Hales CN and Osmond C (1992) The relation of fetal growth to plasma glucose in young men. *Diabetologia* **35**, 444–446.

Robinson JS, Owens JA, de Barro T, Lok F and Chidzanja S (1994) Maternal nutrition and fetal growth. In: *Early Fetal Growth and Development*, ed. Ward RHT, Smith SK and Donnai D, pp. 317–334. Royal College of Obstetricians and Gynaecologists, London.

Robinson JS, Chidzanja S, Kind K, Lok F, Owens P and Owens JA (1995) Placental control of fetal growth. *Reprod. Fertil. Devl.* **7**, 333–344.

Roseboom TJ, van der Meulen JH, Osmond C, Barker DJ, Ravelli AC and Bleker OP (2000a) Plasma lipid profiles in adults after prenatal exposure to the Dutch famine. *Am. J. Clin. Nutr.* **72**, 1101–1106.

Roseboom TJ, van der Meulen JH, Osmond C, Barker DJ, Ravelli AC, Schroeder-Tanka JM, van Montfrans GA, Michels RP and Bleker OP (2000b) Coronary heart disease after prenatal exposure to the Dutch famine, 1944–45. *Heart* **84**, 595–598.

Roseboom TJ, van der Meulen JH, van Montfrans GA, Ravelli AC, Osmond C, Barker DJ and Bleker OP (2001) Maternal nutrition during gestation and blood pressure in later life. *J. Hypertens.* **19**, 29–34.

Rush D (1989) Effects of changes in maternal energy and protein intake during pregnancy, with special reference to foetal growth. In: *Fetal Growth*, ed. Sharp F, Fraser RB and Milner RDG, pp. 203–233. Royal College of Obstetricians and Gynaecologists, London.

Shiell AW, Campbell DM, Hall MH and Barker DJ (2000) Diet in late pregnancy and glucose-insulin metabolism of the offspring 40 years later. *Br. J. Obstet. Gynaecol.* **107**, 890–895.

Shiell AW, Campbell-Brown M, Haselden S, Robinson S, Godfrey KM and Barker DJP (2001) A high meat, low carbohydrate diet in pregnancy: relation to adult blood pressure in the offspring. *Hypertension* **38**, 1282–1288.

Silverman BL, Purdy LP and Metzger BE (1998) The intrauterine environment: implications for the offspring of diabetic mothers. *Diabet. Rev.* **4**, 21–35.

Snow MHL (1989) Effects of genome on fetal size at birth. In: *Fetal growth. Proceedings of the 20th Study Group*, ed. Sharp F, Fraser RB and Milner RDG, pp. 1–11. Royal College of Obstetricians and Gynaecologists, London.

Stein CE, Fall CHD, Kumaran K, Osmond C, Cox V and Barker DJP (1996) Fetal growth and coronary heart disease in South India. *Lancet* **348**, 1269–1273.

Stein Z, Susser M, Saenger G and Marolla F (1975) *Famine and Human Development: the Dutch Hunger Winter of 1944/45*. Oxford University Press, New York.

Stewart RJC, Sheppard H, Preece R and Waterlow JC (1980) The effect of rehabilitation at different stages of development of rats marginally malnourished for ten to twelve generations. *Br. J. Nutr.* **43**, 403–412.

Taylor DJ, Thompson CH, Kemp GJ, Barnes PRJ, Sanderson AL, Radda GK and Phillips DIW (1995) A relationship between impaired fetal growth and reduced muscle glycolysis revealed by ^{31}P magnetic resonance spectroscopy. *Diabetologia* **38**, 1205–1212.

Valdez R, Athens MA, Thompson GH, Bradshaw BS and Stern MP (1994) Birthweight and adult health outcomes in a biethnic population in the USA. *Diabetologia* **37**, 624–631.

Walker SK, Hartwich KM and Seamark RF (1996) The production of unusually large offspring following embryo manipulation: concepts and challenges. *Theriogenology* **45**, 111–120.

Whincup PH, Cook DG, Adshead F, Taylor SJC, Walker M, Papacosta O and Alberti KGMM (1997) Childhood size is more strongly related than size at birth to glucose and insulin levels in 10–11-year-old children. *Diabetologia* **40**, 319–326.

Wills J, Watson JM, Hales CN and Phillips DIW (1996) The relation of foetal growth to insulin secretion in young men. *Diabet. Med.* **13**, 773–774.

8

NUTRITION IN INFANCY

Lawrence T. Weaver and Ann Prentice

LEARNING OUTCOMES

- Breast-feeding is the optimum mode of feeding the newborn infant.

- Human (breast) milk is the sole and sufficient source of energy and nutrients for the infant until about 6 months.

- Human milk contains non-nutritional factors, which provide defence against infection and assist adaptation to life outside the womb.

- All mammals nourish their young on the breast and the composition of the milk of each species reflects the postnatal growth and nutritional requirements of its young.

- Human lactation may last for 2 or 3 years and milk production is largely driven by infant demand: volumes of around 700–800 ml/day are common during established breast-feeding.

- The composition of human milk varies during an individual feed and during the course of lactation, reflecting the nutritional needs of the infant.

- Lactational capacity is relatively resilient and unaffected by maternal nutritional status and dietary intake. Substrate requirements for milk production are relatively small compared with overall maternal needs.

- Energy and nutrient requirements in infancy are defined as dietary reference values based on figures calculated from intakes of breast-fed babies which include factors that account for the difference in bioavailability of some nutrients from formula milks.

- Alternatives to human milk are formulas based on cow's milk. Although these are modified to resemble human milk they cannot reproduce fully the nutrient and non-nutrient components of human milk.

- Breast-feeding is associated with many short-term and long-term health advantages to both mother and baby.

Introduction

Early infancy is a 'critical period', not just for the baby but also for its health thereafter. During the transition from intrauterine to extrauterine nutrition and for the first few months of exclusive breast-feeding, the unique composition of human milk provides and anticipates the nutritional needs of the newborn infant, and through its non-nutritional components assists in adaptation to life outside the womb. Human milk is the best food for babies and contains all the energy and nutrients they need. The bioactive non-nutritional substances, absent from commercial formula milks, confer protection from bacterial and viral infections, and may aid growth and development of the newborn.

The composition of human milk is not constant but changes during feeds, according to the time of day, and during the course of lactation. The total volume of maternal milk production and infant milk intake is variable, depending largely on postnatal age, frequency and effectiveness of suckling, and whether or not formula milk and/or complementary feeds are also being taken. Milk intake by the infant generally increases during the period of exclusive breast-feeding and can reach a plateau of about 750–800 ml per day after about 6 weeks in a singleton, and rises only slightly thereafter. However lactational capacity is relatively plastic and a healthy well-nourished mother is quite capable of providing sufficient milk to feed twins.

The human body undergoes its most rapid phase of growth during infancy and healthy babies double their birth-weight in the first 6 months and triple it in the first year. At the same time body composition changes greatly, particularly the ratio of fat to fat-free mass. Exclusive breast-feeding will fully satisfy the nutritional needs of most infants until about 6 months of age. However, as the baby gets older, bigger and more active, nutritional requirements can no longer be met by breast milk alone. Complementary foods designed to meet the nutritional and physiological needs of the infant are needed to fill the gap between what is provided by breast milk and the total nutritional requirements of the infant. Breast milk is usually the main source of food, and can supply between one-third and one-half of average total energy intake towards the end of the first year. Complementary foods provide *additional* energy and nutrients that should ideally not displace breast milk during the first year. In the developed world where infant formula milks are available, mothers tend to breast-feed for a shorter time than in many parts of the developing world, where they may continue well into the second year and longer. Material in Chapters 3, 6, 9 and 10 should be read in relation to this chapter.

Mammary Gland and Lactation

Comparative aspects

Evolution and function

Mammals owe their success, in addition to the 'amniote egg', which made placentation possible (Morriss, 1975), to the evolution of the mammary gland and to a neonatal gut with complementary morphology and function to make use of the constituents of milk. The mammary gland probably evolved before the placenta, and the provision of protective antimicrobial factors may have been an early feature of its secretions, which helped to defend the infant from the bacterial flora of maternal skin (Long, 1969).

Inverse relations between the supply of immune factors by the lactating mammary gland and the production of these defence agents by the infant are found in all mammals, and coevolution of breast and neonatal gut may have been driven by a common need for protection against infection. The fetus is shielded from most microbial pathogens and therefore does not require a fully developed defence system; energy and nutrients can be directed towards other developing body systems. Delay in immunological maturation is therefore an adaptation that avoids adverse immunological reactions to maternal tissues. A consequence is immature immunological function at birth, which is compensated for by the provision of defence factors in milk (Goldman et al., 1998).

The nutritional value of milk as a primary means of feeding the newborn may have favoured viviparous mammals (that bear young without eggs), and during their diversification and radiation the process of suckling has adapted to serve a variety of neonatal feeding strategies (Pond 1977; 1983). The evolutionary progression to birth of 'immature' mammalian young from well-developed and nutritionally independent reptilian hatchlings was accompanied by a long suckling period. The maternal supply and processing of food made an adult masticatory apparatus and digestive system unnecessary for the neonate, whose gastrointestinal tract and intermediary metabolism became adapted to the utilization of milk. Lactation provides a regulated food supply to the young which is constantly available and of controlled composition. It has permitted the geographical mobility of species unconstrained by the need to seek food for their infants. Mammals have been able to exploit most terrestrial habitats, as well as the skies, seas and inland waters with their diverse food resources, while continuing to provide a uniform source of food to their young.

Although the number of glands differs between species (broadly related to the number of progeny), the structure and function of the breast of all placental mammals (eutheria) are essentially the same. Secreted into the lumen between cells, milk drains via a system of arborizing ducts to a nipple or teat at the skin surface. Each mammary gland is anatomically and functionally independent, and milk secretion is continuous during lactation. The epithelial cells of the alveoli and ducts, which in some species open into sinuses or cisterns, regulate the final composition of milk, like the secretions of other exocrine glands. A network of myoepithelial cells surrounding the alveoli causes milk ejection during suckling. The lactating human breast consists of 10–15 discrete lobes of glandular tissue draining independently to external openings at the nipple (Figure 8.1). It has no storage cisterns, such as are found in the cow and goat, and milk is stored primarily within the alveoli prior to ejection.

Suckling at the breast, while not requiring teeth, allows rapid postnatal growth of the infant skull (and therefore brain) before the appearance of the first dentition. Milk provides many nutrients, especially lactose and some fats, synthesized by the mother and not

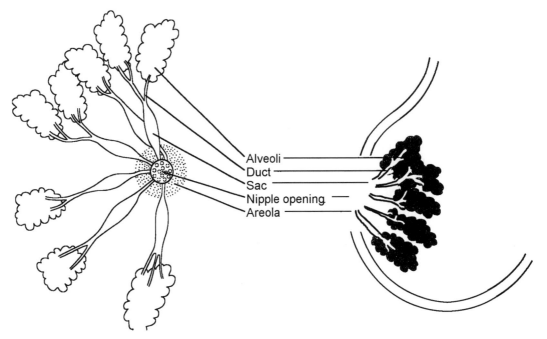

Figure 8.1   The human breast

available in other foods, and essential nutrients such as calcium, which are 'packaged' for secure transfer to and assimilation by the baby. Milk feeding favours a close relationship between mother and young which in the higher mammals, particularly primates, is important for the acquisition of learned behaviour, as well as for protection and nutrition. Mammalian investment in few young that are very likely to survive involves a high nutritional cost (both prenatally and postnatally). However in the overall economy of the mother–infant pair, milk feeding is energetically less expensive than food foraging by either mother or young. In these respects the newborn mammal may be considered an extragestate fetus until weaning, when it becomes truly independent.

Mammalian milks

As the sole food for the suckling newborn, milk contains all the energy and nutrients in appropriate amounts for infant growth and development, as well as many non-nutrient substances essential for perinatal adaptation to neonatal life. The composition and yield of the milk of present-day mammals varies according to maternal size, reproductive rate, litter size and nutrient stores, maturity of the young at birth (altricial or precocial), their metabolic rate, postnatal activity and growth rate (Widdowson, 1981; Table 8.1). Small mammals have higher milk outputs per kg body weight than large animals and in general the smaller the young, the higher their metabolic rate and the richer the milk they receive. With the development of placentation and lactation primitive mammals were able to build up stores of energy and other nutrients for later mobilization and secretion into milk. If it was anything like that of monotremes and marsupials, their milk was probably relatively concentrated.

Milk is nutrients packaged for the journey from breast to gut, and certain aspects of its composition can be explained in the light of

Table 8.1 Milk composition of a selection of mammals (g/100 ml and kcal/100 ml for energy)

Order	Family	Species	Protein	Fat	Carbo-hydrate	Energy
Marsupialia	Macropoditae	Kangaroo	6.7	4.9	9.8	122
Insectivora	Erinaceidae	Northern hedgehog	7.2	10.1	2	142
	Tupaiidae	Tree shrew	8.5	17	2	213
Chiroptera	Vespertilionidae	Little brown bat	7.3	6	3.1	109
Rodentia	Muridae	House mouse	9	13.1	3	184
		Norway rat	8.1	8.8	3.8	142
	Caviidae	Guinea-pig	6.3	5.7	4.8	107
	Capromyidae	Coypu	13.7	27.9	0.6	338
Lagomorpha	Leporidae	Domestic rabbit	10.3	15.2	1.8	206
		Hare	19.5	19.3	0.9	292
Carnovora	Felidae	Domestic cat	10.6	10.8	3.7	174
		Lion	9.3	17.5	3.4	228
	Canidae	Domestic dog	7.5	9.5	3.8	145
		Wolf	9.2	9.6	3.4	154
		Red fox	6.7	5.8	4.6	110
	Ursidae	Polar bear	10.9	33.1	0.3	369
		Brown bear	8.5	18.5	2.3	228
Artiodactyla	Suidae	Domestic pig	5.6	8.3	5	128
		Collared peccary	5.4	3.5	6 5	89
	Hippopotimidae	Nile hippopotamus	6	17.2	2.1	201
	Bovidae	Domestic cow	3.2	3.7	4.6	71
		Domestic goat	2.9	3.8	4.7	70
		Domestic sheep	5	7.1	4.9	113
	Giraffidae	Giraffe	4	4.8	4.9	86
	Cervidae	Red deer	7.1	8.5	4.5	137
	Camelidae	Bactrian camel	3.9	5.4	5.1	92
		Llama	7.3	2.4	6	87
Perissodactyla	Equidae	Horse	1.9	1.3	6.9	50
		Donkey	1.9	0.6	6.1	40
		Plains zebra	2.3	2.1	8.3	65
	Rhinocerotidae	Black rhinoceros	1.4	0.2	6.6	36
Proboscidea		African elephant	4	5	5.3	90
Sea Carnivora	Phocidae	Harp seal	8.7	42.2	0.1	440
	Otariidae	Northern fur seal	10.2	49.4	0.1	515
Cetacea	Delphinidae	Bottlenose dolphin	6.8	33	1.1	348
	Balaenopteridae	Blue whale	10.6	42.3	1.3	458
Primates	Cercopithecidae	Rhesus monkey	1.6	4	7	74
		Baboon	1.5	4.6	7.7	82
	Pongidae	Orangutan	1.5	3.5	6	65
		Chimpanzee	1.2	3.7	7	69
	Hominidae	Man	1.1	4.2	7	73

Adapted from Widdowson (1981).

this function. The principal 'nutritional' carbohydrate in milk is lactose, a disaccharide composed of glucose and galactose. Lactose is found nowhere else in nature apart from in mammalian milks, and is suited for its role as a 'transport' carbohydrate because of its stability, lower osmolality than its component monosaccharides, and resistance to glucose

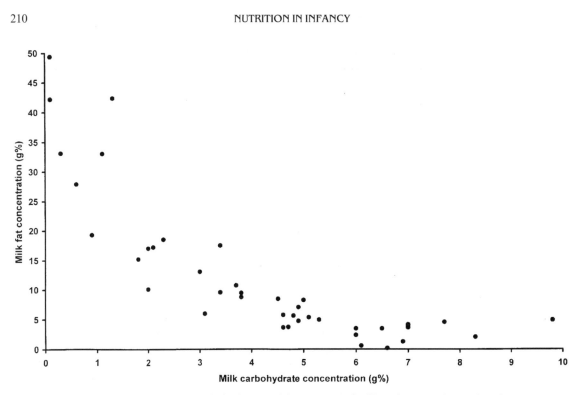

Figure 8.2 Relationship between carbohydrate and fat content of milks of mammals. Each point represents a different species (see Table 8.1)

oxidase. Milk also contains many oligosac-charides, which are thought primarily to be defence factors. The vast majority of the fat in milk is in the form of triacylglycerols. There are also small amounts of free fatty acids, cholesterol and phospholipids. Triacylglycerols offer a convenient means of delivering a variety of different fatty acids in proportions to satisfy the needs of different young, arranged in positional (stereo) configurations that regulate their digestion and uptake. Proteins are of many sizes and structures, and those in milk range from macromolecules to small peptides. They are the principal source of amino acids. Some are antigenic, some not, and they serve a large variety of functions in both breast and gut, many to defend the infant from gastro-intestinal infection.

The milk of species that produce altricial young, which have a rapid postnatal growth rate, is usually rich in protein. The newborn shrew for instance, which doubles its body weight in 24 h, consumes milk with 10 g/l of protein. Immature young also have a poor ability to maintain their body temperature, and their milks are usually energy-dense. In aquatic and arctic mammals insulation demands accu-mulation of substantial adipose tissue and the milk of dolphins and whales is particularly rich in fat. The milk of the newborn seal, for example, has a lipid content of 490 g/l. Milk lipid is also important for nervous system development, particularly during the critical period of brain growth after birth in most species. Precocial mammals, which are rela-tively mature at birth and have acquired substantial energy stores *in utero*, have slow postnatal growth rates, may be reared on milks of low fat and protein content, and can be weaned onto a non-milk diet soon after birth (Table 8.1; Derrickson, 1992; Oftedal, 1980, 1984).

Broadly speaking there is an inverse relation between the fat and carbohydrate content of

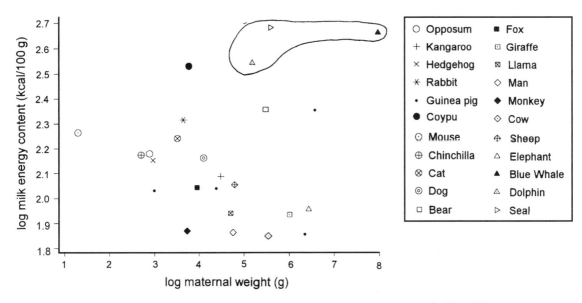

Figure 8.3 Relationship between maternal weight and energy content of milk of 22 mammals

mammalian milks (Figure 8.2), and the lipid fraction is the most variable and the carbohydrate fraction the least (Martin, 1984). Protein content varies with stage of lactation and lipid content varies throughout a feed. Another general feature of milk composition is that energy and protein contents are negatively correlated with maternal body weight (Figure 8.3) and with neonatal weight (except for Arctic species which have high energy demands; Figure 8.4). Primates, including man, however, produce less milk and less milk energy and their milks are lower in fat and protein content and higher in carbohydrate than that of other mammals of comparable size, in relation to both maternal and neonatal weight (Table 8.1, Figures 8.3 and 8.4). Taken with the slow fetal and infant growth rates this suggests that primates, including man, are adapted for limited maternal investment (in terms of energy per unit time) compared with other mammals (Martin and MacLarnon, 1985).

The non-nutritional constituents of milk assist in perinatal adaptation to enteral feeding, provide mucosal protection and compensate for 'immaturities' of neonatal digestive and absorptive function. Their contribution is related to the time that birth occurs in the course of gastrointestinal development (Weaver, 1993). However it is not possible to distinguish precisely between nutrients and non-nutritional substances. Some may serve more than one function, and during evolution, have been selected for another purpose. They may be synergistically interactive and the balance between proteases and anti-proteases and the presence or absence of mechanisms for their uptake, processing and transfer will determine their 'function' in the gastrointestinal tract. A rigid division of the constituents of milk into nutrients and non-nutritional factors does not take account of the dual (sometimes multiple) functions of many milk-borne substances as they pass from mother to infant. For example, up to one-third of the protein of human milk is 'non-nutritional', comprising protective proteins, hormones, growth factors, digestive enzymes etc., while immunoglobulin A (secretory IgA) both provides protection against antigens at mucosal surfaces and is also a source of nitrogen for the newborn (Prentice et al., 1987).

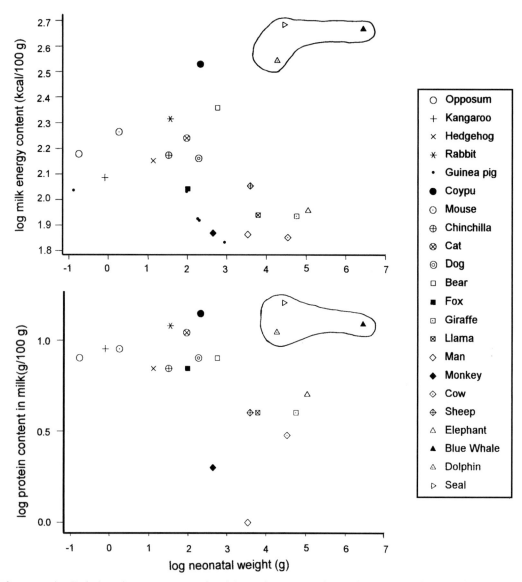

Figure 8.4   Relations between neonatal weight and energy and protein content of milks of 22 mammals

Human mammogenesis

Human breast development occurs in four distinct phases when specific structural and functional changes occur. These are mammogenesis, the period of breast development; lactogenesis, the activation of milk secretion; lactation, the period of copious milk production; and involution, when the lactating breast regresses to a non-functioning state (Neville, 2001).

The mammary gland arises embryologically from an ectodermal ingrowth, which forms a branched system of lactiferous ducts. Mammogensis is signalled first at 35 days gestation by the appearance on both ventrolateral surfaces of the embryo of a thickening of the ectoderm running between the forelimb and hindlimb buds. Two distinctive mammary buds become visible by 49 days. Projections of epithelial cells grow from each bud into the underlying mesenchymal tissue to form the main lactiferous ducts. Secondary and tertiary sprouts develop from each primary sprout and the cells at the centre of each projection die and a canal appears, progressing from the proximal end towards the bud. The nipple and areola develop towards term. The precursors of myoepithelial cells, adipocytes and connective tissue also emerge during fetal life.

The rudimentary structures of the main lactiferous ducts, each with a separate external opening, are well established by birth. The gland is sufficiently developed that, in response to stimulation by maternal and endogenous hormones, newborn babies may produce a milk-like secretion, known as 'witch's milk'. Duct formation and arborization of the ductal tree continue at a slow rate for several months after birth, but the mammary gland is largely quiescent during the rest of childhood. Mammary growth prior to puberty is essentially isometric, paralleling expansion of the whole body.

The main development of the lobular–alveolar system occurs after puberty under the influence of the sex hormones. During adolescence, extensive adipose and connective tissues are deposited, giving rise to the characteristic shape of the human breast. Monthly cyclical changes in breast tissue occur in association with the menstrual cycle. Breast volume increases before menstruation due to fluid retention, alveolar enlargement and accumulation of some secretory material followed by partial regression of the gland after menstruation.

During the first months of pregnancy the glandular tissue in the breast proliferates abundantly, branching of the glandular tree intensifies, mammary blood flow increases and cells differentiate. Numerous alveoli appear at the terminal ends of the ducts, giving rise to the familiar 'bunch of grapes' appearance of mammary tissue (Figure 8.1). The expanding glandular tissue replaces much of the pre-existing adipose and connective tissues of the breast. Distinctive secretory cells become visible in the alveoli clustered around a central, narrow lumen. Interspersed between them are myoepithelial cells with long cytoplasmic projections that extend over and enwrap the surface of the alveolus. The external appearance of the breast also changes during pregnancy, with pronounced increases in overall volume, areola area, and size of various sebaceous glands.

This final phase of mammogenesis is thought to be controlled largely by prolactin and placental lactogen. Pregnancy itself does not appear to be a necessary pre-condition for the final events of mammogenesis; breast development and milk secretion have been reported in men and nulliparous women in response to frequent suckling at the nipple.

Human lactogenesis

Lactogenesis, the onset of milk production, refers to the transition period between the completion of mammary development during pregnancy and the establishment of full lactation. Secretory cells continue to differentiate during the latter half of pregnancy and, under the influence of prolactin, begin to produce small amounts of milk. Milk release, however, is inhibited, probably by high circulating progesterone levels. Secretory products begin to accumulate in the cells and fat droplets and Golgi vacuoles containing protein granules become visible. The fall in progesterone levels which accompanies delivery triggers the rapid increase in milk production and changes in milk composition that occur during the first few days postpartum. Lipid droplets and protein-rich vacuoles accumulate, predominantly in the apical region of the secretory cell. The lateral surfaces of neighbouring cells form tight junctional complexes towards the apical surface, minimizing the flow of substances from the extracellular fluid into luminal milk.

Human lactation

Within the first week or two after birth the quality and quantity of mother's milk stabilizes. Further changes in volume and composition occur during established lactation but at a slow rate. The appearance of breast tissue during lactation resembles that at the end of lactogenesis and few changes are seen until milk production diminishes. The length of the lactation period depends on many factors but can be maintained for several years.

Prolactin is required for the maintenance of lactation and is ensured by its release from the anterior pituitary gland stimulated by suckling. Suckling also stimulates the release of oxytocin by the hypothalamus, which is stored in the posterior pituitary gland and regulates myoepithelial activity and ejection of milk from the breast. Day-to-day changes in milk production are under local control. A small peptide component of breast milk acts as a feedback inhibitor and may be important in the autocrine regulation of breast milk production, matching supply with demand.

Substrates for milk synthesis are supplied from the maternal diet or from maternal stores. In some instances, such as for certain micronutrients, incorporation into milk can be affected by dietary intakes and nutritional status. However, in general, breast milk volume and composition are remarkably resilient to marginal insufficiencies in the maternal diet and production is determined largely by the demands of the infant. The substrate requirements for human lactation are small in comparison to overall maternal requirements, and small adjustments in nutrient retention and metabolism can spare material for milk synthesis. In this respect, human milk production differs from that of many other animal species in which lactational performance is highly dependent on nutrient supply.

Many milk components are manufactured *de novo* within the secretory cell itself. The raw materials for the synthesis of these components and milk constituents that are derived directly from the circulation are sequestered by the secretory cell at the basal membrane; passage of substances into or out of luminal milk via paracellular pathways is thought to occur only during breast engorgement or disease.

Synthesis and secretion of milk fat

Milk lipid consists mainly of triacylglycerols, which are manufactured within the secretory cell from fatty acids and monoacylglycerols. Fatty acids with carbon chain lengths $\leqslant 16$ are synthesized *de novo* from glucose. Fatty acid synthetase orchestrates the construction and elongation of fatty acids until the length of the carbon chain is 10–16, at which point synthesis is arrested by the action of thioesterase II. Fatty acids of chain lengths $\geqslant 16$ and glycerol itself are derived from circulating plasma triacylglycerols by the action of lipoprotein lipase on the endothelial surfaces of mammary capillaries. As a result, the milk lipid profile of these longer chain fatty acids largely reflects that in the mother's diet. Minor components of the fat fraction of milk, such as cholesterol, originate from the circulation or are produced *de novo*.

Once produced, the hydrophobic triacylglycerol molecules coalesce into lipid droplets, which migrate towards the apex of the cell. The droplets are incorporated into the cell membrane and released as membrane-bound globules into the alveolar lumen by exocytosis (Figure 8.5). The globules, which are 1–4 μm in diameter, are dispersed in milk as an emulsion. They often contain small crescents of cytoplasm trapped within the membrane during the passage of the droplet out of the cell, which contribute cytoplasm-derived components to

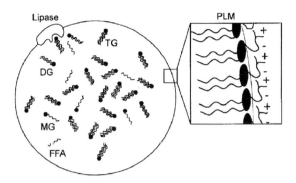

Figure 8.5 Fat globule with core of triacylglycerol (TG), diacylglycerol (DG), monoacylglycerol (MG) and free fatty acid (FFA). A section of the phospholipid membrane (PLM) is shown enlarged. A preduodenal lipase is shown attached to it, acting on TG molecule [from Manson and Weaver (1997) *Arch. Dis. Child.* **76**, F206–211; reproduced by permission of BMJ Publishing Group]

breast milk. The fat globule membrane originates from the apical membrane of the secretory cell globule membrane, is rich in phospholipids and is the major source of these components in breast milk.

Synthesis and secretion of milk lactose

Lactose, the predominant carbohydrate of milk, is a disaccharide of glucose and galactose. It is manufactured from glucose within the Golgi system of the secretory cell, catalysed by lactose synthetase, a multi-enzyme complex comprising alpha-lactalbumin and galactosyl transferase. Lactose, along with milk proteins and some other milk components, is packaged into secretory vesicles, which migrate through the Golgi system the apical membrane of the mammary cell. Water and electrolytes such as sodium and potassium are drawn into the intramembraneous spaces of the Golgi system and into the secretory vesicles by the osmotic effect of lactose transfer. At the apex of the cell the vesicles fuse with the cell membrane and

release their contents into the alveolar lumen by exocytosis.

Synthesis and secretion of milk proteins

Many milk proteins are synthesised *de novo* within the secretory cell. Amino-acid sequences are built up by mRNA transcription on ribosomes in the rough endoplasmic reticulum. The molecules are then transferred to the Golgi system, where some proteins undergo specific post-translational glycosylation, and caseins are phosphorylated and combined with calcium and phosphate to form micelles. The milk proteins are packaged with lactose, water and other components into secretory vesicles for extrusion into the alveolar lumen by exocytosis.

Some blood-borne proteins are incorporated into milk after sequestration from the circulation by receptors on the basolateral membrane of the secretory cell. These proteins enter the cell in endocytic vesicles, which travel either directly to the apical membrane for exocytosis or are transported to the Golgi system for incorporation in secretory vesicles. IgA molecules are synthesized by B-lymphocytes resident in the mammary tissue. The profile of antibody specificities largely reflects maternal exposure to mucosal antigens, as the result of lymphocyte traffic between mucosal sites around the body (entero-mammary circulation; Figure 8.6). IgA molecules enter the secretory cell by endocytosis across the basolateral membrane. The linking of two IgA molecules with secretory component to complete the synthesis of secretory-IgA occurs within the alveolar cell.

Secretion of other milk components

The origins and mechanisms by which other constituents of milk are incorporated into it

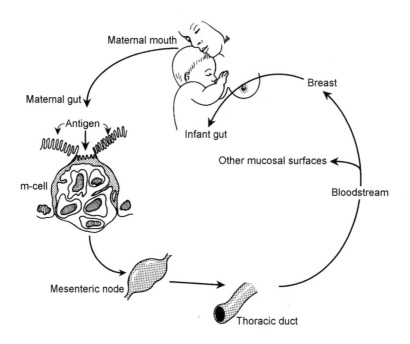

Figure 8.6   Enteromammary immune circulation

are little understood. The uptake of blood-borne components is primarily across the basolateral membrane, by either passive or active transport mechanisms, since paracellular pathways are closed during mature lactation. The absence of paracellular transport prevents modification of milk in the alveolar lumen in the face of the widely different concentrations of many components, notably sodium, potassium and lactose, in milk and extracellular fluid. When paracellular pathways are open, for example during mastitis, the sodium content in milk can be raised many-fold, while lactose, and to some extent potassium, levels are reduced. Other milk constituents may originate from within the secretory cell, where they may have been involved in the biochemistry of milk synthesis or other aspects of cellular metabolism, and become enclosed within secretory vesicles and globules during their production and transportation into milk.

Human mammary gland involution

As lactation ceases the mammary gland regresses to an inactive state. Initially, the decreased amount of milk removed from the breast results in stasis and the disruption of cell junctions. This leads to the characteristic changes in milk composition that are seen at the end of lactation. Milk is slowly resorbed, the secretory cells shrink in volume and the synthetic apparatus disappears. Some secretory cells are preserved in a non-functioning state while others die. The alveoli lose their rounded appearance but the essential alveolar shape is retained and myoepithelial cells are conserved. There is significant diminution of the ductal tree and adipose and fibrous tissues replace the degenerating glandular tissue. However, unlike the pre-pregnant breast, significant numbers of alveoli remain after regression. The resting phase of the breast continues until the next pregnancy when proliferation and differentiation of the glandular tissue occur again. Towards the end of a woman's reproductive life senile involution takes place when the glandular tissue gradually atrophies and is replaced predominantly by adipose tissue.

Composition of Human Milk

General composition

Milk is a complex, multi-phase fluid within which its various constituents, including nutrients, non-nutrients, other chemicals and cells are partitioned. The lipid phase contains triacylglycerols, phospholipids, fat-soluble vitamins, and other lipophilic substances such as sterols and carotenoids. The aqueous phase contains lactose, oligosaccharides, proteins, water-soluble vitamins, minerals and electrolytes. The colloidal phase consists mainly of micellar casein. The composition of breast milk varies between mothers and within the same mother during lactation, in the course of the day and throughout a single breast-feed.

Fat

Fat accounts for approximately one-half of the energy content of human milk and is the vehicle for the transfer of the fat-soluble vitamins A, D, E, K and other lipophilic substances, including prostaglandins. Certain constituents of human milk fat have additional properties to that of a metabolic fuel, for example, linoleic acid (18:2ω6) and linolenic acid (18:3ω3) are essential fatty acids, arachidonic acid (C20:4ω6) and docosahexaenoic acid (C22:6ω3) are vital constituents of brain and neural tissues (Farquarson et al., 1992), and lauric acid (12:0) has antimicrobial properties.

More than 98 per cent of the fat in human milk is present as triacylglycerols; the rest is largely phospholipids and cholesterol (Table 8.2). The fatty acids in the triacylglycerols are medium and long-chain, with carbon chain lengths predominantly >10. Oleic acid (18:1) and palmitic acid (16:0) are particularly abundant, representing more than one-half of the fatty acids (Table 8.8). Over 50 per cent of the triacylglycerols in human milk contain palmitic acid at the central carbon of the glycerol molecule (sn-2 position; Table 8.3), a property which facilitates their digestion and absorption. Triacylglycerols are digested in the infant gut under the influence of lingual and gastric (preduodenal), pancreatic and milk bile-salt stimulated lipases, which together have the range of enzyme specificities to hydrolyse lipids with fatty acids of different chain lengths and positions (Manson and Weaver, 1997; Figure 8.5).

The concentration of fat in human milk increases during a feed and exhibits a marked

Table 8.2 Lipid composition of human milk on different days of lactation

	Lactation day				
	3	7	21	42	84
Total fat (g/dl)	2.0	2.9	3.5	3.2	4.8
Lipid class					
Triacylglycerol (%)	97.6	98.5	98.7	98.9	99.0
Cholesterol (%)	1.3	0.7	0.5	0.5	0.4
Phospholipid (%)	1.1	0.8	0.8	0.6	0.6

Table 8.3 Relative proportions of fatty acids at Sn positions of triacylglycerol molecule

Fatty acid (mol%)	Sn position		
	1	2	3
10:0	0.2	0.2	1.8
12:0	1.3	2.1	6.1
14:0	3.2	7.3	7.1
16:0	16.1	58.2	6.2
16:1	3.6	4.7	7.3
18:0	15.0	3.3	2.0
18:1	46.1	12.7	49.7
18:2	11.0	7.3	2.0
18:3	0.4	0.6	1.6
20:1	1.5	0.7	0.5

diurnal variation. The amount of fat in milk also increases during the course of lactation from about 2 per cent at birth to almost 5 per cent at 12 weeks (Table 8.2), but it is little influenced by maternal diet or nutritional status. However, diet can alter the profile of milk fatty acids. Vegetarian mothers, for example, produce milk with higher proportions of long-chain polyunsaturated fatty acids than omnivores. Women who consume diets that are rich in fat, or who mobilize body fat during periods of food shortage, produce milk which contains 10–17 per cent of fatty acids with chain lengths < 14, whereas the proportion of these endogenously produced fatty acids can reach 25 per cent in women who consume carbohydrate-rich diets.

Carbohydrate

The principal carbohydrate of human milk is lactose, which accounts for about 40 per cent of its total energy. Under the action of lactase in the infant's small intestine, lactose is hydrolysed to glucose, a monosaccharide, which is actively absorbed and is a major energy source, and galactose, a monosaccharide, which is a component of brain tissues and essential for energy transfer. Lactose is efficiently (>90 per cent) digested and absorbed in the small intestine, and that which is not passes to the colon where it is fermented, producing lactic acid. This is absorbed and makes a contribution to energy intake, and reduces colonic pH, enhancing the absorption of calcium. In addition, lactose promotes the growth of lactobacilli and may help to develop a favourable colonic flora that may protect against gastrointestinal infections.

Human milk contains significant quantities of other carbohydrates, mainly monosaccharides, oligosaccharides and protein-bound carbohydrate moieties. The non-lactose fraction represents about 15–20 per cent of total milk carbohydrate. Oligosaccharides amount to around 15 g/l and it is calculated that breast-fed babies daily ingest several grammes of oligosaccharides. Around 40 per cent are excreted in the faeces, and a small percentage with the urine (1–2 per cent). It is probable that part of the remaining percentage is metabolized by the colonic flora to short-chain fatty acids and gases. The oligosaccharides of breast milk may have a function in the defence against viruses, bacteria or their toxins, and in promoting the growth of the intestinal flora, including strains with possible probiotic effects, such as the bifidobacteria.

Protein

Approximately 75 per cent of nitrogen in human milk is contained in a wide variety of proteins. They are relatively rich in cystine, a semi-essential amino acid for the newborn infant. The remaining nitrogen is present as urea, free amino acids, nucleotides and small peptides. There are two distinct protein compartments in human milk: casein, a micellular fraction in which protein subunits are linked by calcium and phosphate ions; and an aqueous whey fraction, containing water-soluble proteins. The ratio of casein/whey in mature human milk is approximately 40:60. The composition of casein is heterogeneous and varies considerably within and between individual mothers. The predominant casein class in human milk is β-casein. The diameter of human milk casein micelles range from 30 to 75 nm. This small micellular volume may be partly responsible for the coagulating properties of human milk casein, which result in a soft, flocculent curd in the infant's stomach, that enhances digestion and may reduce the gastric deactivation of other milk components. Casein, in addition to its role as nutritional protein, may influence the absorption and utilization of calcium and certain casein fragments have been shown to have immuno-stimulatory and opioid-like activities.

The four major proteins in the whey fraction of human milk are α-lactalbumin, lactoferrin, secretory-IgA and serum albumin. These proteins are synthesized and packaged largely within the breast. Two of the major proteins, lactoferrin and secretory-IgA, have antimicrobial properties which protect the breast and, if they survive digestion, the infant's gastro-intestinal and respiratory tracts from infection. Up to 30 per cent of milk secretory-IgA

remains intact in the small intestine of infants older than 6 weeks while 98 per cent of lactoferrin is degraded (Prentice et al., 1987). The proportions of these proteins that survive in younger infants may be higher. A complex and wide variety of proteins are present in small but biologically significant amounts, many of which have important non-nutritional properties (see below and Tables 8.4 and 8.5).

Micronutrients

Human milk contains a full complement of essential vitamins and minerals, which are absorbed with high efficiency by the infant. In general the vitamins originate from the maternal circulation and their concentrations in milk can be influenced by maternal diet and vitamin status. Those that are most affected by the mother's dietary intake are the water-soluble vitamins and, to a lesser extent, the fat-soluble vitamins. With few exceptions, neither dietary maternal intake nor maternal stores affect the amount of minerals secreted in breast milk. Where maternal intake can affect the secretion of micronutrients into milk, there is usually a plateau above which a further

Table 8.4 Non-nutritional factors in human milk that may play a part in neonatal gastro-intestinal defence, function and metabolism

Hormones	Thyroxine (T3, T4), thyroid-stimulating hormone (TSH), thyrotrophin-releasing hormone (TRH), corticosteroids and adrenocorticotropic hormone (ACTH), insulin, somatostatin, luteinizing hormone-releasing factor (LHRF), gonadotropin-releasing factor (GNRF), oxytocin, prolactin, erythropoietin, calcitonin
Trophic factors	Epidermal growth factor (EGF), nerve growth factor (NGF), transforming growth factor (TGF), insulin-like growth factors (IGFs) Somatomedin-C, spermines, nucleotides
Anti-inflammatory agents	Prostaglandin E & F, α-1-antitrypsin and chymotrypsin
Anti-infective agents	Secretory IgA, IgM, IgG, lactoferrin, lysosyme complement, lactoperoxidase, anti-staphylococcus factor, oligosaccharides, bifidus factor
Cytokines	Tumour necrosis factor (TNF), interleukin 1 and 6 (IL1, IL6), interferon
Digestive enzymes	Amylase, bile salt-dependent lipase and esterase

Table 8.5   Protective factors present in human milk

Factor	Function
• Secretory immunoglobulin A	• Protects intestinal epithelium from luminal antigens, and may actively prime the neonate's immune system
• Lactoferrin	• Competes with bacteria for iron
• Lysosyme	• Antibacterial enzyme lyses cell walls
• Bifidus factor	• Stimulates lactic acid bacteria, e.g. bifidobacteria, in the colon
• Macrophages	• Engulf bacteria
• Lymphocytes	• Secrete Igs (B cells) and lymphokines (T cells)
• Protease inhibitors	• Inhibit digestion of bioactive proteins in milk
• Complement	• Assists in bacterial lysis
• Interferon	• Anti-viral agent
• Oligosaccharides	• Inhibitors of bacterial adhesion to epithelium
• B_{12} and folate binding proteins	• Compete with bacteria for these vitamins
• Anti-staphylococcus factor	• Lipid with anti-staph action
• Anti-*Giardia* factor	• Lipid with anti-*Giardia* action

increase in intake will have no further effect in increasing their concentrations in milk. Breast-fed infants rarely show signs of micronutrient deficiencies when maternal intakes are low, unless the mother is severely depleted pre- or postnatally; examples have been reported for vitamin A, vitamin D and folate.

Non-nutritional components

Human milk contains a wealth of constituents which may aid neonatal adaptation to oral feeding, by promoting mucosal defence and function, and by assisting digestion during a period when the infant's own systems are underdeveloped. These factors include anti-microbial and anti-inflammatory agents, digestive enzymes, trophic factors and growth-modulators, cytokines and transport proteins. There are peptides, proteins, oligo-saccharides, nucleotides and macromolecules, and are best classified by their known or supposed actions (Table 8.4).

Biologically active substances in milk are either transported (passively or actively) across the mammary epithelium from the maternal circulation, or are synthesized in the mammary gland. Many are present in concentrations well above those in maternal blood and some are well recognized as true hormones and/or paracrines. Such non-nutritional bioactive substances in milk may therefore transmit signals from mother to young, which may initiate or modulate gastro-intestinal function, may regulate metabolism and may stimulate the immune and endocrine systems of the infant (Koldovsky and Thornburg, 1987).

Protective factors

Protective factors include secretory-IgA, lacto-ferrin, lysozyme, leucocytes and oligosaccharides (Table 8.5). During the neonatal period the infant's mucosal defence systems are immature and these agents act locally in the alimentary canal to defend against infection. Secretory immunoglobulin A acts at mucosal surfaces to protect them from injury by ingested microbial antigens. Lactoferrin is an iron-binding protein that competes with bacteria for iron, reducing bacterial viability and thereby the risk of enteric infections, particularly those caused by *Escherichia coli* and *Staphylococci*. The spectrum of specific activities of secretory-IgA reflects the exposure of the mother to mucosal antigens: via the enteromammary circulation the infant acquires antibodies protective against organisms that pass through the mother's gastrointestinal tract (Figure 8.6). Total IgA secretion by the breast is maintained at around 0.5 g/day throughout the first year of life (Weaver *et al.*, 1998). In addition to supporting the infant's developing mucosal immune system the antimicrobial factors may protect the breast from infection, thereby ensuring a continuing supply of milk. Components in milk may aid the maturation of the child's mucosal defences and may help to establish the characteristic colonic flora of the breast-fed infant. Several proteins may be involved in the transportation and absorption of minerals and vitamins, for example folic acid-binding protein and cobalamin-binding protein. These factors are often bacteriostatic as they deprive bacteria of essential nutrients.

Digestive enzymes

Digestive enzymes may assist in the digestion of milk fat and carbohydrate during the first weeks of life when secretion of enzymes from the infant's pancreas and salivary glands is low. Examples include bile-salt-stimulated lipase, which catalyses the digestion of triacylglycerols at low bile salt concentrations, and amylase, which may assist in the digestion of starch in the first complementary foods.

Trophic factors and nucleotides

Trophic factors, growth promotors and regulators, such as epidermal growth factor, nerve growth factor and taurine, and hormones, such as insulin and prolactin, may be important in the regulation of mucosal function in the infant's gastrointestinal tract and, after absorption, in regulating metabolism and mucosal function at more remote sites. Nucleotides are found in human milk, and in infants with severe intrauterine growth retardation their addition to formula has been associated with accelerated catch-up growth.

Changes in milk composition during lactation

The composition and volume of human milk production are not constant. They vary considerably between individual mothers and within the same mother throughout lactation. Four different phases of milk production are recognized: colostral, transitional, mature and involutional.

Colostrum

Colostrum is the first secretion produced by the breast after parturition. It is rich in whey proteins, particularly secretory-IgA and lactoferrin, and has low concentrations of lactose and fat. Colostrum is also rich in vitamin A. The total volume of colostrum produced is low, of the order of 100 ml/day, and the transfer of nutrients to the baby during the first days of life is relatively small. A notable exception is secretory-IgA which is present in colostrum at such a high concentration that the intake during the first 3 days after birth is superior to that at any other time.

Transitional milk

Milk composition changes rapidly during the first days after parturition. With the onset of lactogenesis on days 3–7, milk volume increases markedly (known as the 'coming in' of breast milk). Milk protein concentrations decrease, the casein/whey ratio increases, lactose and fat concentrations increase and sodium concentrations decrease. The fatty acid profile changes with an increase in the proportion of fatty acids synthesized within the breast. The concentrations of some micronutrients also change. Milk produced between birth and about 14 days postpartum is referred to as transitional milk, although there is no standardized definition. The compositional changes reflect changes in breast structure, which occur at this time, with tightening of the junctions between the secretory epithelial cells preventing direct entry of components from the extracellular space via paracellular pathways. Analysis of a mother's transitional milk composition is a poor predicator of her milk quality in established lactation. After this period the composition of milk stabilizes and concentrations characteristic of the individual mother become evident.

Mature milk

Mature milk is produced from about 14 days postpartum until the number of feeds per day decreases significantly and involutional changes begin to occur in the breast. The period of mature milk production varies; some mothers choose to breast-feed for only a few weeks, others for 2 years or more. Human milk production is determined largely by the demand of the infant and is rarely limited by the mother's innate capacity to synthesize milk. Mothers who suckle twins, for example, produce approximately twice as much milk as mothers nursing singletons. The volume of milk produced by a mother on any particular day depends on factors such as the infant's weight, access to the breast and intake of supplementary and complementary foods.

Peak lactation, the period of maximum milk secretion, generally occurs 3–6 months after birth in women who are fully, but not necessarily exclusively, breast-feeding and declines slowly over successive months. Gradual weaning by the replacement of breast-feeds by other foods leads to a more rapid decrease in milk volume. Typical milk volumes at peak lactation are 750–850 ml/day for mothers who are fully breast-feeding and are broadly similar in different parts of the world. Mothers practising prolonged lactation, such as those in the traditional societies of Africa, produce average volumes of 500 ml/day or more, well into the second year of lactation.

Progressive changes are observed in the composition of mature milk, although these are not as marked as those seen in colostrum and transitional milk. For many constituents, such as protein, fat and calcium, concentrations decline by about one quarter during the first 3–6 months of lactation and then plateau. Some micronutrients, notably zinc, continue to fall throughout lactation and reach very low levels by the end of the first year. Those components with osmoregulatory properties, such as lactose, sodium and potassium, remain essentially constant in mature milk. Only a few components rise in concentration during the mature phase of milk production. Examples include lysozyme, an antimicrobial protein, and some water-soluble vitamins whose concentrations rise steadily during the first year of lactation.

The foremilk, at the beginning of each breast-feed, is more watery, richer in lactose and has a relatively low fat concentration, which rises so that the most energy-dense milk is secreted at the end of the feed. This hind milk therefore makes an important contribution to the infant's energy intake. The low concentrations of many nutrients in mature milk compared with colostrum are counterbalanced by the increase in milk volume, so that for fully breast-fed infants, daily intakes of milk components are greatest at peak lactation. The combination of decreases in milk quality and quantity after peak lactation leads to substantial reductions in nutrient transfer by 1–2 years. However, in countries where the composition of traditional weaning foods is poor, breast milk may remain the predominant source of certain nutrients, especially fat, vitamin A and some other micronutrients during the second year of life. Moreover its lipase and amylase content may assist in the digestion of fat and complex carbohydrates in weaning foods.

Involutional milk

The final changes in milk composition occur when milk production ceases at weaning. Protein, fat and sodium concentrations increase and lactose content decreases. Products of milk synthesis accumulate in the breast and force the tight junctions apart allowing sodium and other extracellular components to enter milk via paracellular pathways. In women who gradually wean the infant, involutional changes occur throughout the process, but are less marked.

Energy and Nutrient Requirements

The term infant is born with reserves of energy and many nutrients that have been acquired during fetal life, particularly in the last trimester of gestation, and these contribute to meeting the nutritional needs of the newborn. Growth during the first two postnatal months is more rapid than at any other time of life, and a much larger proportion of dietary energy and nitrogen is used for this purpose in infancy than later in life (Figure 8.7). Human milk contains all the energy and nutrients needed for the healthy growing infant until about 6 months of life (Table 8.6).

Energy and nutrient requirements are generally defined as dietary reference values (DRV; Department of Health, 1991). Reference nutrient intakes (RNI) are those that should satisfy the needs of around 97 per cent

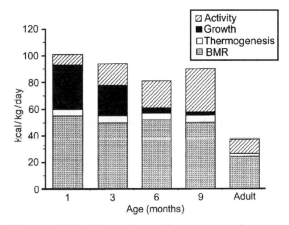

Figure 8.7 Comparison of energy requirements during infancy and adulthood. The greatest proportion is used for growth in the neonatal period [from Michaelsen *et al.* (2000) *Feeding and Nutrition of Infants and Young Children*; WHO Regional Publications, European Series no. 87; reproduced by permission of WHO]

Table 8.6 Composition (per 100 ml) of mature human milk and cow's milk, and compositional guidelines for infant formula

	Mean values for mature human milk	Infant formula	Cow's milk
Energy (kJ)	280	250–315	276
(kcal)	67	60–75	66
Protein (g)	1.3	1.2–1.95	3.2
Fat (g)	4.2	2.1–4.2	3.9
Carbohydrate (g)	7	4.6–9.1	4.6
Sodium (mg)	15	13–39	55
Chloride (mg)	43	32.5–81	97
Potassium (mg)	58	54	140
Calcium (mg)	35	59	120
Magnesium (mg)	3	4	11
Phosphorus (mg)	15	16.3–58.5	92
Iron (μg)	76	325–975	60
Zinc (mg)	0.3	0.3	0.4
Vitamin A (μg)	60	39–117	35
Vitamin C (mg)	3.8	5.2	1.8
Vitamin D (μg)	0.01	0.65–1.63	0.08
Vitamin E (mg)	0.34	1.16	0.09

Adapted from Department of Health (1994) and WHO (2000).

Table 8.7 Estimated average requirements for energy and reference nutrient intakes in infancy

	Units/day	0–3 months	4–6 months	7–9 months
Energy – boys	MJ (kcal)	2.3 (545)	2.9 (690)	3.4 (825)
Energy – girls	MJ (kcal)	2.2 (515)	2.7 (645)	3.2 (765)
Protein	g	12.5	12.7	13.7
Vitamin A	RE	350	350	350
Vitamin B_1	mg	0.2	0.2	0.2
Vitamin B_2	mg	0.4	0.4	0.4
Vitamin B_3	mg	3	3	5
Vitamin B_6	mg	0.2	0.2	0.3
Folate	µg	50	50	50
Vitamin B_{12}	µg	0.3	0.3	0.5
Pantothenic acid	mg	1.7	1.7	1.7
Vitamin C	mg	25	25	25
Vitamin D	µg	8.5	8.5	7
Vitamin E	mg/g PUFA	0.4	0.4	0.4
Vitamin K	µg	10	10	10
Sodium	mg	210	280	320
Potassium	mg	800	850	700
Chloride	mg	320	400	500
Calcium	mg	525	525	525
Magnesium	mg	55	60	75
Phosphorus	mg	400	400	400
Iron	mg	1.7	4.3	7.8
Zinc	mg	4	4	5
Selenium	µg	10	13	10
Copper	mg	0.3	0.3	0.3
Iodine	µg	50	60	60

From Department of Health (1991), Garrow (1999) and Michaelsen *et al.* (2000).

of infants. Energy needs are usually expressed as an estimated average requirement (EAR). For most nutrients the DRVs of infants that are not wholly breast-fed represent at least the same amount of each nutrient from milk formulas and other foods as the fully breast-fed infant of the same age would consume. The amount of any nutrient ingested can be calculated from its concentration in breast milk and volume consumed, but the efficiency of absorption of energy and some nutrients from milk formulas is less than from breast milk. The DRVs for infants that are formula-fed therefore exceed those that might be expected to be derived from breast milk.

While there is broad consensus as to these figures, there is some variation in those used in different countries around the world. The recommended energy and reference nutrient intakes for infants during the first 9 months of life are shown in Table 8.7 (Michaelsen *et al.*, 2000).

Alternatives to Human Milk

It is generally accepted that human milk is the best food for the newborn human infant and WHO/UNICEF recommend exclusive breast-feeding in the healthy infant to about 6 months. They also recommend that breast-feeding should continue for up to 2 years and possibly for longer. Evidence supporting the continuation of breast-feeding into the second year of life is strongest in settings where hygiene is poor and infection rates are high. In these conditions, breast-feeding for up to 2–3 years has been found to be protective against infectious disease and to have a positive association with child survival. In industrialized countries the benefits of prolonged breast-feeding are less evident (Elsom and Weaver, 1999).

There are situations where it may be preferable or necessary to substitute breast milk with an alternative. These include certain medical contraindications and situations where the mother, despite efforts to continue breast-feeding, is unable to maintain lactation that is sufficient to meet the infant's nutritional requirements fully. When alternatives to breast-feeding are considered, the risk of feeding other than breast milk should be less than the potential risks associated with continued breast-feeding. The following issues are relevant:

- *nutritional requirements* – other methods of feeding need to provide all the infant's nutritional requirements as completely as possible, however no substitute fully replicates the nutrient content of human milk;
- *infections* – breast milk substitutes lack the properties of human milk which protect against infections; bacteria may contaminate breast milk substitutes during preparation, and even when hygiene is good, artificially fed infants suffer a significantly higher rate of gastrointestinal and respiratory infections than breast-fed infants;
- *cost* – the use of breast milk substitutes is expensive and it has to be borne by individual families and translates into costs to communities, with an impact at the population level; in addition to the need to purchase formula milk, the associated costs of fuel, water and health-care need to be taken into account;
- *family planning* – women who do not breast-feed lose the benefits of lactational amenorrhoea; in populations where contraceptives are not readily available, this can translate into short birth intervals, reduced infant survival and compromised maternal health;
- *psycho-social stimulation* – not breast-feeding can affect mother–infant bonding, which may result in lack of stimulation for the infant, unless efforts are made for the infant to receive as much attention as it would had it been breast-fed.

Animal milks

Milks derived from other mammals, particularly the cow, have been used for centuries to feed the human infant. The composition of cow's milk differs in many important respects from human milk (Table 8.6) and this affects its nutritional value, digestibility, the bioavailability of micronutrients and the delivery of potentially important non-nutritional agents to the infant.

There are many notable differences. The protein content of cow's milk is three times higher than that of breast milk. Moreover, human milk is whey-predominant, whereas cow's milk is casein-predominant with only 20 per cent whey proteins. The major whey protein found in cow's milk is β-lactoglobulin, which is not present in human milk and can evoke an adverse antigenic reaction in some infants. The predominant casein class is α-casein, rather than β-casein, which alters the micellar and coagulation properties of the milk. Lactoferrin, a major whey protein in breast milk with antimicrobial propertied, is present in only small amounts in cow's milk, and IgG is the predominant immunoglobulin. The concentrations of the electrolytes sodium, potassium and chloride, and of the minerals calcium, phosphorus and magnesium are three to four times greater in cow's milk than in breast milk. The higher protein and sodium concentrations can cause renal solute overload in the newborn baby and cow's milk needs to be modified before being fed to young infants.

Compared with cow's milk, human milk has a greater proportion of unsaturated fatty acids and a higher concentration of essential fatty acids (Table 8.8). Furthermore, the long-chain polyunsaturated fatty acids (LCPUFAs) in breast milk are better absorbed than those in cow's milk. Evidence suggests that LCPUFAs are essential for normal neurodevelopment and visual cortical function. Because LCPUFAs cannot be synthesized by the fetus and the newborn's capacity to convert essential fatty acids to LCPUFAs is limited during the first few months of life, infants rely on the efficient transfer of LCPUFAs from the mother, prenatally via the placenta and postnatally from breast milk (Farquarson *et al.*, 1992).

Commercial infant formula milks

Most commercial infant formula milks are based on cow's milk, and have been designed to mimic the nutrient composition of human milk. Thus, the concentrations of protein and electrolytes such as sodium, potassium and chloride are lower than those in cow's milk, while, as a result of fortification, the levels of certain minerals, primarily iron and to a lesser extent zinc, are higher. Commercial infant formula milks usually lack the non-nutritional, bioactive components of human milk and the quality of their proteins and lipids (amino acid and fatty acid profiles) may not be optimal for the needs of the baby. There is evidence, for example, that the phospholipid fatty acid composition of the brains of infants is in part determined by the essential fatty acid composition of the milk they receive. The addition of non-nutrient components such as lactoferrin,

Table 8.8 Differences in fatty acid composition of human and cow's milk

Fatty acid	Mature human milk (%)	Unmodified cow's milk (%)
10:0	1.4	3.5
12:0	5.4	4.1
14:0	7.3	12.0
16:0	26.5	31.3
16:1	4.0	1.3
18:0	9.5	9.2
18:1	35.5	21.7
18:2	7.2	1.6
18:3	0.8	0.4
20:0	0.2	0.2
20:4	0.3	0.1
Total fat (g/l)	42	38

From Manson and Weaver (1997).

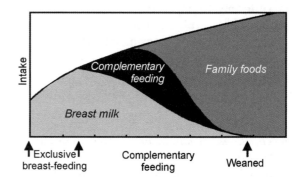

Figure 8.8 Gap between intake and requirements that must be filled by complementary feeds during infancy

oligosaccharides, nucleotides, specific immunoglobulins and enzymes to formula milks is a further development in the production of human milk substitutes.

The composition of infant formula milk (Table 8.6) varies between manufacturers, but should conform to specifications drawn up by regulatory bodies. Many milks, particularly those marketed in Europe, are modified by the addition of demineralized whey to give casein/whey ratios similar to that found in human milk. The predominant whey protein, however, remains β-lactoglobulin, a protein, which is not present in human milk except as a minor constituent originating from the maternal diet. The addition of demineralized whey lowers the total protein, sodium and calcium concentrations while raising the lactose content, thus making the composition closer to that of human milk. Vegetable fats and oils are often added to, or completely replace, milk fat to achieve fatty acid profiles that resemble that of human milk. The concentrations of certain micronutrients, particularly vitamins, are adjusted by fortification. The bioavailability of many of the minerals in formula milks is generally inferior to that in human milk. The concentrations of many of the factors with putative non-nutritive roles are often considerably lower in formula milks than in human milk and in general it is not clear whether their biological activity survives the manufacturing process.

Used under optimal conditions, commercial infant formula milks can provide a satisfactory alternative to breast milk as a sole source of nutrition to young infants up to around 6 months of age (Figure 8.8). Even after the introduction of complementary foods, in these circumstances formula milk can continue to make a major contribution to infant energy and nutrient requirements, and *in the absence of breast-feeding* it should be the main fluid in the diet for the first 9 months and possibly beyond. Infants should not be given unmodified cow's milk *as a drink* before at least the age of 9 months. If infants are formula-fed, cow's milk can be gradually introduced into the infant's diet between 9–12 months. However, if there are no economic constraints it may be better to continue with formula until 12 months.

Breast-feeding and Health

The advantages of breast-feeding to mother and baby are numerous and long lasting (Table 8.9). In addition to its nutritional benefits, breast-feeding confers a number of non-nutritional advantages to young infants. These include protection against various acute and chronic illnesses, and enhanced physiological and behavioural development. Although the evidence for a beneficial effect of each may be small, together they add up to give the breast-fed infant a significant health advantage over the formula-fed baby.

The growth and development of infants can be influenced by choice of milk given in the neonatal period, and by feeding practices later in infancy. There is evidence that nutrition in early postnatal life may affect childhood neurobehavioural development and performance, and even have long-lasting effects in determining the risk of some chronic diseases in adulthood. However little is known about the mechanisms by which perinatal nutrition may programme metabolism, endocrine and immune function in early life, and reduce the risk of cardiovascular disease. Breast-feeding favours early bonding between mother and infant which plays a role in the development of optimal parental caring behaviours.

Health advantages to the infant (Table 8.9)

Protection against infection

Breast-feeding protects infants from infections by two mechanisms. First it lowers or eliminates exposure to bacterial pathogens transmitted by contaminated food and fluids. Second, human milk contains antimicrobial factors and other substances (Tables 8.4 and 8.5), which strengthen the immature immune system and protect the digestive system of the newborn infants, and thereby confer protection against infections, particularly those of the gastrointestinal and respiratory tracts. Formula-fed infants therefore enjoy less protection against infection. Colostrum is especially rich in protective proteins, but the concentrations

Table 8.9   Health advantages of breast-feeding for infants and mothers

Infant
- Reduced incidence and duration of diarrhoeal illnesses
- Protection against respiratory infection
- Reduced occurrence of otitis media and recurrent otitis media
- Possible protection against neonatal necrotizing enterocolitis, bacteraemia, meningitis, botulism and urinary tract infection
- Possible reduced risk of auto-immune disease (diabetes mellitus type 1, inflammatory bowel disease)
- Reduced risk of sudden infant death syndrome
- Reduced risk of developing cow's milk allergy
- Possible reduced risk of adiposity later in childhood
- Improved visual acuity and psychomotor development, which may be due to polyunsaturated fatty acids in milk, particularly DHA
- Higher IQ scores in breast-fed infants, which may be the result of factors present in milk, or to better stimulation of breast-fed infants
- Reduced malocclusion due to better jaw shape and development

Mother
- Early initiation of breast-feeding after childbirth:
  - promotes maternal recovery from childbirth
  - accelerates uterine involution, reduces risk of postpartum haemorrhage, reducing maternal mortality
  - reduced blood loss preserves maternal haemoglobin stores leading to improved iron status
- Breast-feeding prolongs period of postpartum infertility leading to increased spacing between successive pregnancies
- Possible accelerated weight loss and return to pre-pregnancy body weight
- Reduced risk of maternal pre-menopausal breast cancer
- Possible reduced risk of maternal ovarian cancer
- Possible improved bone mineralization and thereby reduced risk of osteoporosis

Adapted from Heinig and Dewey (1996; 1997).

of anti-infective substances in breast milk are sustained beyond the first year of life. They continue to offer protection against infection thereafter and infants who are breast-fed into their second year have significantly improved survival compared with those who have ceased breast-feeding.

There is abundant evidence that exclusive breast-feeding for about the first six months reduces both infant morbidity and mortality, and these beneficial effects are more pronounced where infection rates are greatest and hygiene and sanitation are poor (Elsom and Weaver, 1999). In addition, infants tend to continue to accept breast milk during episodes of diarrhoea whereas consumption of non-breast milk foods and fluids may decrease.

Breast-feeding therefore both diminishes the negative impact of illness on nutritional status and provides a clean source of fluid to counter dehydration.

The evidence that breast-feeding is protective against infectious disease is greatest for diarrhoeal disease: formula-fed infants suffer a significantly higher number of diarrhoeal episodes than infants who are breast-fed. The risk of necrotizing enterocolitis is also greater in formula-fed infants than in infants receiving human milk, and the protective effects of human milk remain, at a reduced level, even when infants are only partially breast-fed. There is evidence that breast-feeding also protects against lower respiratory disease including pneumonia, especially in the first months of life. Furthermore, a number of studies have demonstrated a protective effect of breast-feeding against otitis media. Breast-feeding may also be protective against bacteraemia and meningitis, botulism and urinary tract infection, although the evidence is less strong (Heinig and Dewey, 1996).

Most of the protective effects of breast-feeding against infectious disease are passive: immuno-protective factors in breast milk protect the mucosal surfaces of the gastrointestinal and respiratory tract and thereby decrease the risk of infections. However, there is also evidence that breast milk has an active positive influence on the infant's immune system.

Non-infectious and chronic diseases

Studies investigating the impact of infant feeding on chronic illness are limited by their unavoidable retrospective design. An inverse relationship between insulin-dependent diabetes mellitus (IDDM) and breast-feeding duration has been reported. Early exposure (<4 months of age) to cow's milk protein may also act as a trigger for early-onset IDDM. There is also some evidence that breast-feeding may be protective against Crohn's disease, ulcerative colitis and childhood cancer. Breast-feeding may be protective against adiposity later in childhood.

It is thought likely that breast-feeding is protective against atopic and allergic disease, firstly because human milk provides immunological factors that may protect the infant from exposure and reaction to antigens, and secondly because breast-feeding results in delayed exposure to many potentially allergenic substances present in foods. Breast-feeding protects against the development of cow's milk allergy, but whether it protects against other allergic diseases and whether protection against the symptoms of food allergy extends beyond the period of exclusive breast-feeding remains unresolved. In several studies, lack of

breast-feeding has been a significant risk factor for sudden infant death syndrome.

Failure to thrive and nutrient deficiencies

The period of early infancy is a critical period when growth rate is at its maximal and the infant is potentially vulnerable to growth faltering, deficiencies of certain nutrients, and their clinical consequences. However in exclusively breast-fed infants failure-to-thrive, growth faltering and specific nutrient deficiencies are rare until the first introduction of complementary foods and thereafter they are particularly common in the developing world. This is one of the reasons why WHO and UNICEF recommend exclusive breast-feeding until about 6 months of age for healthy term babies. Complementary feeding and problems associated with it are addressed in Chapter 9.

Health advantages to the mother (Table 8.9)

Anaemia, cancer, osteoporosis and obesity

Breast-feeding can have positive effects on maternal health in both the short and long term. Maternal mortality may be reduced, haemoglobin stores preserved and the risk of premenopausal breast cancer is lower in women who breast-fed than in those who bottle-fed their babies. The reduction in cancer risk is greatest in women who practise prolonged breast-feeding. It is also possible that breast-feeding reduces the risk of ovarian cancer. Lactation was considered to be a factor in the aetiology of osteoporosis because of the high rate of transfer of calcium from mother to the fetus and baby, but this is no longer considered likely because lactational changes in calcium and bone metabolism are reversed in the later stages of lactation and after weaning. Indeed, recent studies suggest that lactation may ultimately result in increased bone mineralization, which may reduce the risk of later osteoporosis. In well-nourished women lactation promotes a loss of excess weight accrued during pregnancy and helps to maintain a healthy body weight, although there is no evidence that it protects against subsequent obesity (Heinig and Dewey, 1997).

Lactational amenorrhoea

Lactational amenorrhoea refers to the inhibitory effects of breast-feeding on ovulation during the postpartum period. The duration of postpartum infertility is lengthened by breast-feeding, the more so the greater the frequency and duration of infant suckling. The cause of suppression of fertility is suckling stimulation, which increases the secretion of prolactin, and inhibits that of gonadotrophin releasing hormone (GnRH). The interaction between prolactin and GnRH prevents the resumption of the normal pre-ovulatory surge in luteinizing hormone, thereby suppressing ovulation.

Reducing maternal fertility extends the intervals between successive pregnancies and leads to a decrease in the number of births, if other forms of contraception are not used. Increasing the space between births so that infants are conceived 18–23 months after a previous live birth, is strongly associated with improved child health and survival and has a number of positive effects on maternal health. The Bellagio Consensus Statement on the use of breast-feeding as a family planning method estimated its contraceptive effect to be over 90 per cent for the first 6 months postpartum, in women who are amenorrhoeic and either fully or nearly fully breast-feeding on demand. Exclusive breast-feeding on-demand for up to 6 months therefore represents a valuable method of contraception where other methods are not readily available or acceptable. It is promoted not only for the direct advantages it confers to the infant in terms of nutrition and protection from disease, but also for the indirect effects it exerts on maternal fertility and consequently child spacing, and the health and survival of future children.

Conclusion

Nourishment of the young on milk is one of the defining characteristics of mammals: human (breast) milk is for babies, cow's milk is for calves. The composition of the milk of each species reflects the postnatal growth and nutritional requirements of its young. Sound child health is the foundation of sound adult health, and optimal nutrition during early life has both immediate and long-term positive health consequences. Breast-feeding is the optimum mode of feeding of the newborn infant, and human (breast) milk is the sole and sufficient source of energy and nutrients for the infant until about 6 months. As well as containing nutrients in the amounts and forms suited to the needs of the newborn, human milk also contains a range of non-nutritional factors, which provide defence against infection and assist adaptation to life outside the womb.

Human milk production is largely driven by infant demand: volumes of over half a litre per day are usual during established breast-feeding, which can be sustained for well over 2 years. The composition of human milk varies during an individual feed and during the course of lactation, reflecting and anticipating the nutritional needs of the infant. There comes a time, at about 6 months of age in the healthy term baby, when milk alone is insufficient to meet the nutritional needs of the growing infant. This is the time for the introduction of complementary (weaning) food, which should be added to rather than substituted for, milk.

Substrates for milk synthesis are supplied by maternal diet and stores. Lactational capacity is relatively resilient and unaffected by maternal nutritional status and dietary intake, and substrate requirements for milk production are relatively small compared with overall maternal needs. Energy and nutrient requirements in infancy are defined as dietary reference values based on figures calculated from intakes of breast-fed babies that include factors that account for the difference in the bioavailability of some nutrients from formula milks. Alternatives to human milk are formulas based on cow's milk. Although these are modified to resemble human milk, they cannot reproduce the nutrient and non-nutrient components of human milk. Breast-feeding is associated with many short-term and long-term health advantages to both mother and baby.

Acknowledgements

We are grateful to Shona Hutchison for Figures 8.2, 8.3 and 8.4, to Jean Hyslop for preparing the figures and to Kim Michaelsen, Aileen Robertson and Francesco Branca, co-authors with Lawrence Weaver of *Feeding and Nutrition of Infants and Young Children* (WHO, Geneva, 2000).

References

Department of Health (1991) *Dietary Reference Values for Food Energy and Nutrients for the United Kingdom.* HMSO, London.

Department of Health (1994) *Weaning and the Weaning Diet.* HMSO, London.

Derrickson EM (1992) Comparative reproductive strategies of altricial and precocial eutherian mammals. *Funct. Ecol.* **6**, 57–65.

Elsom R and Weaver LT (1999) Does breastfeeding beyond one year benefit children? *Fetal Matern. Med. Rev.* **11**, 163–174.

Farquarson J, Cockburn F, Patrick W, Jamieson E and Logan R (1992) Infant cerebral cortex phospholipid fatty acid composition and diet. *Lancet* **340**, 810–813.

Garrow JS *et al.* (1999) *Human Nutrition and Dietetics.* Churchill Livingstone, London.

Goldman AS, Chheda S and Garofalo R (1998) Evolution of immunologic functions of mammary gland and the postnatal development of immunity. *Pediatr. Res.* **43**, 155–162.

Heinig MJ and Dewey KG (1996) Health advantages of breastfeeding for infants: a critical review. *Nutr. Res. Rev.* **9**, 89–110.

Heinig MJ and Dewey KG (1997) Health advantages of breastfeeding for mothers: a critical review. *Nutr. Res. Rev.* **10**, 35–56.

Koldovsky O and Thornburg W (1987) Hormones in milk. *J. Pediatr. Gastroenterol. Nutr.* **6**, 172–196.

Long CA (1969) The origin and evolution of mammary glands. *Bioscience* **19**, 519–523.

Manson WG and Weaver LT (1997) Fat digestion in the neonate. *Arch. Dis. Child.* **76**, F206–211.

Martin RD (1984) Scaling effects and adaptive strategies in mammalian lactation. *Symp. Zool. Soc. Lond.* **51**, 87–117.

Martin RD and MacLarnon AM (1985) Gestation period, neonatal size and maternal investment in placental mammals. *Nature* **313**, 220–223.

Michaelsen KF, Weaver LT, Branca F and Robertson A (2000) *Feeding and Nutrition of Infants and Young Children.* WHO Regional Publications, European Series no. 87. WHO, Copenhagen.

Morriss G (1975) Placental evolution and embryonic nutrition. In: *Comparative Placentation*, ed. Steven DH, pp. 87–107. Academic Press, London.

Neville MC (2001) Anatomy and physiology of lactation. *Pediatr. Clin. N. Am.* **48**, 13–34.

Oftedal OT (1980) Milk in mammalian evolution. In: *Comparative Physiology: Primitive Animals*, ed. Schmitz-Nielson K, Bolis L and Taylor CR, pp. 31–42. Cambridge University Press, Cambridge.

Oftedal OT (1984) Milk composition, milk yield and energy output at peak lactation: a comparative review. *Symp Zool. Soc. Lond.* **51**, 33–85.

Pond CM (1977) The significance of lactation in the evolution of mammals. *Evolution* **31**, 177–199.

Pond CM (1983) Parental feeding as a determinant of ecological relationships in Mesozoic terrestial ecosystems. *Acta Palaeontol. Polon.* **28**, 215–224.

Prentice A, Ewing G, Roberts SB, Lucas A, MacCarthy A, Jarjou LM and Whitehead RG (1987) The nutritional role of breast milk IgA and lactoferrin. *Acta Paediatr. Scand.* **76**, 592–598.

Weaver LT (1993) Egg, placenta, breast and gut: comparative strategies for feeding the young. *Endocr. Regul.* **27**, 95–104.

Weaver LT, Arthur HMC, Bunn JEG and Thomas JE (1998) Human milk IgA concentrations during the first year of lactation. *Arch. Dis. Child.* **78**, 235–239.

Widdowson EM (1981) *Feeding the Newborn Mammal.* Carolina Biology Readers Decker, Burlington, NC.

9

COMPLEMENTARY FEEDING FOR THE FULL-TERM INFANT

Nilani Sritharan and Jane Morgan

LEARNING OUTCOMES

- The importance of complementary feeding – the key role of infant feeding in the maintenance of growth and awareness of the relationship between poor growth, malnutrition and morbidity, e.g. lowered cognitive development in children has been linked to poor iron status in infancy.

- When to introduce complementary (solid) foods – understanding of the complications associated with early and late weaning, the difficulties in prescribing a precise age for weaning onset for a population, and understanding that each infant has a 'window of opportunity' during which solid feeding should begin.

- Suitable complementary (solid) foods – the types of foods that are commonly fed to infants in the UK, market trends in infant feeding, and understanding the importance of both the quantity and quality of complementary foods.

- National and international guidelines for complementary feeding – what these are and the differences between them, e.g. interorganizational differences in the recommended age of weaning onset.

- Areas of evidence-based research – the uncertainties associated with complementary feeding; e.g. optimal fat quality and NSP recommendations; understanding that many recommendations are based on adult studies.

- Controversial aspects of infant feeding – the implications of the lack of research in certain aspects of complementary feeding; examples include the age of introduction of cow's milk as a drink.

Introduction

Definitions

Complementary feeding (also known as weaning or transitional feeding) is defined as 'the process of expanding the diet to include foods and drinks other than breast milk or infant formula' (DOH, 1994a) and therefore will influence the growth potential and health of the infant. Since the publication of this report by the Department of Health, UK, other organizations have reconsidered the definition of weaning. The World Health Organization (WHO, 1998) state that, for developing countries. 'The period during which other foods or liquids are provided along with breast milk is considered the period of complementary feeding. Any nutrient-containing foods or liquids other than breast milk given to young children during the period of complementary feeding are defined as complementary foods.' The WHO document went further and highlighted the fact that the term *weaning* is often used in a limited sense to indicate complete cessation of any breast-feeding. Consequently, the WHO now avoids using the term 'weaning foods' so as not to imply that complementary foods are intended to displace breast milk or initiate the withdrawal of breast-feeding. As this change has not been adopted formally in the UK, we shall use the terms 'complementary feeding' and 'weaning' interchangeably, in accordance with the DOH (1994a) definition.

The feeding of mature human milk in sufficient amounts normally meets the nutritional needs of the human infant, but he/she inevitably outgrows its provision. The gradual introduction of foods other than milk is essential to meet the increasing nutritional requirements. However, the introduction of solid foods is a complex event and evidence-based opinion on three fundamental aspects should be considered: the age of weaning onset; the nutritional composition of weaning foods at each transitional stage; and the

influence of the infant diet on adult disease outcomes. In addition to these concepts, we must also be aware of the social, psychological and cultural influences that the mother brings to this equation.

Formulating feeding guidelines is further complicated by the current lack of consensus or lack of research into some aspects of the weaning process. For example, there is little evidence-based research on which to base recommendations for complementary feeding in the preterm infant. Practical advice for complementary feeding of the preterm infant is reviewed by King (2001).

Good clinical judgement has to be the principal guiding source. As Figure 9.1 illustrates, the multidimensional nature of weaning means that infant feeding guidelines must continually be reviewed. It is the role of health professionals to maintain an awareness of consensus and practice in this area, and to suggest or to implement any changes where justifiably appropriate.

Historical trends

In 1974 Fomon reviewed the literature regarding trends in the feeding of 'bekoist' (the German term for foods other than breast or formula milk for the young infant). Until the 1920s solid foods were seldom offered to young children (from Holt's *The Diseases of Infancy and Childhood*, published from 1897 to 1953). Up until 1911 green vegetables were not recommended before 3 years of age! By the 1940s, however, there were reports in the UK of infants being given fish at 4–6 weeks and solids within the first few days of life. In the 1960s and 1970s the early introduction of solids (often a wheat-based cereal mix) with milk (inside as well as outside a bottle) was popular. The increased availability of commercial 'weaning' foods coincided with the trend towards the earlier introduction of solids. By the 1970s (DHSS, 1974) concern about possible hazards

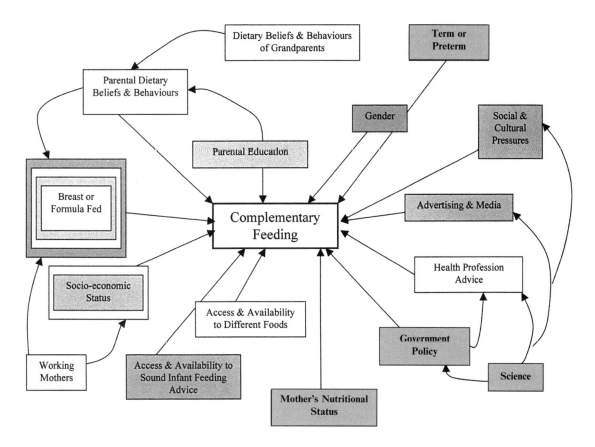

Figure 9.1 The multidimensional nature of complementary feeding

from the early introduction of solid foods, for example obesity, resulted in the recommendation that the introduction of cereals and other solid foods should be discouraged before 3 months of age.

The British Nutrition Foundation Briefing Paper 'Nutrition in Infancy' (Wharton 1997a) describes the secular changes in the weaning diet in the UK from 1975 to 1990. Table 13 of that report shows that in the early 1970s 40 per cent of infants had received some solid foods at 6 weeks of age, and by 4 months 97 per cent of infants had begun the weaning process. However, it was not so long ago that health professionals were advising mothers to introduce complementary foods before one month

of age (Akre, 1989). By the 1990s the situation was a little better, and many mothers were following advice from the Department of Health (DOH). Currently the DOH (1994a) advice is 'The majority of infants should not be given solid foods before the age of four months, and a mixed diet should be offered by the age of six months'. This advice is given for the breast-fed and formula-fed infant.

Growth

Poor growth (in particular poor weight gain) in infancy reflects an inadequate nutritional intake and as such is a convenient indicator of malnutrition. Since weight gain is most

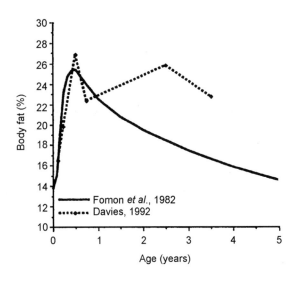

Figure 9.2 Contemporary measurements of body fatness in young male children: a comparison with Fomon's reference data [reproduced from Davies (1995) *Essays on Auxology*, by permission of Castlemead Publications]

rapid during the first year of life, particularly during the first 6 months when body fat is being deposited, energy intakes in infancy are especially important. However, our knowledge of body fatness in young children is open to question (Davies, 1995) and as new data are published, the accepted norms are refined. It is clear from Figure 9.2 that there is accelerated deposition of fat between 0 and 6 months of age (coinciding with the onset of the weaning process) from 14 to 25 per cent of total body weight, declining to around 22 per cent by 12 months.

Growth (discussed in greater detail in Chapter 1) should be maximized as far as possible because growth impairment, for example, is strongly associated with delayed mental development, reduced intellectual achievement at school and impaired functionality in the workplace in adulthood (De Onis *et al.*, 2000; Pollitt *et al.*, 1993; Mendez and Adair, 1999; Spurr *et al.*, 1977).

Growth in infancy and young childhood must be safeguarded because it signifies nutritional adequacy and also because poor growth has been associated with increased risk of ill health in adult life (Barker, 1990).

'Growth faltering' is commonly associated with late weaning because it frequently follows a period of undernutrition. Breast or formula milk alone is unable to meet the nutritional and in particular the energy, vitamin D, zinc, copper and iron requirements for most infants beyond 6 months (DOH, 1994a). As a result, beyond 6 months, the majority of infants cannot afford to use the limited energy intake imposed by late weaning, for growth, since energy is also needed for the infant's metabolic activity and so he/she becomes (at least in the short-term) malnourished. As the infant grows he/she becomes fatter and contains less water. However, growth velocity slows in late infancy. The composition of the body changes with the accretion of protein, the mineralization of the skeleton and with the appearance of teeth. Moreover the type of milk fed, whether human or formula, can alter the percentage of fat in the body of the young infant. There are no similar data on the effect of the age of weaning on subsequent body fat proportions.

Detailed information on growth-related infant disorders such as failure-to-thrive can be found elsewhere (Shaw and Lawson, 2001). Material in Chapters 1, 7, 8 and 10 should be read in relation to this section.

Age of Introduction of Complementary Feeding

During the first 10 days of postnatal life the infant's diet is dominated by colostrum; the transitional period is completed when mature human milk is fed (Figure 9.3). After a while human milk inevitably becomes physiologically and nutritionally inadequate (in particular energy and dietary iron) and the next major

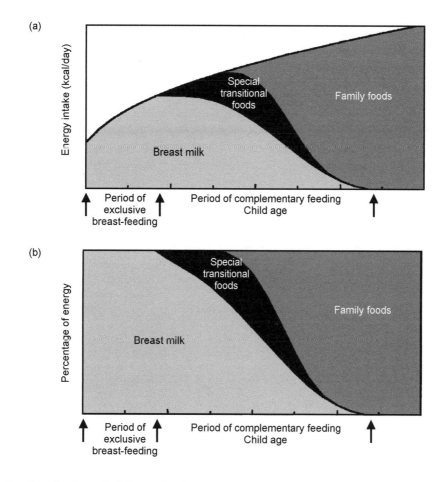

Figure 9.3 Contribution of different food sources to young children's energy intake in relation to age [reproduced from WHO (1998) *Complementary Feeding of Young Children in Developing Countries: a Review of Current Scientific Knowledge*, by permission of WHO]

change in feeding patterns occurs. Deficiency of dietary iron (resulting in anaemia) is unlikely to occur in the breast-fed infant if a solid food, with an iron source, is introduced at between 4 and 6 months and cow's milk introduction is postponed to 1 year (Williams, 1991).

The past decade has seen a dramatic upturn in attitudes towards issues of infant nutrition, the duration of breast-feeding and the age of weaning onset. Barker (discussed further in Chapter 7) hypothesized that nutrition during pregnancy and early childhood could exert

metabolic changes that 'programmed' a baby's risk of developing chronic diseases in adulthood, suggesting that nurture might be as important as nature.

Research into this phenomenon, commonly known as the 'Barker Hypothesis', has since demonstrated, among other things, a direct link between the duration of breast-feeding and arterial distensibility (Leeson *et al.*, 2001). This is consistent with the findings of Fall *et al.* (1992), who found that breast-feeding to 1 year was associated with an increased risk of ischaemic heart disease (IHD) 60 years later.

Table 9.1 Time of introduction of complementary foods into the infant's diet [reproduced from Michaelsen *et al.* (2000) *Feeding and Nutrition of Infants and Young Children*, WHO Regional Publications no. 87, by permission of WHO Regional Office of Europe]

Country	Average age of introduction			
	<3 months	3–4 months	5–6 months	>6 months
Baltic countries				
Lithuania	Fruit, berries, vegetable juice		Curd, egg yolk, oil, butter, cereals	Meat, broth
Central Asian republics (CAR)				
Uzbekistan	Vegetables, fruit	Broth	Poultry, fish, eggs, meat, flour, potatoes	Family food
Commonwealth of Independent States (excluding CAR)				
Armenia			Fruit, porridge, vegetables, potatoes, biscuits	
Azerbaijan		Potatoes, cereals, soup, milk, porridge, biscuits		
Russian Federation		Fruit	Vegetable purée, cereals	Meat
Southern Europe				
Italy		Rice, porridge, fruit, parmesan	Meat, pasta, vegetables	Eggs, fish, rice, pulses
Spain			Cereals, fruit	Bread, vegetables, yoghurt, meat, fish, eggs, pulses

Kallio *et al.* (1992), found that infants weaned between 2 and 6 months had lower low-density-lipoprotein cholesterol (LDL-C) and total cholesterol concentrations than exclusively breast-fed infants of the same age, although this probably reflects the lower fat content of the weaning diet compared with that of breast milk.

As Table 9.1 shows, complementary feeding recommendations are highly variable across the globe. Problems concerning the appropriate time for weaning result from the narrow window that lies between early and late weaning, the variation between infants' needs and the complications associated with each. Full-term infants do appear to be able to adapt to the premature introduction of solids. If starch (cereal) is fed before the gut matures, i.e. at around 4 months of age, sufficient gastric and pancreatic enzymes can be secreted to aid the digestion of food in the gut lumen. There is also compensation by an increased salivary amylase activity and intestinal glycoamylase (Lebenthal and Lee, 1980). Early weaning, however, is associated with many undesirable effects such as increased coughs and chestiness in the short term (Forsyth *et al.*, 1993) and, questionably, obesity (Akre, 1989) in the longer term. The early introduction of complementary foods may also reduce nutritional sufficiency by displacing the intake of breast milk with foods of an inappropriate nutrient profile, particularly those low in energy and iron. The recommendation to delay the introduction of solid foods to very young children has been cited as the reason for an increase in the age of onset of coeliac disease. (DOH, 1994a; for more information on allergies in infancy, see Chapter 5).

Delaying the onset of weaning can be detrimental to the child's health (see previous section on growth faltering). The delayed intake of solid foods can also delay the development of psychomotor function and reflexes that are important to both feeding and speaking in the young infant (Wharton, 1997b).

Current recommendations

This subject was reviewed by Brown (2000), Wharton (2000) and others at a workshop organized by the International Paediatric Association (IPA) and the Committee on Nutrition of the European Society of Paediatric Gastroenterology, Hepatology, and Nutrition (ESPGHAN), entitled 'Research Priorities in Complementary Feeding'.

Is there sufficient evidence to revise the current recommendations? A systematic review of 300 relevant published research papers was undertaken by Lanigan et al. (2001). Thirty-three studies were included in the systematic review, which fulfilled strict inclusion criteria and which examined outcome measures in relation to the age of introduction of complementary feeding in the full-term infant. The authors found substantial methodological flaws in more than half of the studies included and no study met all methodological criteria. Of the 13 papers which were comparable, no evidence-based conclusions could be drawn in support of the modification of existing UK guidelines, which advocate that weaning should commence

at between 4 and 6 months for the majority of infants, irrespective of milk feeding.

However, an expert Consultative Panel, facilitated by the World Health Organization (WHO) undertook their own review of the literature on the introduction of complementary feeding in the full-term infant after an expert consultation and global peer review of the information. The Expert Consultation recommended 'Exclusive breast feeding for 6 months, with introduction of complementary foods and continued breast feeding thereafter' (WHO, 2001).

The WHO press release (WHO, 2001) on the optimal duration of exclusive breast-feeding recognized that there is no one solution to the problem. Attempts to provide feeding guidelines that are appropriate for both the developed and developing worlds must therefore be a compromise. Whilst their revised recommendations seem appropriate for developing countries, where the incidence of microbial infections associated with the introduction of complementary foods is high, there are also pitfalls to this advice. The introduction of whole cow's milk before 12 months, for example, is known to be a risk factor for iron deficiency (Mira et al., 1996). Other deficiencies including a failure to thrive may also prevail in exclusively breast-fed infants whose mothers have a poor dietary intake, such as those in developing countries and among low income groups in the developed world.

Whether the UK will adopt these recommendations remains the subject of much discussion. The arguments for the provision of a separate set of recommendations for the introduction of complementary foods to the exclusively formula-fed infant is outside the scope of this chapter.

Perhaps the question should not be one of amending UK guidelines on when to wean; rather we should focus our efforts on understanding why mothers continue to disregard government advice on weaning. One possible reason is that breast milk may actually be less

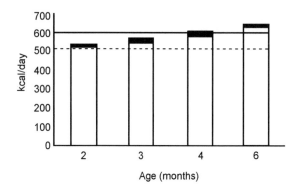

Figure 9.4 Energy requirement of infants (grey bars), assuming the energy density of breast milk to be 70 kcal/100 ml (solid line) or 58 kcal/100 ml (dashed line); data derived from Butte (1996) [reproduced from Morgan (1998) *BNF Nutr. Bull.* **23**(Suppl. 1), by permission of BNF]

energy dense than was previously thought: 58 kcal/100 ml (Lucas and Davies, 1990) as against 70 kcal/100 ml. Within the context of weaning, this could help to explain why mothers choose to wean their infants so early, as it would appear that at 58 kcal/100 ml breast milk becomes energy-insufficient much earlier than 6 months (Figure 9.4, Morgan, 1998).

Other reasons, such as the influence of an increased food intake on the infant's propensity to sleep (anecdotal evidence), or the rise in the number of mothers returning to work after maternity leave (Mintel Market Intelligence, 2000; WHO, 1998) might also account for mothers' persistent attitudes.

Nutrient Profile of Complementary Foods

The report *Weaning and the Weaning Diet* (DOH, 1994a) provides extensive advice and recommendations on the nutritional composition of the infant diet. This report gives advice on both the macronutrient and micronutrient intakes suitable for infants and is required

reading by manufacturers of baby foods and by health professionals. In the following section our knowledge of dietary energy, dietary fat, non-starch polysaccharide (NSP) and protein in relation to weaning will be addressed.

Dietary energy

Details of dietary energy requirements in infancy are to be found in Chapter 8.

Homo sapiens are most sensitive to energy intakes during infancy because this is the time when growth, which is dependent on a sufficient intake of energy, is most rapid. Both the Food and Agricultural Organization/World Health Organization (FAO/WHO 1985) and the Department of Health, UK (DOH, 1991) have published recommended intakes for dietary energy in infancy. However these values have been questioned by some experts in the field. Methods of measuring desired intakes were originally based on the assumption that dietary energy intakes were equivalent to the energy needs of the infant and that the physiological processes that regulate appetite in the hypothalamus would regulate these intakes. More recently, the doubly labelled water technique has been adapted for use in infants and is viewed as a more accurate assessment of energy requirements. This method estimates energy expenditure of the infant and, when compared with the FAO/WHO (1985) recommendations, suggests that they were unnecessarily overinflated (Butte, 1996; Butte *et al.*, 2000). Whilst the results of Butte's meta-analysis called for changes to the recommendations, they have not yet been altered amid fears that energy intakes would drop below those required for growth. Figure 9.5 illustrates the divide between the 1985 FAO/WHO recommendations compared with Butte's own data.

There is convincing evidence that energy intakes (and thus requirements) in infants have

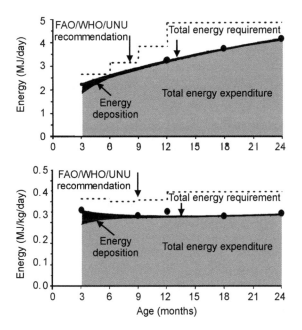

Figure 9.5 Total energy expenditure, energy deposition and total energy requirements of children aged 3–24 months compared with the 1985 FAO/WHO/UNU recommendations [reproduced from Butte *et al.* (2000) *Am. J. Clin. Nutr.* **72**, 1558–1569, by permission of the *American Journal of Clinical Nutrition.* © *Am. J. Clin. Nutr.* American Society for Clinical Nutrition]

significantly declined over the past 25 years; certainly data from English children provide such evidence. The paradox is that young children are becoming fatter, despite this phenomenon of lower energy intakes. In 1988 Prentice and co-workers suggested that we should consider whether our energy recommendations are a 'prescription for overfeeding' or whether, rather than lowering current recommendations, we should consider the potential consequences of a less active baby.

Davies (1995) has proposed a number of explanations for this paradox:

- less physical activity – children watch TV and are carried around in cars;
- families are generally smaller in number and therefore play less;

- central heating has led to a reduction in energy needs to maintain body temperature;
- improved control of infantile paediatric diseases, again lowering the need for energy;
- the lowered energy content of modern infant formulas.

Dietary energy recommendations

What is perhaps more worrying is the proportion of babies who are receiving insufficient energy after weaning because of the use of inappropriate foods such as fruit and vegetable purées (Stordy *et al.*, 1995). These foods, whilst 'single-ingredient' foods, are very low in fat and often form the basis of the educational, and sometimes the transitional diet too. In these infants, milk (either breast or formula) frequently remains the main source of energy after solid foods are introduced. There are no official guidelines for a minimum (or maximum) level of energy (kcal/100 g) in commercial infant foods. If there were, it might be reasonable to use the average energy content of human breast milk (usually stated as 70 kcal/100 ml) as the minimum value.

Dietary fat

Fat is the most energy-dense nutrient available to the infant and is therefore one of the best means of providing sufficient energy to ensure maximum growth, within a volume that can be managed by the infant's small gastric capacity. It is also a source of fat-soluble vitamins (vitamin A, D, E and K), essential fatty acids and exogenous cholesterol, each of which is needed by the infant, to some degree. Fat also improves the palatability of food, providing enhanced taste and texture (Michaelsen *et al.*, 2000). With mothers being encouraged to use single-ingredient foods in the early stages of weaning (to improve the chances of identifying specific allergies), the challenge to provide desirable high-energy foods is great. Estimated requirements for total fat in infancy and the fatty acid profile that this should comprise, however, remains controversial and will be discussed here.

Knowledge that fatty plaques in the arterial wall, which may progress to atherosclerosis during adolescence or adult life and form as early as the first weeks of infancy (Pesonen et al., 1990), has prompted increasing concern over the fat content of the weaning diet. Opinion is varied, however, over the benefits of introducing a low-saturated-fat diet at a very young age, and this is reflected in the lack of government guidance on this issue world-wide. It is not known whether the presence of neonatal fatty streaks or the progression of these fatty streaks to atherosclerotic plaques during adolescence is the greater threat to the development of cardiovascular disease (CVD). Recommendations from the Netherlands (Michaelson and Jorgensen 1995) permit 'fat restriction' (in this instance the fat *quality* not *quantity* is meant) as early as 7 months of age, whereas recommendations from the UK and USA do not advise such a diet before the age of 2 years and the Canadians do not advocate it until adolescence (Zoltkin, 2000). Whilst introducing good eating habits from an early age may make a child more likely to adopt healthy eating regimens in adult life (Law, 2000), so too might the infant become nutrient-deficient (if fed a diet designed for adults) and suffer from growth impediment with a risk of developing certain chronic adult diseases, thus compromising the aim of introducing such a diet in infancy.

There is a lack of consensus regarding fat intakes in infancy. The DOH (1994a) currently advises minimum levels for polyunsaturated fat intakes (1 per cent dietary energy as linoleic acid and 0.2 per cent dietary energy as α-linolenic acid) as the desirable fat quality of the weaning diet. General recommendations on fat quantity are vague and state that fat should not be restricted in children under the age of 2 years

and that the dietary reference values for fat should not be implemented before 5 years of age (DOH, 1991, 1994a,b). The profile of fats [i.e. the ratio of polyunsaturated fatty acids to monounsaturated fatty acids to saturated fatty acids (SFA)], as well as target amounts (as a percentage of energy intake), are not available from national or international authorities so far. However, evidence is accumulating from randomized controlled intervention trials into the effect of dietary fat [36 per cent fat energy ratio (FER)] on cardiovascular risk factors in infancy (Fuchs et al., 1994), although these studies are short-term in nature. Their findings illustrate that the fat composition of an infant's diet can indeed influence the serum lipid and lipoprotein profile. The implication of these findings and their public health message are still under review.

The Finnish Special Turku Coronary Risk Factor Intervention Project for babies (STRIP) studies (Lapinleimu et al., 1995; Niinikoski et al., 1997a,b; Simell et al., 2000) are randomized intervention trials that have attempted to address the issue of optimal fat quantity and quality in infancy. Researchers controversially introduced a low-SFA, energy-matched diet in infants aged 7 months and compared these against a control group where there was no fat restriction The infants in the intervention group were closely monitored to ensure that they did not become growth impaired and that their energy intakes did not drop to levels that were significantly different from their control counterparts. They found no significant difference in the growth velocities of the control and intervention groups. On a population basis, however, such close-monitoring of infants would be costly and impractical to employ. Advice to restrict the SFA content of the infant diet might also risk exposure to a 'macrobiotic'-type diet (Dagnelie et al., 1989a,b) in which infants could become deficient in several nutrients and, hence, growth-faltered. Infants may also be at risk of being fed diets that are either excessively high in sugar (Nicklas et al., 1992)

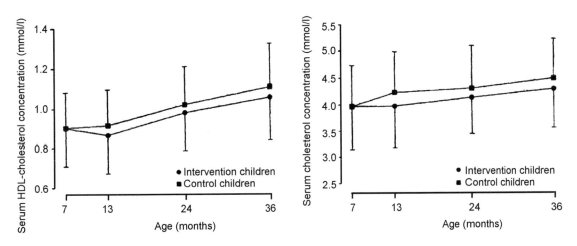

Figure 9.6   The effect in infants of a low-SFA and -cholesterol diet on serum cholesterol (right) and serum HDL (left) in the intervention group, compared with the control group [reproduced from Simell *et al.* (2000) *Am. J. Clin. Nutr.* **72**(Suppl.), 1316S–1331S, by permission of the *American Journal of Clinical Nutrition.* © *Am. J. Clin. Nutr.* American Society of Clinical Nutrition]

or fibre (Wharton 1997b). If saturated fat was replaced with unsaturated fats it is plausible that molecular changes to the phospholipid bilayer would ensue, thus increasing membrane fluidity. Widdowson *et al.* (1975) reported that, in infants, triglycerides in adipose tissue can be altered by the type of fat in the milk consumed. The consequences of this are not known to be either detrimental or beneficial based on current knowledge.

Furthermore, if the unsaturated fatty acid content of the diet becomes proportionally greater, as in the diet of the STRIP studies, an increased susceptibility to oxidative modification is probable. This would not only raise the requirement for antioxidant-rich foods, but it might also reverse the desired effect by increasing the prevalence of fatty streaks in infancy.

The STRIP studies also highlight the problem of 'optimal' plasma high-density lipoprotein cholesterol (HDL-C) concentration in infancy (Figure 9.6). If the HDL-C levels had dropped significantly, this may have impaired the reverse transport (and excretion) of cholesterol in the blood. As a result, lipoprotein metabolism would have been altered and these infants would have been at an increased risk of

developing heart disease or atherosclerosis. The HDL-C concentrations in the serum of the intervention group at the end of the trial were not given. However, should these fall below 2 mmol/l (adult cut-off point, there are no similar data for infants; Griffin B, personal communication), this would confer an increased CVD risk and thus invalidate the intended effect.

Dietary fat recommendations

There are many issues governing appropriate recommendations on fat quality and quantity in infancy for which there are at present no answers. Until the situation improves, we should proceed with caution, but maintain an awareness that advice is subject to refinement in the future. In the mean time, since FER is 40–50 per cent of total energy for breast-fed infants from birth to 4–6 months (DOH, 1994a) and the Government advocate that the FER for all formula and follow-on milks is between 30 and 56.6 per cent (CEC, 1991), it seems reasonable to recommend that the FER should not be less than 30 per cent

Table 9.2 Advisable intake of selected nutrients in infancy [reproduced from Wharton (1997a) *Nutrition in Infancy*, by permission of the British Nutrition Foundation]

	Reference nutrient intake per day			Advisable intake per 100 kcal
	0–3 months	4–6 months	7–9 months	0–12 months
Energy (kcal)	530	670	790	0–4 months 100–110 kcal/kg
				4–12 months 80–100 kcal/kg
Protein (g)	13	13	14	2.25–3.0
Fat (g)				3.6–6.5
Carbohydrate (g)				7–14
Vitamin A (µg)	350	350	350	60–180
Vitamin D (µg)	9	9	7	1–2
Vitamin C (mg)	25	25	25	5 or more
Vitamin K (µg)	10	10	10	2.5–15
Calcium (mg)	525	525	525	45 or more
Phosphorus (mg)	400	400	400	25–90
Sodium (mg)	210	280	320	1.0–2.6
Iron (mg)	2	4	8	0.5–1.5
Zinc (mg)	4	4	5	0.3–1.0
Iodine (µg)	50	60	60	5 or more

dietary energy. It is advised that skimmed milk and semi-skimmed milk should not be introduced before the age of 5 and 2 years, respectively, and that whole cow's milk be avoided before 1 year of age (DOH, 1994a). Formula milks or breast milk are better sources of iron for the infant and, because 'many children's diets are capricious' (DOH, 1994a), fat intakes should average a FER of 40 per cent to help maintain energy intakes. This is achievable through a daily intake of formula or breast milk.

With respect to the type of fat used in the diet, there is currently insufficient evidence upon which to base any recommendations and, as the fatty acid composition of breast milk will reflect the mother's diet, it would be inappropriate to use this as the gold standard. Providing a mother does not interpret a low-SFA diet as a low-fat one, there seems to be no case against its use, although it seems wise to await further evidence before promoting such a diet for infants. Wharton (1997b) has devised advisable intakes of selected nutrients, includ-

ing fat in infancy, and these have been reproduced in Table 9.2.

Existing guidelines on fat intakes are proving to be inadequate and have resulted in a misunderstanding of what constitutes a healthy diet for infants. Some mothers falsely believe that a low-fat diet is appropriate for their infants (Morgan *et al.*, 1995), and such mothers may be depriving their infants of the energy that they need. As we recently found in our analysis of popular infant cookbooks (Sritharan 2001, unpublished findings), several authors are promoting a 'low animal fat' diet without adequate evidence to support such advice. Whilst 'fat restriction' in infancy may prove, in the future, to be correct, particularly if the carbohydrate, protein, vitamin and mineral intakes are maintained, evidence is at present lacking. Greater research is needed to investigate suitable fat profiles and quantities. Any recommendations must balance the requirement of energy for growth against the need to develop good eating habits and minimize future disease risk.

Non-starch polysaccharide

The NSP content of complementary food is, like dietary fat, a contentious issue. Found in two forms, soluble and insoluble, predominantly in vegetables, fruit and cereals, fibre became a popular component of Western diets in the 1970s because of its satiating and health-giving properties.

Dietary Fibre Hypothesis

Diets rich in foods containing plant cell wall material in a relatively natural state are protective against a range of diseases that are prevalent in western affluent communities, for example, diabetes, coronary heart disease, obesity, gall bladder disease, diverticular disease and large bowel cancer (Southgate and Johnson, 1994).

However, whilst NSP remains an important component of healthy adult dietary guidelines, it has been suggested that fibre should not be given to infants at the expense of energy-rich foods (DOH, 1994a; Michaelsen *et al.*, 2000). Infants have a high growth velocity and it would be difficult to meet these energy demands through a bulky and early-satiating fibre-predominant diet because infants have a limited gastric capacity. The detrimental influence of fibre on fat absorption and mineral availability is also a cause for concern: soluble fibres bind fatty acids and cholesterol in the gut, making them unavailable for micelle formation and thus prevent their absorption, forcing their excretion via the bile (Groff and Gropper, 1999). If the diet is especially abundant in cereals and legumes, the infant is likely to have a raised phytate intake. Phytates, in high concentrations, can limit the intestinal uptake of several nutrients, including iron (DOH, 1994a), and, since infants have especially poor iron stores during the initial stages of weaning due to the low (although highly bioavailable) iron content of breast milk, this fact is particularly worrying. Thus, mothers who ignore advice and wean

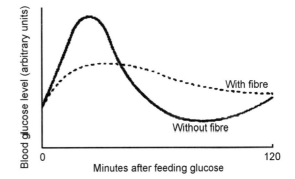

Figure 9.7 Glycaemic effect of NSP on blood insulin and glucose levels [reproduced from Gibney (1986) *Nutrition Diet and Health*, by permission of Cambridge University Press]

their infants onto a diet that consists largely of legumous and wholegrain cereal-based foods risk growth failure in their children, with deficits in several micronutrients and the symptoms of 'Muesli-Belt Malnutrition'.

NSP does have several physiological benefits that might justify its inclusion, in low amounts, as part of the complementary diet in infancy. Firstly, NSP can increase stool weight and help to reduce intra-abdominal pressure, and, secondly, it is also known to flatten the glucose and insulin 'spike' that results from a starchy, carbohydrate intake (see Figure 9.7).

This effect is due to the low glycaemic index of fibre-rich foods (see Foster-Powell and Brand Miller, 1995, for a full list of glycaemic indices) and has been used in adults for the management of diabetes and blood lipid control. This effect may bring potential advantages to the growing infant, but its importance remains to be established.

NSP recommendations

Besides the recommendation that infants should not consume NSP-rich foods at the expense of energy-dense foods and that children require proportionately less fibre than adults due to their smaller body size, there is limited guidance on the age of introduction, quantity (either minimum or maximum) and the type of NSP that should be consumed during complementary feeding. Research into the timing, quantity and quality of fibre in the weaning diet is not sufficient to make any recommendations. Agostoni *et al.* (1995) found that fibre-rich foods 'lower the caloric and proteic density of meals' and concluded that whole cereals and leguminous matter could be 'routinely introduced during the weaning process to achieve better nutritional balance and accustom children to diets with fibre contents.' Whilst it is important that a child adopts healthy dietary habits from an early age, the energy-depriving effect of a high-fibre weaning diet could have detrimental consequences, leading to malnutrition and impaired growth.

The fibre content of typical UK weaning foods is already relatively high. Assuming an average weight at 4 months is 6.35 kg for a male infant (FAO/WHO 1985):

> RNI for NSP = 18 g/day for a 70 kg adult male
> so, $18/70 = $ g NSP/kg/day
> $\therefore$ 1.6 g/day is calculated for an average 4-month-old male infant based on adult recommendations.

If Heinz babyrice = 2 g fibre/100 g and one apple, stewed = 1.5 g/100 g (Englyst method), and since an infant is likely to consume both a fruit purée and babyrice in a day, it is easy to exceed the adult, weight-adjusted NSP RNI in a 4-month-old infant, if he/she consumes 100 g/day of fruit or rice.

Protein

The issue of the protein composition of complementary foods – quantity and quality – is less contentious than that of fat or NSP, certainly with respect to the developed world; a typical mixed weaning diet contains more than adequate amounts of protein provided by milk, eggs, meat and pulses. Dietary surveys on infants consistently illustrate higher than average intakes of protein when compared with the RNI (Mills and Tyler, 1992).

However, undernutrition, which is not related to morbidity, may be the result of an inappropriate nutrient intake and could be associated with inappropriate use of milk formulas, e.g. prolonged partial breast-feeding without adequate addition of complementary foods; excessive juice intake; the offering of inadequate foods because of perceived food 'allergens'; or the inappropriate provision of a milk-free diet that is low in protein (Michaelsen *et al.*, 2000).

Devising appropriate weaning foods with respect to their fat, energy protein and NSP quality and quantity therefore requires careful consideration, supported by evidence-based research.

The Types of Complementary Foods

The popularity of home-prepared weaning foods rose sharply during the early 1990s after a succession of media-provoked health scares such as those of genetic modification and BSE contamination of foods. Indeed, by 1995 41 per cent of infants were receiving home-prepared foods compared with only 12 per cent in 1990 (Foster *et al.*, 1997), although Mintel Market Intelligence (2000) proposed that this might actually reflect an interest in 'home-assembly,' i.e. prepared foods that require input from the consumer (such as pasta sauces that need to be added to pasta), rather than home-cooked infant foods *per se*. By 1999 this trend began to reverse with two-thirds of mothers returning to work once maternity leave had ceased (Mintel Market Intelligence 2000). 'Time' was driving the up-turn in the sales of commercially prepared infant foods, especially sales of organic brands. It seems that organic manufactured baby foods are sufficiently able to satisfy maternal desires to provide safe and nutritious foods within a convenient, easy-to-prepare form, so much so that sales of organic baby foods have seen a 5-fold rise since 1995 (Mintel Market Intelligence, 2000):

What's driving the organic market for babies?

- Healthy eating concerns
- Consecutive food scares
- An increased awareness by consumers of food safety issues

Despite this trend, or perhaps in parallel to it, there is a rise in the number of infant cookbooks, indicative of the continued interest in home-cooked weaning foods. Contrary to popular belief, these are not necessarily nutritionally superior for infants compared with commercial baby foods. Whilst they are probably cheaper than commercial foods (a large sachet of babyrice costs approximately £1.70) and may make it easier for the infant to adapt to family foods towards late infancy

(DOH, 1994a), such foods can reflect the dietary misconceptions and potentially sodium- and sucrose-rich tastes of a child's parents.

Commercial vs home-prepared foods

Stordy *et al.* (1995) and Wharton (1997a) have each considered the nutritional value of weaning foods; the first based their comparative analysis by chemical analysis techniques and the latter on food composition tables (Figure 9.8). On average the results suggested that home-made infant foods were lower in fat, iron and vitamin D and higher in sodium compared with commercially prepared foods. Possible explanations for this may lie in the fact that commercial infant foods must comply with UK government legislation, *The Processed Cereal-Based Foods and Baby Foods for Infants and Young Children Regulations (1997)* (refer to Table 9.3 for UK fat regulations). This

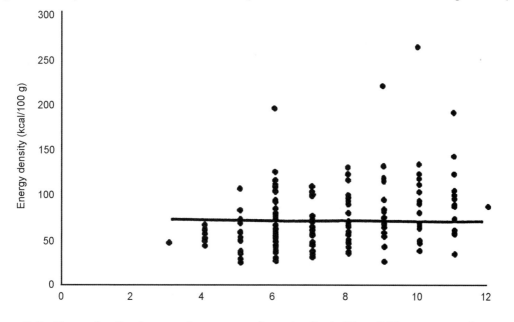

Figure 9.8 Energy density of savoury home-prepared weaning foods. The solid line represents the mean energy content of mature human milk of 70 kcal/100 ml [reproduced from Stordy *et al.* (1995) *Acta Paediatr.* **84**, 733–741, by permission of Taylor & Francis]

Table 9.3 UK regulations for the fat content of baby foods (modified from *The Processed Cereal-Based Foods and Baby Foods for Infants and Young Children Regulations*, 1997)

Product	Fat content should not exceed
Simple cereals (reconstituted with milk)	3.3 g/100 kcal
Cereals with added high-protein food (reconstituted with water)	4.5 g/100 kcal[a]
Pastas (after cooking)	No regulations
Rusks and biscuits (with addition of water or other liquids)	3.3 g/100 kcal

[a]Profile of fatty acids is also regulated if total exceeds 3.3 g/100 kcal.

suggests the need for greater guidance to help mothers wishing to provide nutritionally sound home-made weaning foods for their infants.

We recently investigated the dietary composition of recipes suitable for home cooking in five popular infant nutrition books. The nutritional discrepancies of home-prepared weaning foods (reported above) were again apparent in the recipes suggested in these books. The results of this analysis also highlighted the current trend to promote low-fat, (especially low-saturated-fat) foods and, in several cases, these books provided shockingly incorrect nutrition advice. Such information frequently reflected concern over the perceived influence of infant diets on adult disease, most notably coronary heart disease. We also noted a failure of many of these diets to meet the energy requirements of the infant. In one case the authors actually promoted a vegan diet that consisted of little more than fruit and vegetable purées up to the age of 9 months, and encouraged wheat-containing juices for infants as young as 6 months. An infant consuming such a diet would receive so little energy and such an imbalance of micro- and macronutrients that growth impairment would undoubtedly ensue at this very crucial time of life. Unfortunately there are no guidelines on how

the information in these books should conform to good nutritional practice at present.

Suitable complementary foods

Infants receiving commercial weaning foods do not appear to be at any nutritional disadvantage compared with their 'family food'-fed counterparts (Wharton, 1997b). In fact, they might actually be at an advantage because of the more balanced nutrient profile of manufactured baby foods (Morgan *et al.*, 1995) and the strict legal codex to which they must comply. There are nonetheless some issues relating to the suitability of some foods for infants of which we must be aware (Table 9.4):

Non-wheat cereals, fruit, vegetables and potatoes are suitable first weaning foods. Salt should not be added and additional sugars should be limited to that needed for the palatability of sour fruits. By the age of one year the diet should be mixed and varied (DOH, 1994a).

It has been advised that 'pureed vegetables and fruit are not suitable first weaning foods because they are low in energy, low in fat and low in many micronutrients' (Morgan, 1998), but that the energy deficit of these foods can be overcome by 'the addition of a fat source, for example olive oil, to puréed vegetables, as is done by some mothers in Spain (Van den Boom *et al.*, 1997). However, the WHO (Michaelsen *et al.*, 2000) and DOH (1994a; see quotation above) state that first foods should be 'single-ingredient' foods such as fruit and vegetables. In this way, mothers will be able to detect any allergies with greater certainty.

Good examples include non-wheat cereals... soft thick porridge made from traditional cereal foods such as oats, and pureed vegetables and fruit (Michaelsen *et al.*, 2000).

Table 9.4 Nutrient profile of human milk and 'first complementary foods'

	Colostrum	Mature human milk	Babyrice[a] (reconstituted)	Carrots
Energy (kcal/100 g)	56	69	66	22
Fat (percentage energy)	42	53	23	<1
Protein (percentage energy)	14	8	12	10
Carbohydrate (percentage energy)	44	39	65	80
Iron (mg/100 g)	0.07	0.07	1	0.4
Vitamin D (µg/100 g)	N[b]	0.04	1	0

[a]Manufacturer's information.
[b]No reliable information.

The following section, addressing the suitability of complementary foods, has been modified from the WHO publication on infant feeding (Michaelsen et al., 2000).

During the first few weeks and months of weaning (4–6 months), feeding allows the infant to develop the skills to eat from a spoon and introduces new textures and tastes. In this way, the mother should be able to supplement their infant's milk diet with solid foods. For this reason it is recommended that first foods should be offered after the infant has been breast-fed to avoid replacing breast milk with solid foods. However, complementary foods are frequently low in fat and therefore, as breast milk intake declines, a lower energy intake than is currently recommended will result. Reasons for this are likely to relate to the effect of fat and starch on the viscosity of infant solids. Michaelson et al. (2000) explain that starch granules (which could improve the energy density of the food) often gelatinize when heated, for example in porridge (which is the main staple for many infants of the developing world), making it difficult for the infant to consume and digest the food. Similarly foods rich in solid fats (such as lard) will also increase the viscosity such that the infant cannot easily consume the food. Fat-rich foods are also likely to compromise the protein and micronutrient content of the complement, both of which are essential for

growth and the prevention of micronutrient deficiency at this stage. Complement that is energy-poor, whilst being easier to consume, will result in the infant having to feed more frequently and to consume greater volumes to satisfy his/her energy requirements. In practice this can be difficult to achieve because of the infant's small gastric capacity. The addition of oil (as suggested by Van den Boom et al., 1997) or a suitable full-fat milk (Michaelsen et al., 2000; breast milk or infant milk formula) to solids can help overcome these problems, but this is often not well-recognized by mothers who are preparing foods in the home.

Infants who are being weaned should also be encouraged to try different tastes, although food acceptance is unlikely to occur before 8–10 exposures to that food. Research suggests that breast-fed infants are more inclined to try new foods than their formula-fed counterparts because they have been exposed to an increased variation in tastes via their mother's milk. Parents should be aware of the fact that infants also have a preference for sweet foods and that a child's preference for certain foods is related to the frequency of exposure to certain tastes. Exposure to sugary foods should thus be limited in an infant's diet as this also has implications for dental health. Salt intakes should also be kept to a minimum and mothers are advised to avoid adding salt to home-prepared meals.

Timetable for introducing complementary foods

The 'timetable for weaning' varies considerably depending on the reference source; different authorities provide conflicting advice on the appropriate stages at which certain foods are introduced. The timetable for the inclusion of full-fat cow's milk as a drink is an example of this confusion. In the UK, the DOH (1994a) recommends 'pasteurised whole cow's milk should only be used as a main milk drink after the age of one year.' On the other hand, recommendations from the WHO (Michaelsen et al., 2000) state that, 'from 9–12 months, cow's milk can be gradually introduced into the infant's diet as a drink.'

Perhaps more intriguing is the advice given by the official textbook for dietitians in the UK (Talbot, 2001) where, in the 'Timetable for Weaning', Stage 1 (the initial stage), it is recommended that the introduction of first solid foods should occur *before* the first 4–6 months of age (described as Stage 2). An example of the 'Timetable for Weaning' can be found in Michaelson et al. (2000).

Good Infant Feeding Practices

Interest in the relationship between diet and CVD leading to the promotion of a low-fat, high-NSP diet, as appropriate for a healthy heart in adults, appears to have confused many mothers into believing that this diet is best for infants too. Such parental misconceptions have been outlined as a cause of both failure-to-thrive and hypothyroidism with short stature (Pugliese et al., 1987; Labib *et al.*, 1989), both of which significantly influence growth outcomes and later health.

Parental misconceptions

It is not uncommon to find a mother who is attempting to feed her infant a diet that is very low in fat and potentially energy-deficient. For example, whilst 95 per cent of mothers considered a wide variety of foods to be 'important' or 'very important', more than 80 per cent of mothers attached the same degree of importance to a low-fat (88 per cent), fibre-rich (83 per cent) diet as being appropriate for infants (Morgan *et al.*, 1995). This finding has been supported elsewhere (Hobbie *et al.*, 2000) and suggests that mothers have a poor understanding of infant nutrition which in some cases can be highly detrimental to the health of their child.

Mothers who are described as 'food restrictors' illustrate the full extent to which psychological and sociological factors can influence the food intake of their offspring. For example,

Table 9.5 US Mothers attitudes towards infant feeding practices (Hobbie *et al.*, 2000)

Question asked	Disagree or strongly disagree (%)	Neutral or do not know or did not answer (%)	Agree or strongly agree (%)
Cow's milk can be introduced into a baby's diet when the baby begins to take solids	60	21	19
Fruit juice provides babies with nutritional benefits unavailable in infant formula or breast milk	61	22	17
Fruit juice is a necessary part of the baby's diet	44	21	35
The best time to wean babies from the breast is when they start to develop teeth	46	25	30

Table 9.6 Nutritional composition of a day's menu using recipes taken from five infant nutrition cookbooks, suitable for infants aged 6–9 months (Sritharan, unpublished data)

Nutrient	Book 1	Book 2[a]	Book 3[a]	Book 4	Book 5
Energy (kcal)	745	420	1060	465	510
Fat (g)	71	25	52	57	38
NSP (g)	8	6	7	7	2
Sugars (g)	90	60	64	83	91

[a]Organic recipe books.

mothers with a history of eating disorders have been linked to infants with eating difficulties as well as infants that restrict their food intake.

Pugliese *et al.* (1987) reported that a mother's fear of obesity, fear of atherosclerotic disease and a desire for a healthy diet were all potential causes of failure-to-thrive in children, but that parental intentions were not to 'deprive' their children, rather to give them what they believed to be best. Further evidence of this phenomenon comes from Stein *et al.* (1994, 1995), who investigated the cause of eating disorders in infants; they found that 'conflict arose because maternal eating disorder psychopathology interfered with aspects of responsible parenting and, that feeding disturbances in children are specifically associated with disturbed eating habits and attitudes among mothers.'

At the other end of the spectrum the behavioural traits of obese women may also differ from the norm in the manner in which they feed their infants. This could have important public health implications, as obesity is increasing rapidly in children and adults. Work from Drewett and Parkinson (1999) suggests that obese mothers encourage their babies to eat when they (the babies) are not hungry, thus attempting to override a child's own appetite control mechanisms. This could then predispose the child to overeat and become obese later in life (Johnson and Birch, 1994).

These examples illustrate the importance of the mother understanding and implementing appropriate infant feeding practices; they also demonstrate the potential harm in trying to apply health guidelines for the whole population to the infant population.

We have examined the nutrient content of a day's menu based on recipes taken from five infant nutrition cookbooks currently available on the market. We found great discrepancies in the total energy intakes and the fat profiles of these menus, some showing alarmingly low levels of energy compared with the dietary reference value. Interlinked to this is the apparent misconceived belief that a low-fat diet is appropriate for infants (Table 9.6).

A public health approach

Food-based dietary guidelines for adults were recommended for use by the FAO and WHO in an attempt to better educate the adult public on aspects of healthy eating (website of the FAO). Current schematics class nutrients according to their food group classifications, i.e. fat, carbohydrates etc. (Figures 9.9 and 9.10), yet fail to address the fact that many foods in Western diets comprise several nutrient groups and also fail to include commonly consumed foods in their illustrations. Fraser (1994) stresses that the use of individual foods would be of greater benefit in the long term, partly because some foods contain biochemically active compounds that can promote health.

These nutrition tools, whilst widely used, are only intended for children over the age of 2 years and adults (Buiten and Metzger, 2000),

The Balance of Good Health

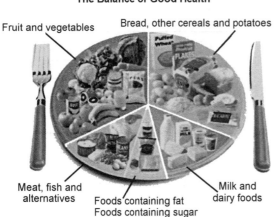

Fruit and vegetables

Bread, other cereals and potatoes

Meat, fish and alternatives

Foods containing fat
Foods containing sugar

Milk and dairy foods

Figure 9.9 Balance of Good Health – the UK nutrition healthy eating education tool [reproduced from the BNF website www.nutrition.org.uk, by permission of the Food Standards Agency]

although awareness of this fact appears to be poor. Such food-based dietary guidelines are not available for infants but should be a consideration for the future. An Australian dietitian has identified this need and developed

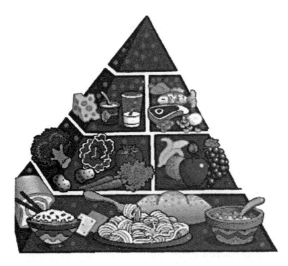

Figure 9.10 USDA food pyramid (2–6 years). The uppermost tip of the pyramid represents fats and sugars [reproduced from USDA and US Department of Health and Human Services (1992) *The Food Guide Pyramid*, Home and Garden Bulletin no. 252]

a set of simple, consumer-focused guidelines for infant feeding (Figure 9.11). These are similar in concept to the UK's 10 guidelines for healthy eating but, like these, the Australian tool does not address all parental misconceptions or all aspects of the infant diet. The schematic also uses terms such as 'low-fat' which are poorly understood by the public and uses terms which require a good understanding of the nutrient composition of food, e.g. 'serve foods containing iron'. This is, however, a step in the right direction and should be used as a framework for a UK equivalent to educate mothers about optimal infant feeding practices.

Recognition of this problem of a lack of guidelines for infants led to the WHO's *Health21* (2000) initiative for the new millennium which hopes to introduce 'the development of food-based dietary guidelines and infant/young child feeding strategies, as an integral part of national health policies'.

Evaluations of the effectiveness of these dietary guidelines for children are sparse and difficult to quantify. One study, however (Brady *et al.*, 2000), found that a high percentage of children failed to meet the recommended

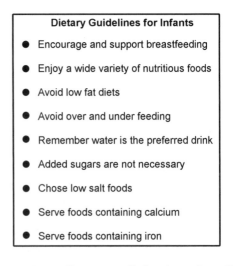

Dietary Guidelines for Infants

- Encourage and support breastfeeding
- Enjoy a wide variety of nutritious foods
- Avoid low fat diets
- Avoid over and under feeding
- Remember water is the preferred drink
- Added sugars are not necessary
- Chose low salt foods
- Serve foods containing calcium
- Serve foods containing iron

Figure 9.11 Summary of the Australian dietary guidelines for infants [reproduced from Gibbons (1998) *Dietary Guidelines for Infants*, by permission of K. Gibbons]

servings from each of the food groups that appear in the US Food Guide Pyramid (USDA and US Department of Health and Human Services, 1992), but, as the authors suggest, it is foolish to assume absolute compliance. What can be extracted from this study is the question 'should a nutrition tool for infants be introduced?' Its efficacy would depend on it being supported by other public health interventions that are, in turn, dependent on appropriate authorities providing sufficient financial backing.

Conclusion

The provision of an optimal diet in infancy is crucial to the survival and long-term health of a child, and is one of several factors that can influence infant growth and therefore later health. Undernutrition in infancy still accounts for a large proportion of infant mortality worldwide, both directly and through an increased susceptibility to disease. As a compensatory mechanism, growth may also be retarded and this has since been shown to have a lifelong influence on that individual's health.

It is apparent that there is a worrying lack of evidence-based research upon which to develop appropriate infant feeding practices post exclusive milk-feeding. We have therefore been unable to give a definitive guide on the optimal age and dietary intake for complementary feeding, but we have reviewed the literature and highlighted where the strengths and weaknesses lie. The challenge of identifying an 'ideal' first, single-ingredient complementary food which is high in energy, whilst not compromising the total nutrient profile, is for the future; we must endeavour to move away from the heavy reliance on fruit and vegetable purées which are perceived to be 'healthy'.

Whatever the future unfolds, we believe that any guidelines should inherently include an element of flexibility to reflect the cultural, economic and physiological diversity of infants in the global context. Feeding during infancy is, whilst still poorly understood, a determinant of the health and productivity of a person. Establishing optimal infant feeding guidelines will inevitably contribute to the success and wealth of a nation.

Acknowledgements

The authors would like to acknowledge the assistance of Nutricia, the Institute of Grocery Distribution (IGD) and Liz Read for their valued contributions to this chapter.

References

Agostoni C, Riva E and Giovannini M (1995) Dietary fibre in weaning foods of young children, Pediatrics **96**(5), 1002–1005.

Akre J (1989) Infant feeding: the physiological basis. *Bull. WHO* **67**(Suppl.), 1–108.

Barker DJP (1990) The fetal and infant origins of disease. *Br. Med. J.* **301**, 1111.

Brady LM, Lindquist CH, Herd SL and Goran MI (2000) Comparison of children's dietary intake patterns with US dietary guidelines. *Br. J. Nutr.* **84**, 361–367.

Brown KH (2000) WHO/UNICEF Review on complementary feeding and suggestions for future research: WHO/UNICEF guidelines on complementary feeding. *Pediatrics* **106**(Suppl. 5), 1290.

Buiten C and Metzger B (2000) Childhood obesity and risk of cardiovascular disease: a review of the science. *Pediatr. Nurs.* **26**(1), 13–18.

Butte NF (1996) Energy requirements of infants. *Eur. J. Clin. Nutr.* **50**(Suppl. 1), S24–36.

Butte NF, Wong WW, Hopkinson JN, Heinz CJ, Mehta NR and Smith EO (2000) Energy requirements derived from total energy expenditure and energy deposition during the first 2 years of life. *Am. J. Clin. Nutr.* **72**, 1558–1569.

CEC (1991) Directive on infant formulae and follow-on formulae. 91/321/EEC. *Off. J. Eur. Communities* **L175**, 35–49.

Dagnelie PC, van Staveren WA, Vergote FJ, Burema J, van't Hof MA, van Klaveren JD and Hauvast JG (1989a) Nutritional status of infants aged 4 to 18 months on macrobiotic diets and matched omnivorous control infants: a population-based mixed-longitudinal study II. Growth and psychomotor development. *Eur. J. Clin. Nutr.* **43**, 325–338.

Dagnelie PC, van Staveren WA, Verschuren SA and Hauvast JG (1989b) Nutritional status of infants aged 4 to 18 months on macrobiotic diets and matched omnivorous control infants: a population-based mixed-longitudinal study I. Weaning pattern, energy and nutrient intake. *Eur. J. Clin. Nutr.* **43**, 311–323.

Davies PSW (1995) Measurement of body composition in children. In: *Essays on auxology*, ed. Hauspie R, Lindgren G and Falkner F. Castlemead, Welwyn Garden City.

De Onis M, Frongillo EA and Blossner M, (2000) *Is Malnutrition Declining? An Analysis of Changes in Levels of Child Malnutrition since 1980.* World Health Organisation, Geneva.

DHSS (1974) *Present Day Practice in Infant Feeding.* Department of Health and Social Security. Report on Health and Social Subjects no. 9. HMSO, London.

DOH (1991) *Dietary Reference Values for Food Energy and Nutrients for the United Kingdom.* Department of Health. Report on Health and Social Subjects, no. 41. HMSO, London.

DOH (1994a) *Weaning and the Weaning Diet.* Department of Health. Report on Health and Social Subjects, no. 45. HMSO, London.

DOH (1994b) *Nutritional Aspects of Cardiovascular Disease*, Department of Health. Report on Health and Social Subjects, No. 46. HMSO, London.

Drewett RF and Parkinson KN (1999) Maternal obesity and child feeding practices in the late weaning period. *Arch. Dis. Child.* **80**, A6.

Fall CHD, Barker DJP, Osmond C, Winter PD, Clark PMS and Hales CN (1992) Relation of infant feeding to adult serum cholesterol concentration and death from ischaemic heart disease. *Br. Med. J.* **304**, 801–805.

FAO/WHO (1985) *Energy and Protein Requirements.* Report of a Joint FAO/WHO/UNU Expert Consultation, Technical Report series no. 724. WHO, Geneva.

Fomon SJ (1974) *Infant Nutrition*, 2nd edn. WB Saunders, Philadelphia, PA.

Forsyth SJ, Ogston SA, Clark A, Florey C du V and Howie PW (1993) Relationship between early introduction of solid foods to infants and their weight and illness during the first two years of life, *Br. Med. J.* **306**(6892), 1572–1576.

Foster F, Lader D and Cheeseborough S (1997) *Infant Feeding 1995.* Publication no. 97-106. HMSO, London.

Foster-Powell K and Brand Miller J (1995) International tables of glycaemic index. *Am. J. Clin. Nutr.* **62**, 871S–893S.

Fraser GE (1994) Diet and coronary heart disease: beyond dietary fats and low density lipoprotein cholesterol. *Am. J. Clin. Nutr.* **59** (Suppl. 5), 1117S–1123S.

Fuchs GJ, Farris RP, DeWier M, Hutchinson S, Strada R and Suskind RM (1994) Effect of dietary fat on cardiovascular risk factors in infancy. *Pediatrics* **93**, 756–763.

Gibbons K (1998) Chief Dietitian, Royal Children's Hospital, Melbourne. *Dietary Guidelines for Infants.* Educational brochure. Available at: www.healthyeating.club.com/info/articles/diet-guide/infant -dg.htm (access date 22 June 2002).

Gibney M (1986) *Nutrition, Diet and Health.* Cambridge University Press, London.

Groff JL and Gropper SS (1999) *Advanced Nutrition and Human Metabolism*, 3rd edn. Wadsworth Thomson Learning, London.

Hobbie C, Baker S and Bayerl C (2000) Parental understanding of basic infant nutrition: Misinformed Feeding Choices. *J. Pediatr. Health Care* **14**(1), 26–31.

Johnson SL and Birch LL (1994) Parent's and children's adiposity and eating style. *Pediatrics* **84**, 653–661.

Kallio MJ, Salmenpera L, Siimes MA, Perheentupa J and Miettinen TA (1992) Exclusive breast-feeding and weaning: effect on serum cholesterol and lipoprotein concentrations in infants during the first year of life. *Pediatrics* **89**(4), 663–666.

King C (2001) *Preterm infants.* In: *Manual of Dietetic Practice*, 3rd edn, Chapter 3.2, ed. Thomas B. Blackwell Science, Oxford.

Labib M, Gama R, Wright J, Marks V and Robins D (1989) Dietary maladvice as a cause of hypothyroidism and short stature. *Br. Med. J.* **298**, 232–233.

Lanigan JA, Bishop JA, Kimber AC and Morgan J (2001) Systematic review concerning the age of introduction of complementary foods to the healthy full-term infant. *Eur. J. Clin. Nutr.* **55**, 309–320.

Lapinleimu H, Viikari J, Jokinen E, Salo P, Routi T, Leino A, Ronnemaa T, Seppanen R, Valimaki I and Simell O (1995) Prospective randomised trial in

62 infants of diet low in saturated fat and cholesterol. *Lancet* **345**, 471–476.

Law M (2000) Dietary fat and adult diseases and the implications for childhood nutrition: an epidemiologic approach. *Am. J. Clin. Nutr.* **72**(Suppl.), 1219S–1226S.

Lebenthal E and Lee RDC (1980) Glucoamylase and disaccharidase activities in normal subjects and in patients with mucal injury in the small intestine. *J. Pediatr.* **97**, 389.

Leeson CPN, Katterhorn N, Deanfield JE and Lucas A (2001) Duration of breastfeeding and arterial distensibility in early life: population-based study. *Br. Med. J.* **322**, 643–647.

Lucas A and Davies PSW (1990) Physiologic energy content of human milk. In: *Breastfeeding, Nutrition, Infection and Infant Growth in Developing and Emerging Countries*, ed. Atkinson SA, Hanson LA and Chandra RK. ARTS, St John's, Newfoundland.

Mendez MA and Adair LS (1999). Severity and timing of stunting in the first two years of life affect performance on cognitive tests in late childhood. *J. Nutr.* **129**, 1555–1562.

Michaelson KF and Jorgensen MH (1995) Dietary fat content and energy density during infancy and childhood: the effect on energy intake and growth. *Eur. J. Clin. Nutr.* **49**, 467–483.

Michaelsen KF, Weaver L, Branca F and Robertson A (2000) *Feeding and Nutrition of Infants and Young Children*. WHO Regional Publications, European Series, No. 87. World Health Organisation Regional Office for Europe, Copenhagen.

Mills A and Tyler H (1992) *Food and Nutrient Intakes of British Children aged 6–12 Months*. MAFF/HMSO, London.

Mintel Market Intelligence (2000) *Baby Food and Drink*. Mintel International Group, London.

Mira M, Alperstein G, Karr M, Ranmuthugala G, Causer J, Niec A and Lilburne AM (1996) Haem-iron intake in 12–36 month-old children depleted in iron: case-control study. *Br. Med. J.* **312**, 881–883.

Morgan JB (1998) Weaning: when and what. *BNF Nutr. Bull.* **23**(Suppl. 1).

Morgan JB, Redfern AM and Stordy BJ (1995) Healthy eating for infants – mother's attitudes. *Acta Paediatr* **84**, 512–515.

Nicklas TA, Webber LS, Koschak ML and Berenson GS (1992) nutrient adequacy of low fat intakes for children: the Bogalusa Heart Study. *Pediatrics* **89**, 221.

Niinikoski H, Lapinleimu H, Viikari J, Ronnemaa T, Jokinen E, Seppanen R, Terho P, Tuominen J,

Valimaki I and Simell O (1997a) Growth until 3 years of age in a prospective, randomised trial of a diet with reduced saturated fat and cholesterol. *Pediatrics* **99**, 687–693.

Niinikoski H, Viikari J, Ronnemaa T, Helenius H, Jokinen E, Lapinleimu H, Routi T, Lagstom H, Seppanen R, Valimaki I and Simell O (1997b) Regulation of growth of 7- to 36-month-old children by energy and fat intake in the prospective, randomised STRIP baby trial. *Pediatrics* **100**, 810–817.

Pesonen E, Norio R, Hirvonen J, Karkola K, Kuusela V, Laaksonen H, Mottonen M, Nikkari T, Raekallic J, Viikari J, Herttuala S and Åkerblom HK (1990) Intimal thickening in the coronary arteries of infants and children as an indicator of risk factors for coronary heart disease. *Eur. Heart J.* (Suppl E 11), 53–60.

Pollitt E, Gorman KS, Engle PL, Martorell R and Rivera J (1993) Early supplementary feeding and cognition. *Monogr. Soc. Res. Child Devl.* **58**: 1–99.

Prentice AM, Lucas A, Vasquez-Velasquez L, Davies PS and Whitehead RG (1988) Are current dietary guidelines for young children a prescription for overfeeding? *Lancet* **2**(8619), 1066–1069.

Pugliese MT, Weyman-Daum M, Moses N and Lifshitz F (1987) Parental health beliefs as a cause of non-organic failure to thrive. *Pediatrics* **80**, 175–182.

Shaw V and Lawson M (2001) *Clinical Paediatric Dietetics*, 2nd edn. Blackwell Science, Oxford.

Simell O, Niinikoski H, Ronnemaa T, Lapinleimu H, Routi T, Lagstrom H, Salo P, Jokinen E and Viikari J (2000) Special Turku Coronary Risk Factor Intervention Project for Babies (STRIP). *Am. J. Clin. Nutr.* **72**(Suppl.), 1316S–1331S.

Southgate DAT and Johnson IT (1994) *Dietary Fibre and Related Substances*. Chapman and Hall, London.

Spurr GB, Barac-Nieto M and Maksud MG (1977) Productivity and maximal oxygen consumption in sugar cane cutters. *Am. J. Clin. Nutr.* **30**, 316–321.

Stein A, Woolley H, Cooper SD and Fairburn CG (1994) An observational study of mothers with eating disorders and their infants. *J. Child. Psychol. Psychiat.* **35**, 733–748.

Stein A, Stein J, Walters EA and Fairburn CG (1995) Eating habits and attitudes among mothers of children with feeding disorders. *Br. Med. J.* **310**, 228.

Stordy BJ, Redfern AM and Morgan JB (1995) Healthy eating for infants – mother's actions. *Acta Paediatr.* **84**, 733–741.

Talbot D (2001) Infants. In: *Manual of Dietetic Practice*, 3rd edn, Chap. 3.3, ed. Thomas B. Blackwell Science, Oxford.

The Processed Cereal-Based Foods and Baby Foods for Infants and Young Children Regulations (1997) SI 1997 No. 2042. HMSO, London.

USDA and US Department of Health and Human Services (1992) *The Food Guide Pyramid*. Home and Garden Bulletin no. 252. US Government Printing Office, Washington, DC. Available at: www.nalusda.gov/faic/fpyr/guide.pdf (access date 22 June 2002).

Van den Boom SAM, Kimber AC and Morgan JB (1997) Nutritional composition of home-prepared baby meals in Madrid. Comparison with commercial products in Spain and home-made meals in England. *Acta Paediatr.* **86**, 57–62.

Wharton BA (1997a) *Nutrition in Infancy*. Briefing Paper. BNF, London.

Wharton BA (1997b) Weaning in Britain: practice, policy and problems. *Proc. Nutr. Soc.* **56**, 105–109.

Wharton BA (2000) Patterns of complementary feeding (weaning) in countries of the European Union: topics for research. *Pediatrics* **106**(5 Suppl.), 1273.

WHO (1998) *Complementary Feeding of Young Children in Developing Countries: a Review of Current Scientific Knowledge*. WHO/NUT/98.1. WHO, Geneva.

WHO (2000) *Health21 Nutrition Programme Plans*. Available at: www.who.int/wha-1998/pdf98/ea5.pdfwww.whosea.org/ pdf/rdoc/NUT-146.pdf.

WHO (2001) *The Optimal Duration of Exclusive Breastfeeding: Results of a WHO Systematic Review*. Available at: www.who.int/inf-pr-2001/en/note2001-07.html.

Widdowson EM, Dauncey MJ, Gairdner DM, Jonxis JH and Pelikan FM (1975) Body fat of British and Dutch infants. *Br. Med. J.* **1**, 653–655.

Williams AF (1991) Lactation and infant feeding. In: *Textbook of Paediatric Nutrition*, ed. McLaren DS, Burman D, Belton NR and Williams AF, 3rd edn, Churchill Livingstone, Edinburgh.

Zoltkin S (2000) Canadian recommendations. *Pediatrics* **106**(Suppl.), 1272.

10

NUTRITION OF THE LOW-BIRTH-WEIGHT AND VERY-LOW-BIRTH-WEIGHT INFANT

Caroline King and Michael Harrison

LEARNING OUTCOMES

- Enteral feeding requirements of both the term and preterm infant.

- Different energy and nutrient requirements in low-birth-weight and term infants.

- Various methods and routes of feeding the preterm infant.

- Understanding of the methods and importance of monitoring growth in the preterm infant.

- To understand the concept of failure to thrive and be able to institute a plan of management.

Introduction

Low birth weight babies are usually defined as those born less than 2500 g at any gestation, the vast majority worldwide being born at term. Very low-birth-weight infants (VLBWI) are those less than 1500 g at birth, the majority of these being born preterm. Both categories of babies are at risk of increased morbidity and mortality compared with appropriately grown term babies, and the latter have the added problem of immaturity and are at greater risk.

One of the most difficult tasks is the achievement of adequate nutrition, as these babies have higher requirements than their term counterparts, but poorer tolerance both enterally and parenterally. The higher requirements are due to the very much higher growth rate of the healthy VLBWI, the last trimester of pregnancy being the most important for growth and accumulation of nutrients (Ziegler et al., 1976). For example a 26 week gestation baby will consist of only a few per cent body fat, whereas a term infant will have attained approximately 30 per cent. Likewise bone mineralization is very poor at 26 weeks, with only an average of 6 g total body calcium, rising to 30 g at term.

Material in Chapters 1, 3, 7, 8 and 9 should be read in relation to this chapter.

Enteral Nutrition

Enteral nutrition for the preterm baby is a complex issue with quite marked changes in practice and recommended intakes of nutrients over the last two decades. In addition to decisions on type of feed, it must also be carefully considered when to start and whether to add supplements, rate of increase and how to deliver the feed, although not all of these areas can be discussed in this chapter.

Requirements

The most recent and comprehensive guidelines are those of Tsang et al. (1993), although some formula manufacturers still use those of ESPGAN (1987).

Energy

Energy is the most important of nutrients but one with the largest variation between and within different individuals. Table 10.1 shows some of the major influences on energy requirements. It can be seen that requirements can more than double over the first few postnatal weeks and potentially vary by up to 50 per cent at any point in time. In practice such extreme variations should be rare with minimal handling and nursing in a thermo-neutral environment. As discussed by Tsang et al. (1993) requirements increase with age, nutrient intake and growth rate; however, they give a fairly narrow recommendation of 110–120 kcal/kg. This can only be used as a

Table 10.1   Breakdown of energy requirements (kcal/kg/day)

	Acute phase	Intermediate phase	Convalescence
Resting energy expenditure (REE)[a]	45	50–60	50–70
Cold stress	0–10	0–10	5–10
Activity/handling[b]	0–10	5–15	5–15
Stool losses[c]	0–10	10–15	10–15
Specific dynamic action[d]	0	0–5	10
Growth	0	20–30	20–30
Total	50–80	85–135[e]	105–150[e]

[a]The lower level applies to babies with normal REE, upper limit to those with diseases associated with increased REE, e.g. cardiac abnormalities or chronic lung disease.
[b]Zero if paralysed/heavily sedated.
[c]Zero if on total PN.
[d]Ten per cent of energy given (Brooke et al., 1979).
[e]Upper limit probably not physiological and should not be necessary.

guideline and assessment of individual energy needs must be made. In practice this can only be achieved by feeding to theoretical requirements and then titrating against growth once all other influences on growth have been taken into account (see below in causes of failure to thrive).

Protein

Tsang *et al.* suggest higher protein intakes for smaller less mature babies, namely 3.6–3.8 g/kg for those < 27 weeks and < 1000 g and 3.0–3.6 g/kg for those 28–34 weeks and > 1000 g. Previous guidelines have not made this distinction, which in practice can be difficult to apply as the smallest babies often have poorer nutrient tolerance.

Composition of weight gain

The composition of weight gain is dependent on the ratio of energy and protein (see below in 'Parenteral amino acids'). At a given protein intake, increasing the energy intake above needs leads to an increased fat deposition. In well-growing infants given sufficient protein, feeding 100 kcal/kg results in 16 per cent of weight gain as fat, and when fed 130 kcal/kg around 40 per cent of weight gain is fat (Reichman *et al.*, 1981, 1983; Putet *et al.*, 1984; Tsang *et al.*, 1993, chapter 20). The former represents weight gain *in utero*, whereas the latter is similar to the composition of a term neonate; it is still uncertain which is preferable.

Lipids

In formula feeds, lipids should supply around 50 per cent of total energy, comparable to human milk. Initially, preterm babies are likely to suffer some fat malabsorption due to reduced bile salt pool (Putet *et al.*, 1984; Signer

et al., 1974), and reduced pancreatic lipase activity (Forget *et al.*, 1995; Hamosh, 1987). This affects saturated more than unsaturated fats. To overcome this, medium chain triglycerides (MCT) have been added to preterm formulas in varying amounts, as they do not require emulsification prior to absorption. However this has not led to growth advantages (Hamosh *et al.*, 1991; Sulkers *et al.*, 1992). Tsang *et al.* state that there is no clear advantage in feeding more than 1 per cent energy as MCT, but do not suggest an upper limit. Another strategy has been the incorporation of 'structured lipids' formulated to resemble those in human milk; although improved calcium absorption has been shown, total fat absorption has not (Lucas *et al.*, 1997).

There are guidelines for the essential fatty acids linoleic and α-linolenic, namely 4–15 and 1–4 per cent fat energy or 5 and 1 per cent total energy, respectively (Tsang *et al.*, 1993). However, there is much debate around the provision of their long chain polyunsaturated (LCP) derivatives arachidonic and docosahexaenoic acids (AA and DHA, respectively). Some agencies claim that they are conditionally essential in neonates (BNF, 1992; ESPGAN, 1991; Food and Agriculture Organization, 1994), and others suggest that more evidence is needed to prove this and that possible harm cannot be ruled out (Hay *et al.*, 1999). Details relevant to this topic may be found in Chapter 5. A recent systematic review concludes that LCP supplementation gives more rapid early visual maturation, but no long-term benefits have been shown as yet (Simmer, 2000). Tsang *et al.* advise that babies of < 1750 g consuming < 100 kcal/day enterally may benefit from a supplement of 0.25 per cent total energy each as DHA and AA.

Vitamin A

Many preterm babies are born with low vitamin A stores (Mupanemunda *et al.*, 1994;

Shenai et al., 1990). A correlation has been demonstrated between gestation at birth and vitamin A status (Mupanemunda et al., 1994); others have not seen this, but have shown levels approaching those of term babies in those born at 36 weeks (Brandt et al., 1978). Some appear to need very high enteral intakes to overcome poor absorption (Landman et al., 1992) which is probably due to the lipid malabsorption seen in many preterm babies (Ojeda et al., 1994). Vitamin A is needed for normal epithelial growth and regeneration and thus has been given in supplementation studies to evaluate its role in prevention and ameliora- tion of chronic lung disease (CLD). A protocol giving 5000 IU intramuscularly, three times a week for the first 4 postnatal weeks showed a small but significant decrease in risk of CLD (Tyson et al., 1999). One study giving 5000 IU enterally showed no effect (Wardle et al., 2001). In the latter vitamin A status was not evaluated and the dose may have been too low to compensate for large enteral losses due to lipid malabsorption. This evidence was not available at the time Tsang et al. made their recommendation for enteral intakes of 1500– 2800 IU for those with CLD and 700–1500 IU for those without. A recent systematic review agrees that prophylactic intramuscular vitamin A gives a small but significant reduction in risk of oxygen dependence at 36 weeks, which is a marker of chronic lung disease of prematurity, but recommends that the intravenous route be investigated to avoid the need for repeated intramuscular injections (Darlow and Graham 2000). A good review of the subject has recently been published (Shenai, 1999).

Vitamin D

Vitamin D levels in the neonate depend on maternal stores, which vary greatly depending on maternal diet and exposure to ultraviolet light. This has lead to studies using different levels of supplementation, some quite high

(Evans et al., 1989). However, these high doses did not give any advantage over lower ones and it appears that 400 IU/day is adequate for the vast majority of babies (Backstrom et al., 1999) and is recommended by Tsang et al. Mothers who are at high risk of vitamin D deficiency should be strongly advised to take a supplement themselves, especially if they are providing breast milk.

Vitamin E

Tsang et al. recommend a minimum of 0.7 IU (mg)/100 kcal (420 kJ) and a maximum of 25 IU (mg)/day. Pharmacological doses have been investigated in the hope that they will protect against diseases, which many believe are caused in part by oxidative stress. Unfortu- nately such doses have been associated with increased risk of sepsis and necrotizing entero- colitis (NEC; Johnson et al.., 1985; Raju et al., 1997). The former authors have gone on to report an improved outcome in infants supple- mented once retinopathy has been diagnosed rather than before (Johnson et al., 1995). If larger than recommended doses of iron are given there may be depression of serum vitamin E levels (Rudolph et al., 1994), in which case it may be useful to give additional vitamin E.

Water-soluble vitamins

Tables 10.5 and 10.6 give intakes recommen- ded by Tsang et al. It is of interest that it remains policy on many neonatal units to give folic acid supplements despite the fact that preterm formulas have always contained ade- quate amounts.

Calcium, phosphorus and magnesium

Mineral accretion is maximal during the last trimester, leaving the preterm baby vulnerable

Table 10.2 Calcium and phosphorus requirements in human milk-fed preterm babies

	Calcium (mmol/kg)	Phosphorus (mmol/kg)
Daily intrauterine accretion last trimester	3.5	2.4
Human milk fed at 200 ml/kg	1.6	1.0
Maximum absorbed from milk	1.0	0.9
Protoplasmic requirements	Minimal	0.6
Remaining for bone	1.0	0.3
Used for bone formation	0.5	0.3
Excreted in urine	0.5	0

to deficiency (Ziegler *et al.*, 1976). A manifestation of this is bone disease, particularly in babies on unsupplemented human milk. Where this was once thought to be due to poor vitamin D status it has now been attributed to mineral deficiency (Evans *et al.*, 1989). Table 10.2 shows an outline of the fate of calcium and phosphorus ingested by a preterm baby fed human milk, clearly showing its inability to provide sufficient mineral when unsupplemented. Provision of sufficient magnesium is essential both for adequate bone formation and soft tissue needs; however, as only 0.12 mmol/kg/24 h is needed to match late gestation accretion rates, deficiency is rare.

Iron

Preterm and low-birth-weight babies have lower endogenous stores than term and appropriate birth-weight babies, and therefore become depleted earlier, i.e. at around 8 weeks (Olivares *et al.*, 1992). The early anaemia of prematurity (before 8 weeks), is not ameliorated by iron supplements (Shaw, 1982). The timing of supplementation remains contentious, with some concerned that iron given early may increase the risk of infection due to

promotion of the growth of iron-requiring bacteria (Michie and Raffles, 1990). This remains a theoretical risk not borne out in studies where iron was given early (Hall *et al.*, 1993; Melnick *et al.*, 1988). Tsang *et al.* recommend supplementation at any time between birth and 8 weeks. Iron is one of the components of preterm formulas which can vary significantly between products (see Tables 10.5 and 10.6). This should be taken into consideration when devising an iron supplementation policy.

Studies suggest that an enteral intake of 2 mg iron/kg prevents iron deficiency and this remains the latest recommendation (Ehrenkranz, 1994; Tsang *et al.*, 1993). It is advised that this intake be continued throughout the first year, although there is some work showing that lower intakes after hospital discharge also maintain good iron status (Griffin *et al.*, 1999).

Zinc

Tables 10.5 and 10.6 show the recommended levels in formula milk, whereas for human milk-fed babies a supplement of 0.5 mg/kg/day after the first 4–6 weeks is suggested (Tsang *et al.*, 1993). Others feel that an input of 1.2 mg/100 ml formula is needed (Friel and Andrews, 1994); however, one study showed impairment of immune function in malnourished babies receiving a formula with 1.5 mg/100 ml (Schlesinger *et al.*, 1993). Doses higher than those recommended by Tsang *et al.* should not be given unless there is a strong suspicion of zinc deficiency such as persistent peri-oral and nappy rash, often preceded by an abnormally low serum alkaline phosphatase (Weismann and Hoyer, 1985).

Selenium

Preterm babies have a low selenium status at birth, which continues to fall in the absence of supplementation (Lockitch *et al.*, 1989). There is some evidence that poor selenium status and poor respiratory outcome are associated (Darlow *et al.*, 1995), although not all supplementation studies show any benefit (Huston *et al.*, 1996).

Conditionally Essential Nutrients

β-Carotene

Although there are no recommendations for addition to formula at present, many manufacturers are already adding β-carotene. The rationale has been that it is needed for its antioxidant and pro-vitamin A properties, although the latter is unnecessary if the guidelines for addition of preformed vitamin A are followed. It is also cited as desirable because of its presence in human milk; however, it only comprises approximately 25 per cent of total carotenoid activity and levels vary considerably depending on the stage and number of lactations (Patton *et al.*, 1990). The possible hazards of supplementation must be further evaluated, namely the risk of reduced absorption of other carotenoids in human milk if it is fed mixed with a β-carotene-supplemented formula (Gaziano *et al.*. 1995), and that of other pathologies such as cancer, which have been associated with adult supplementation studies (Rowe, 1996).

Nucleotides

Demand for nucleotides by the immune system is maximal when cell turnover is high, e.g. during sepsis and rapid growth. If supply depends on *de novo* synthesis at these times it may lag behind needs, therefore a preformed source may be beneficial (Rudolph, 1994). Tsang *et al.* gave no recommendation for the

addition of nucleotides in 1993; however, more encouraging work has been published since then. In term babies there are reports of reduced risk of diarrhoea (Pickering *et al.*, 1996), and improved growth (Cosgrove *et al.*, 1996) and in preterm babies there may be enhancement of lipoprotein synthesis (Sanchez Pozo *et al.*, 1995), although there are contradictory studies. Many formula manufacturers have already added nucleotides, but more work needs to be done to get the optimal balance (Leach *et al.*, 1995; Quan *et al.*, 1990).

Glutamine

Both the immune system and the intestine use glutamine preferentially as a fuel (Powell-Tuck, 1993) and it has proved of benefit in studies on adults and preterm babies (Lacey *et al.*, 1996; Neu *et al.*, 1997) and may be useful in short gut syndrome (Byrne *et al.*, 1995; King, 2001). However, routine supplementation is not yet recommended (Tsang *et al.*, 1993; Tubman and Thompson, 2000) and more data are needed on lack of toxicity (Neu *et al.*, 1996).

Type of Feed

Human milk

This area has undergone some of the most profound changes with much research in the field. Consensus has moved from human milk to formula (both term and preterm) and back to human milk as the preferred feed. Current debate centres round the use of breast milk fortifiers.

Human milk is the preferred choice both for its non-nutritional as well as nutritional advantages (Schanler *et al.*, 1999a). It has been shown to reduce the risk of infection in a dose-dependent manner (el-Mohandes *et al.*, 1995;

Schanler et al., 1999b; Uraizee and Gross, 1989) and of necrotizing enterocolitis (Beeby and Jeffrey, 1992; Lucas and Cole, 1990; Schanler et al., 1999b). It is also usually better tolerated than formula, leading to more rapid tolerance of full enteral feeds (Uraizee and Gross, 1989). This has implications for a reduction in requirements for, and thus reduced complications of, parenteral nutrition, including line sepsis and cholestasis. It may also result in improved developmental scores compared to formula as shown in preterm babies (Amin et al., 2000; Horwood et al., 2001; Lucas et al., 1992b, 1994, 1998) and term babies (Anderson et al., 1999), with possible mechanisms explored (Amin et al., 2000), although the methodology of some of the studies has been challenged (Jacobson et al., 1999).

There may also be a benefit with reduction in incidence of allergic reactions in those infants with a strong family history of atopy (Lucas et al., 1990) and reduced blood pressure at 13–16 years of age (Singhal et al., 2001).

Donor milk

Should mother's own milk not be available it is recommended that donor human milk be used to initiate feeds. All donor milk in the UK is subject to rigorous screening to reduce risk of contamination and is then pasteurized at 62°C according to national guidelines (UKAMB, 1999). This heat treatment is sufficient to destroy HIV while preserving many of the bio-active immune components. Unfortunately, live cells and the enzyme, bile salt-stimulated lipase, are destroyed – the result of the latter being significantly reduced fat absorption (Williamson et al., 1978). It is for this reason that the majority of babies need to be re-graded onto appropriate formula milk once full feeds of donor milk are tolerated to ensure adequate energy. However, where there is a very high risk of NEC and sufficient donor milk is available it should be continued a little longer (Lucas and Cole, 1990), while ensuring appropriate mineral and vitamin supplements.

Nutritional Adequacy of Human Milk

Energy

As discussed previously, donor milk will not provide the theoretical needs of the rapidly growing preterm baby. The situation is less clear with maternal expressed breast milk (MEBM), as the nutritional composition can vary quite considerably between women and between milk expressions (Hibberd et al., 1982). Lactose content tends to be consistent, but the fat content can be very variable as measured by the creamatocrit (Lucas et al., 1978; Wang et al., 1999). For example, in one study the energy value of the highest fat milk was over 40 per cent higher than the lowest (Warner et al., 1998). If the breast is fully expressed to remove all the high-fat hind milk, energy levels should be maximized. However, there are potentially very great fat losses in the container and tubing when human milk is fed continuously via nasogastric tube (Greer et al., 1984). This can be overcome by positioning the syringe to allow the fat portion to be delivered first (Narayanan et al., 1984). A systematic review evaluating the effect of adding fat to human milk concluded that there was insufficient evidence to support this practice; however, there was a recommendation for further research in the context of a multinutrient fortifier (Kuschel and Harding, 2000a).

Protein

Although early preterm human milk in general has more protein than mature milk, the range is very large, with up to 100 per cent variability between samples; however, over the first few weeks the levels fall to those of mature term milk (Lucas and Hudson, 1984). The levels found in mature milk will be inadequate for most babies less than 1500 g and many babies less than 2000 g, even when fed at maximum tolerated volumes (i.e. >200 ml/kg). In the UK, assessment of the macronutrient composition of human milk is not done routinely, except, rarely, the creamatocrit which is used to estimate energy content (Lucas *et al.*, 1978; Wang *et al.*, 1999). Assessment of protein has been reported to be of use, however the delay between milk sampling and the receipt of results led to a delay in manipulation of the protein levels (Polberger *et al.*, 1999). An alternative is the use of serum urea levels to indirectly assess the amount of protein a baby is getting (Polberger *et al.*, 1990). Serial measurements are necessary to see the trend, and it is important to take into account other factors which may affect urea levels (i.e. state of hydration, renal function and steroid use).

It is probably wise to start adding additional protein before a baby starts to 'fail to thrive' because of inadequate nitrogen intake, a guide being once serum urea levels have fallen to around 3 mmol/l. However, maximum volumes tolerated should be achieved first as there are potential problems associated with the addition of breast milk fortifier (BMF; see below). Supplementation with protein has been assessed in a systematic review which concluded that it leads to improvements in anthropometric measurements, but there were not enough data to assess any possible adverse side effects (Kuschel and Harding, 2000b). The most suitable format for supplementation is probably as a multinutrient fortifier often termed 'breast milk fortifier'.

Lipids

The lipid content of human milk is very variable both in overall amount and types of fatty acids, the amount depending on time of day and stage of each individual feed, the types depending on maternal diet (Neville, 1989). However, despite very different diets some investigators have pointed out how consistent the presence of AA and DHA is across many countries (Koletzko *et al.*, 1992).

Vitamins

Vitamin levels in human milk will be inadequate in certain respects. Once intravenous vitamins via parenteral nutrition have been stopped and before a BMF is started, an oral supplement containing 10 μg vitamin D (400 IU) per day and at least 210 μg/kg (63 IU)/24 h vitamin A should be given – in practice a standard multivitamin is often used.

Minerals

Most preterm babies fed unfortified human milk will need supplements of sodium and phosphorus. Expressed human milk can have higher sodium content as a by-product of breast inflammation (McKiernan and Hull, 1982). Babies less than 32 weeks' gestation will be likely to need a sodium supplement to avoid hyponatraemia and poor growth (Chance *et al.*, 1977; Haycock, 1993).

With respect to bone growth, phosphorus becomes the first limiting nutrient, see Table 10.2. Supplements have been shown to reduce the incidence of bone disease of prematurity (Holland *et al.*, 1990); 0.5 mmol twice a day was given in this study, but in practice needs can vary quite considerably and supplementation to maintain plasma levels >1.5 mmol/l while maintaining an appropriate serum calcium:phosphorus ratio is advisable. If BMF is delayed, a calcium supplement will also be needed. The importance of avoiding inadequate mineral input is beginning to be revealed in longer-term studies showing shorter stature in ex-prematures who had higher alkaline phosphatase levels in the neonatal period (Fewtrell *et al.*, 2000a). This may have implications for later bone mass as it appears to be positively related to height (Fewtrell *et al.*, 2000b).

Iron stores will be exhausted more rapidly than in term babies, and it is recommended that all preterm babies receive 2 mg/kg by 8 weeks of age whether they are on human milk or formula (Tsang *et al.*, 1993).

Breast milk fortifiers

The most practical format for redressing the nutritional shortfall of human milk is probably through the addition of a BMF. These have been evaluated in a systematic review and been shown not only to improve anthropometric measurements, but also to lead to greater bone mineral and nitrogen accretion without an increase in adverse side effects (Kuschel and Harding, 2000b). Further research is needed into long-term outcomes following supplementation with BMF. Tables 10.3 and 10.4 show the composition of those available in the UK and USA. They are designed predominantly to supplement the protein, mineral and vitamin levels of human milk, however some still need vitamin supplements to comply with recommended intakes. They do not contain iron so a supplement must be started before 8 weeks. Although they provide some energy, it is not the most important component as at intakes of at least 180 ml/kg there is evidence that protein rather than energy is the growth-limiting nutrient (Boehm *et al.*, 1990; Polberger *et al.*, 1989).

However, there are potential problems when any additions are made to human milk. Feed tolerance may be affected (Ewer and Yu, 1996), although the clinical significance of this is debatable (Moody *et al.*, 2000). Furthermore there is a reduction in immune components (Quan *et al.* 1994), increased osmolarity (De Curtis *et al.*, 1999) and

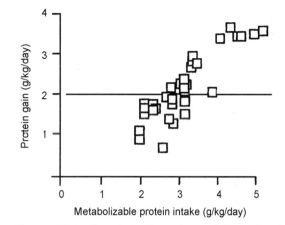

Figure 10.1 Protein intake and growth [reproduced from Tsang *et al.* (1993) *Nutritional Needs of the Preterm Infant: Scientific Basis and Practical Guidelines*, by permission of Digital Educational Publishing]

increased bacterial growth (Jocson *et al.*, 1997). These problems occur with prolonged storage of fortified milk so it is advisable to make up only the minimum amount possible at a time. Due to the extremely high variability in content of different mother s milk, use of a BMF should be accompanied by a detailed policy for nutritional monitoring of individual needs, and responses to fortification (see King, 1999). Some unit policies advise routine addition of a fortifier once a particular enteral volume has been reached, regardless of blood biochemistry; however, this will only serve to further accentuate differences in nutritional input between babies and may subject individuals to unacceptably high levels of some nutrients. Early studies to assess protein needs found formulas providing levels >4 g/kg were associated with toxic effects (Goldman *et al.*, 1974), and it is unlikely that there will be growth benefits (see Figure 10.1).

Preterm formulas

Since their first use and evaluation, there has been continual development of formulas for

Table 10.3   Composition of human milk fortifiers in the UK

Composition of recommended dose	NUTRIPREM breast milk fortifier (Cow & Gate)	Eoprotin (Milupa)	SMA breast milk fortifier (SMA)[a,b]	FM85 (Nestle)
Recommended dose (g/100 ml)	3	3	4	5
Protein (g)	0.7[d]	0.6	1.0	0.8[d]
Casein:whey	60:40	60:40	0:100	0:100
Energy (kcal)[c]	10	11	15	18
Minerals (mmol)				
Calcium	1.5	1.0	2.25	1.3
Phosphorous	1.3	0.8	1.45	1.0
Magnesium	0.15	0.06	0.12	0.08
Sodium	0.3	0.8	0.8	1.0
Potassium	0.1	0.03	0.6	0.2
Chloride	0.2	0.3	0.5	0.5
Trace elements (µg)				
Zinc	300	–	200	–
Copper	26	–	–	–
Manganese	6	–	4.6	–
Iodine	11	–	–	–
Vitamins (µg)				
Vitamin A	130	22.5	270	–
Vitamin C (mg)	12	11	40	–
Vitamin D	5	–	6.6	–
Vitamin E	2600	250	3000	–
Vitamin K	6.3	0.15	11	–
Biotin	2.5	–	–	–
Folic acid	5.0	–	–	–
Niacin	2500	–	3600	–
Vitamin, B_{12}	0.2	–	0.3	–
Pyridioxine, B_6	110	–	260	–
Riboflavin, B_2	170	–	260	–
Thiamin	130	–	220	–
Pantothenate acid, B_5	750	–	–	–
Presentation	1.5 g sachets powder	400 g tins powder	2 g sachets powder	200 g tins powder

[a]Available on request to company.
[b]SMA BMF contains β-carotene.
[c]All contain carbohydrate only as energy source.
[d]Hydrolysed protein.
Only correct at time of publication – please check with manufacturers.

preterm babies, much of the important work being carried out by Alan Lucas and his team. Review of their papers shows that early growth is highly significantly improved by the use of a nutrient-rich preterm formula compared with either a term formula or unfortified human milk (which was a combination of mother's own and banked) (Lucas et al., 1984). Follow-up has revealed that, by 8 years of age, the latter groups caught up with respect to anthropometric measurements (Morley and Lucas, 2000), but that the preterm formula group held

Table 10.4 Composition of human milk fortifiers in the USA

Composition of recommended dose	Enfamil (Mead Johnson)	Similac (Ross)	Similac Natural Care[a] (Ross)
Recommended dose (g/100ml)	4	3.6 (4 sachets)	100 ml (Dilute: 1:1 with breast milk)
Protein (g)	0.7	1	2.2
Casein:whey	60:40	60:40	60:40
Energy (kcal)	14	14	81
Minerals (mmol)			
Calcium	2.25	2.9	4.25
Phosphorous	1.4	2.1	2.7
Magnesium	0.04	0.3	0.4
Sodium	0.3	0.6	1.5
Potassium	0.4	1.6	2.7
Chloride	0.5	1.0	1.8
Trace elements (µg)			
Zinc	714	1000	1200
Copper	62	170	200
Manganese	4.7	7.2	9.6
Iodine	–	–	4.8
Vitamins (µg)			
Vitamin A	285	186	163
Vitamin C (mg)	11.6	25	30
Vitamin D	5.2	3	3
Vitamin E	4500	3200	3200
Vitamin K	4.4	8.3	9.6
Biotin	2.7	26	30
Folic acid	25	23	30
Niacin	3000	3570	4000
Vitamin, B_{12}	0.18	0.64	0.68
Pyridoxine, B_6	114	211	200
Riboflavin, B_2	210	417	496
Thiamin, B_1	151	233	200
Pantothenate acid, B_5	730	1500	1500
Presentation	1 g sachets powder	Sachets powder	Liquid

[a]Contains taurine, inositol, choline and selenium.
Only correct at time of publication – please check with manufacturers.

a neuro-developmental advantage compared with the term formula-fed group (Lucas *et al.*, 1998). This advantage was most marked in males but blunted by the use of human milk, despite the low energy content of the banked mostly 'drip' milk. This highlights one of the many advantages of human milk due to (as yet) undetermined factors, and the concept of 'programming' (Lucas, 1994). Tables 10.5 and 10.6 show comparisons of preterm formulas available in both the UK and USA.

All babies with a birth-weight less than 2000 g should receive a preterm formula if human milk is not available, and this should continue until a weight of 2500 g is reached or discharge, whichever is sooner. Transfer to a term formula sooner is likely to compromise growth (Friel *et al.*, 1993; Cooke *et al.*, 1999).

Table 10.5 Composition of preterm formulas in the UK

Nutrients per 100 ml	Recommendations of Tsang (1993) based on 80 kcal/100 ml	Nutriprem (Cow & Gate)	Osterprem (Farley's)	Pre-Aptamil (Milupa)	LBW (SMA)	Pre-Nativa (Nestle)
Energy (kcal)	80	80	80	80	82	80
Protein (g/kg)		–	–	–	–	–
< 1000 g	3.6–3.8					
> 1000 g	3.0–3.6					
Protein (g)		2.4	2.0	2.4	2.0	2.3
Fat (g)	3.5–4.8 (tentative)	4.4	4.6	4.4	4.4	4.2
MCT (✓) percentage of total fat	N.S.				(✓ 15%)	(✓ 26%)
LCP	Conditionally essential	AA/DHA/ GLA	DHA/GLA	AA/DHA/ GLA	AA/DHA	AA/DHA/ GLA
Linoleic acid (g)	0.35–1.36	0.57	0.54	0.73	0.7	0.64
Linolenic acid (g)	0.09–0.35	0.06	0.06	0.06	0.07	0.07
Carbohydrate (g)	N.S.	7.8	7.6	7.8	8.6	8.6
Minerals						
Sodium (mg)	30–46	41	42	41	35	33
Potassium (mg)	52–80	80	72	80	85	95
Chloride (mg)	47–71	48	60	48	60	51
Calcium (mg)	80–154	100	110	100	80	99
Phosphorus (mg)	48–112	50	63	50	43	53
Ca:P ratio (by weight)	N.S.	2:1	1.7:1	2:1	1.9:1	1.8:1
Magnesium (mg)	5–10	10	5	10	8	8.3
Iron (mg)	2.0 (/kg)	0.9	0.04	0.9	0.8	1.2
Zinc (mg)	0.7	0.7	0.9	0.7	0.8	0.6
Copper (µg)	80–100	80	96	80	83	70
Iodine (µg)	20–40	25	8	14	10	20
Manganese (µg)	5	10	3	8	10	5.2
Selenium (µg)	0.9	1.9	×	×	×	×
Vitamins						
Vitamin A (µg)[a]	CLD: 450–840 µg/kg No CLD: 210–450 µg/kg	227	100	108	74	84
Vitamin D (µg)[a]	2.4–6.4 (min 10/day)	5.0	2.4	2.4	1.5	2
Vitamin E (TE; mg)	4–8 IU (max 25 IU/day)	3.0	10	3.0	1.2	1.4
Vitamin K (µg)	5.3–6.7	6.6	7.0	6.6	8.0	6.4
Thiamin B_1 (mg)	0.12–0.16	0.14	0.1	0.14	0.12	0.56
Riboflavin B_2 (mg)	0.16–0.24	0.2	0.18	0.2	0.2	0.12
Niacin (mg)	2.4–3.2	3.0	1.0	2.5	1.3	0.8
Panthothenic acid (mg)	0.8–1.2	1.0	0.5	1.0	0.45	0.36
Pyridoxine, B_6 (mg)	0.1–0.14	0.12	0.1	0.12	0.07	0.06
Folic acid (µg)	17–34	48	50	48	49	56
Vitamin B_{12} (µg)	0.2	0.2	0.2	0.2	0.3	0.24
Biotin (µg)	2.4–4.0	3.0	2.0	3.0	2.4	1.8
Vitamin C (mg)	12–16	16	28	16	11	13
Choline (mg)	N.S.	10	5.6	10	13	12

(continued)

Table 10.5 (*continued*)

Nutrients per 100 ml	Recommendations of Tsang (1993) based on 80 kcal/100 ml	Nutriprem (Cow & Gate)	Osterprem (Farley's)	Pre-Aptamil (Milupa)	LBW (SMA)	Pre-Nativa (Nestle)
Vitamins (*continued*)						
Taurine (mg)	3–6.0	5.5	5.1	5.5	7.0	6.4
Inositol (mg)	22–54	30	3.2	30	4.5	5.2
Carnitine (mg)	N.S.	2.0	1.0	2.0	2.9	1.7
Nucleotides	N.S.	✓	×	×	×	×
β-Carotene (μg)	N.S.	40	24	×	2.5	×
Osmolality (mOsmol/kg/ H₂O)	N.S.	293	300	312	277	325
Estimated renal solute load (mOsmol/l)	N.S.	148	134	148	134	143

N.S., not specified; CLD, chronic lung disease; MCT, medium chain triglycerides; AA, arachidonic acid; DHA, docosahexaenoic acid; GLA, gamma linolenic acid.
[a]Conversion factors: vitamin A, μg ÷ 0.3 = IU; vitamin D, μg × 40 = IU. 1 IU vitamin E = 1 mg D, Lα tocopherol acetate.
Only correct at time of publication – please check with manufacturers.

Nutrient-enriched postdischarge formulas

These have been developed over the last few years in response to the realisation that many babies changed to term formula at discharge might struggle to take in the volumes needed to achieve catch-up growth. Postdischarge some babies have been observed to take well over 200 ml/kg of term formula (Lucas *et al.*, 1992a). Improving nutrient intake with the use of a nutrient-enriched postdischarge formula has been shown to improve growth (Lucas *et al.*, 1992c; Cooke *et al.*, 1999), bone mineral content (Bishop *et al.*, 1993) and possibly neuro-development (Carlson *et al.*, 1994).

Initiation of Enteral Feeds

Although there have been completely opposing views on the optimal time to start enteral feeding over the last few decades, there are now many studies showing the advantage of early minimal (or trophic) enteral feeds (Berseth, 1992, 1996; Bissett *et al.*, 1989; Dunn *et al.*, 1988; Lucas *et al.*, 1986; McClure and Newell, 1999, 2000; Meetze *et al.*, 1992; Schanler *et al.*, 1999c). Human milk is better tolerated than formula for initiation of enteral feeds and also appears to aid tolerance of full oral feeds (McClure and Newell, 2000). Unfortunately a systematic review could only identify two studies designed in such a way as to allow strict comparisons according to set criteria, leading to a conclusion that there was insufficient evidence to say whether feeds should be started early or not (Kennedy *et al.*, 2000). However most clinicians now acknowledge the wealth of other data and will attempt to start feeds early.

Another systematic review could not identify an advantage to either continuous or bolus feeds (Premji and Chessell, 2001). However, if, as recommended, the feed is human milk, there is risk of significant energy loss with continuous feeding as discussed previously. There is also a risk of sedimentation of additives, e.g. BMF.

Table 10.6 Composition of Preterm Formulas in the USA

Nutrients per 100 ml	Recommendations of Tsang (1993) based on 80 kcal/100 ml	Enfamil Premature 20 (Mead Johnson)	Enfamil Premature 24 (Mead Johnson)	Similac Special Care 20 (Ross)	Similac Special Care 24 (Ross)
Energy (kcal)	80	68	81	67	80
Protein (g/kg)					
< 1000 g	3.6–3.8				
> 1000 g	3.0–3.6				
Protein (g)		2	2.4	1.8	1.8
Fat (g)	3.5–4.8 (tentative)	3.5	4.1	3.6	4.3
MCT (✓) percentage of total fat	N.S.				
LCP	Conditionally essential	N.S.	N.S.	✓	✓
Linoleic acid (g)	0.35–1.36	0.77	0.9	0.47	0.47
Linolenic acid (g)	0.09–0.35	0.11	0.13	✓	✓
Carbohydrate (g)	N.S.	7.5	9	7.1	8.5
Minerals					
Sodium (mg)	30–46	26	32	29	29
Potassium (mg)	52–80	70	84	87	87
Chloride (mg)	47–71	57	69	54	54
Calcium (mg)	80–154	112	134	121	121
Phosphorus (mg)	48–112	56	67	67	67
Ca:P ratio (by weight)	N.S.	2:1	2:1	1.8	1.8
Magnesium (mg)	5–10	4.6	5.5	8.1	8.1
Iron (mg)	2.0/kg	0.17 (with Fe 1.22)	0.2 (with Fe 1.46)	0.24 (with Fe 1.2)	0.24 (with Fe 1.2)
Zinc (mg)	0.7	1	1.22	1.0	1.0
Copper (µg)	80–100	85	101	168	168
Iodine (µg)	20–40	17	20	4	4
Manganese (µg)	5	4.3	5.1	8.1	8.1
Selenium (µg)	0.9	1.22	1.46	1.2	1.2
Vitamins					
Vitamin A (µg)[a]	CLD: 450–840 µg/kg No CLD: 210–450 µg/kg	2830	3366	3333	3333
Vitamin D (µg)[a]	2.4–6.4 (min 10/day)	4.5	5.5	2.5	2.5
Vitamin E (TE) (mg)	4–8 IU (max 25 IU/day)	4.3	5.1	2.7	2.7
Vitamin K (µg)	5.3–6.7	5.4	6.5	8.1	8.1
Thiamin, B_1 (mg)	0.12–0.16	0.135	0.162	0.169	0.169
Riboflavin, B_2 (mg)	0.16–0.24	0.2	0.24	0.418	0.418
Niacin (mg)	2.4–3.2	2.7	3.2	0.169	0.169
Panthothenic acid (mg)	0.8–1.2	0.8	0.97	1.282	1.282
Pyridoxine, B_6 (mg)	0.1–0.14	0.1	0.122	0.025	0.025
Folic acid (µg)	17–34	24	28	25	25
Vitamin B_{12} (µg)	0.2	0.17	0.2	0.37	0.37
Biotin (µg)	2.4–4.0	2.7	3.2	25	25
Vitamin C (mg)	12–16	13.5	16.2	25	25
Choline (mg)	N.S.	8.1	9.7	6.7	6.7

(continued)

Table 10.6   (*continued*)

Nutrients per 100 ml	Recommendations of Tsang (1993) Based on 80 kcal/100 ml	Enfamil Premature 20 (Mead Johnson)	Enfamil Premature 24 (Mead Johnson)	Similac Special Care 20 (Ross)	Similac Special Care 24 (Ross)
Vitamins (*continued*)					
Taurine (mg)	3–6.0	4.1	4.9	N.S.	N.S.
Inositol (mg)	22–54	11.5	13.8	3.7	3.7
Carnitine (mg)	N.S.	1.3	1.6	N.S.	N.S.
Nucleotides	N.S.	×	×	7.2	7.2
Beta-carotene (µg)	N.S.	×	×	N.S.	N.S.
Osmolality (mOsmol/kg/ H$_2$O)	N.S.	260	310	235	280
Estimated renal solute load (mOsmol/l)	N.S.	125	150	N.S.	N.S.

N.S., not specified; CLD, chronic lung disease; MCT, medium chain triglycerides; AA, arachidonic acid; DHA; docosahexaenoic acid; GLA, gamma linolenic acid.
[a]Conversion factors: vitamin A, µg÷0.3=IU; vitamin D, µg×40=IU. 1 IU vitamin E=1 mg D, L α tocopherol acetate.
Only correct at time of publication – please check with manufacturers.

Parenteral Nutrition

During intrauterine life, the foetus receives nourishment via the parenteral route, and part of successful adaptation to extrauterine life is the change to enteral feeds. In most babies of VLBW and less than 30 weeks, full feeding via the enteral route is both difficult and dangerous and parenteral nutrition (PN) has been developed to provide full nutritional requirements. The aim of PN is to achieve the intravenous administration of a nutritionally complete formulation in a volume compatible with the babies' clinical state. The first published report of PN in a baby was that of Dudrick *et al.* (1968), where they describe the long-term administration of a hypertonic parenteral solution to a baby with small bowel atresia. Further progress over the last 30 years has resulted in the ability to deliver prolonged PN to VLBW babies, although in practice nutrition is rarely provided exclusively by PN, as there are many benefits to small trophic enteral feeds started early on as discussed in the last section. A recent review of more detailed theoretical needs and practical guidelines for PN is available (King, 1998).

Indications for Initiation

Parenteral nutrition should be considered in the following infants:

- less than 30 weeks' gestation;
- less than 1500 g birth-weight;
- major gut anomalies;
- post-major gut surgery with or without short gut syndrome;
- for 'gut rest', i.e. for conservative treatment of NEC;
- intractable diarrhoea.

Nutrient Composition

Energy

The energy intake required in a preterm babies is about 100 kcal/kg/day. Table 10.1 summarizes the different components making up total energy expenditure and their ranges. Without the provision of exogenous energy the baby will rapidly lose weight due to tissue catabolism. Babies nursed within current guidelines and in modern incubators should not have an energy expenditure of more than 50–60 kcal/kg/24 h, thereby requiring an additional 60–70 kcal/kg/24 h for adequate growth (Heimler et al., 1993).

Carbohydrate

Studies have shown that neonatal hypoglycaemia (blood glucose <2.6 mmol/l) adversely affects both mortality and morbidity. Glucose is the carbohydrate source of choice and should supply the majority of the non-protein energy. In addition to energy supply, glucose primes the Krebs's cycle and theoretically exerts a protein-sparing effect by stimulation of insulin production (Woolfson et al., 1979). The use of exogenous insulin has been suggested to promote growth with only short-term objectives in sight; however long-term outcome must be assessed as insulin is a powerful agent with the potential to down-regulate endogenous receptors if administered exogenously (Goldman and Hirata, 1980). The majority of infants tolerate an increase in glucose over 24–48 h to 10 mg/kg/min, equivalent to 15 g/kg/24 h infused at a constant rate over 24 h. There is evidence to suggest that babies of less than 1200 g birthweight may have a glucose demand inversely related to their weight, increased demand being provided for by increased rate of gluconeogenesis (Keshen et al., 1997).

Lipids

Intravenous lipid (IVL) is required in parenteral nutrition that is running for more than a few days for a number of reasons. IVL provides the essential fatty acids required,

acts as the optimal medium for the delivery of fat-soluble vitamins and is a relatively low volume isotonic energy store. Essential fatty acid deficiency is biochemically detectable within 72 h after birth in the smallest babies on a lipid-free regimen (Cooke et al., 1985; Foote et al., 1991); however, it can be prevented with as little as 0.5 g lipid/kg/24 h (Cooke et al., 1987) and this should ideally be started within 48 h of birth. In addition to this, the joint administration of glucose and amino acids rather than glucose alone has been shown to accelerate the development of essential fatty acid deficiency (Anderson et al., 1979) possibly due to increased growth. It has been shown that the energy requirements of parenterally fed babies are significantly reduced if at least 25 per cent of the non-protein energy is provided by lipid; without a lipid source, lipogenesis occurs from glucose and this consumes significantly more energy than direct use of parenterally infused lipid (MacFie et al., 1983; Van-Aerde et al., 1989).

Amino acids

Newborn babies, and particularly sick VLBW preterm babies, undergo substantial negative nitrogen balance without the provision of exogenous energy, and although intravenous glucose can reduce this, growth involving nitrogen accretion and the laying down of lean body mass cannot occur without an exogenous nitrogen source, i.e. amino acids. Intolerance frequently occurs with glucose and lipid intakes, which often have to be temporarily reduced, thus reducing the amount of nitrogen that can be layed down (Duffy et al., 1981; Zlotkin et al., 1981). With sufficient non-protein energy, nitrogen accretion increases in a linear fashion up to an intake of 4 g protein/kg. Unless there is substantial catch-up growth to be made, no further accretion is seen at higher nitrogen intakes (see Figure 10.1).

A number of previous trials have demonstrated a significant improvement in protein synthesis and nitrogen accretion when starting amino acids on day one of birth compared with delaying a few days (Saini *et al.*, 1989; van-Lingen *et al.*, 1992).

Vitamins

Recommendations for intravenous vitamins need to take into account losses due to interactions with tubing, photo-degradation and increased renal wasting. Water-soluble include vitamins C, B_1, B_2, B_6, niacin, pantothenate, biotin, folic acid and B_{12}. These vitamins can be delivered as Solivito-N at 1 ml/kg/24 h. Fat-soluble vitamins are vitamins A, E, K and D and can be delivered as Vitilipid Infant at 4 ml/kg/24 h to a total maximum of 10 ml/24 h (Greene *et al.*, 1988).

Minerals and trace elements

Although published a while ago, the most comprehensive review remains that of Greene *et al.* (1988). Table 10.7 summarizes some of these recommendations.

Future Developments

Glutamine

Glutamine has a number of key functions including involvement in energy metabolism, hepatic urea production and acting as a fuel for both the small intestine and the immune system (Powell-Tuck, 1993). Although there is some evidence that VLBW enterally fed babies are able to produce glutamine endogenously (Darmaun *et al.*, 1995), it may become a conditionally essential AA in the stressed baby. However, a recent systematic review

Table 10.7 Recommendations for parenteral trace elements and minerals in preterm infants

Recommended dose per kg/24 hr	Preterm, Greene *et al.* (1988)	Peditrace 1 ml/kg
Zinc (µg)[a]	400	250
Copper (µg)[a]	20	20
Selenium (µg)[b]	2.0	2.0
Chromium (µg)	0.2	–
Manganese (µg)[a]	1.0	1.0
Molybdenum (µg)[b]	0.25	–
Iodine (µg)	1.0	1.0
Fluoride (µg)[c]	–	57
Iron (µg)[d]	–	–
Magnesium (mmol)	0.25–0.37	–
Sodium (mmol)	3–5	–
Potassium (mmol)	1–2	–
Phosphorous (mmol)	1.5–2.2	–
Calcium (mmol)	1.5–2.2	–
Chloride (mmol)	3–5	–

[a]Omit in patients with obstructive jaundice.
[b]Needed only with long-term PN, omit in patients with significant renal dysfunction.
[c]Firm recommendations for routine inclusion cannot be made; 500 µg daily in infants over 3 months on exclusive PN should be considered.
[d]Not required until 6 weeks or at doubling of birth-weight in preterm; then dose of 200 µg/kg (100 µg/kg at 3 months in term babies). Concerns over the pro-oxidative effects of i.v. iron remain.

concluded that there was no evidence to support the routine use of parenteral or enteral glutamine supplementation in preterm babies (Tubman and Thompson, 2000).

Carnitine

Carnitine is an essential co-factor in the transfer of long-chain fatty acids across the inner mitochondrial membrane to the site of β-oxidation. It can be synthesized *de novo* in adults and older children, but not in babies (Olson *et al.*, 1989; Penn *et al.*, 1980) and it has been postulated that carnitine deficiency may impair fatty acid oxidation. A recent systematic review could find no evidence at present to support the routine use of carnitine in parenterally fed preterm babies (Cairns and Stalker, 2000).

Inositol

Inositol is an essential nutrient for cell survival and has been shown to be important in surfactant production. A recent systematic review concluded that there may be significantly reduced respiratory morbidity associated with its addition to PN solutions (Howlett and Ohlsson, 2000). The evidence is based on very few studies and more work is needed in this area.

Monitoring Tolerance

The clinical condition of the baby should be regularly assessed while on PN. It has been shown that, in enterally fed babies, blood urea levels can give an indication of protein adequacy (Polberger et al., 1990), and that a serum urea of between 2 and 8 mmol/l would indicate that protein requirements had been met (Kashyap and Heird, 1994). Daily urea, electrolytes and liver function tests should be measured until the PN regimen is well established, after which twice weekly is adequate. Triglycerides and cholesterol should be measured prior to increasing fat to 3.5 g/kg/day and then weekly thereafter. For babies requiring PN for more than 2 weeks, with very little enteral intake, a weekly aminogram is advisable. Although the plasma amino acids usually reflect the composition of the infusate (Anderson et al., 1977), it will indicate whether potentially neurotoxic amino acids such as phenylalanine and tyrosine are building up to undesirable levels.

Complications

Catheter infection, both bacterial and less commonly fungal, is a major cause of morbidity on a neonatal unit. The prevalence of infection secondary to central venous access varies dramatically between neonatal units with staff training playing a major role in its prevention (Puntis et al., 1991). Other technical problems include extravasation, central vein thrombosis, pulmonary embolism and rarely cardiac tamponade. Metabolic complications include electrolyte disturbances, acid–base abnormalities, essential fatty acid deficiency, hypo- and hyperglycaemia, cholestatic jaundice and prerenal uraemia. Haematological complications include anaemia and thrombocyte and neutrophil dysfunction.

Transition to enteral feeding

As discussed above, minimal enteral feeding has numerous benefits for the baby who can tolerate it, while the majority of the nutritional input is provided parenterally.

Failure-to-Thrive and Catch-up Growth

Early poor growth has been associated with adverse outcomes in preterm babies (Georgieff et al., 1985; Powls et al., 1996; Ross et al., 1983). Those with high perinatal risk fare worse at 2 years if they are more poorly grown (Connors et al., 1999). However, as these studies were not randomized trials testing nutrient interventions, it is impossible to conclude that improved nutrition would have improved outcome. With respect to neurodevelopmental outcome, growth may not be as important a factor as use of human milk.

Early severe malnutrition has been associated with reduced brain cellularity (Winick and Rosso, 1969). There could be more immediate adverse effects on respiratory and immune function as demonstrated in older subjects (Ong et al., 1998; Suskind et al., 1976).

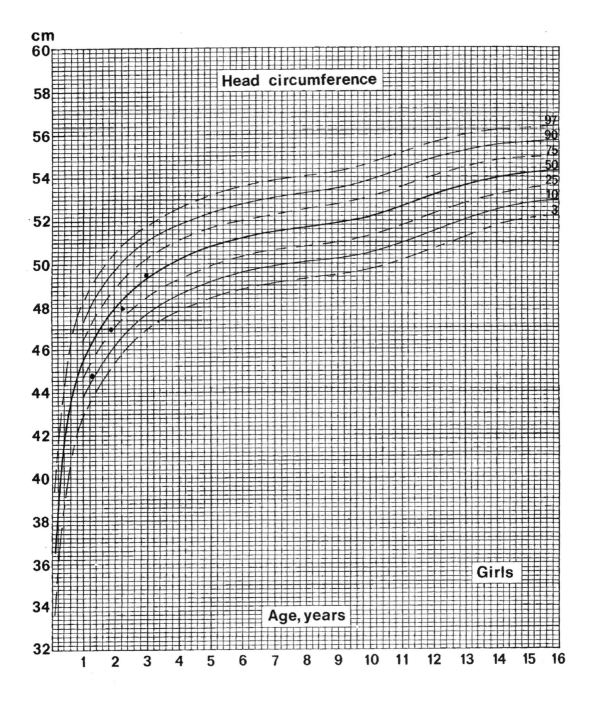

Figure 10.2a Catch-up growth (NB, the growth charts used are no longer recommended). © Castlemead Publications

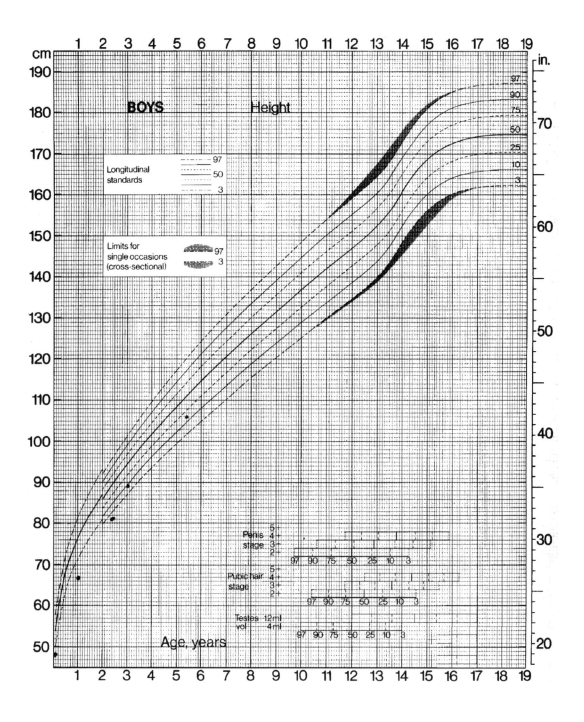

Figure 10.2b.   © Castlemead Publications

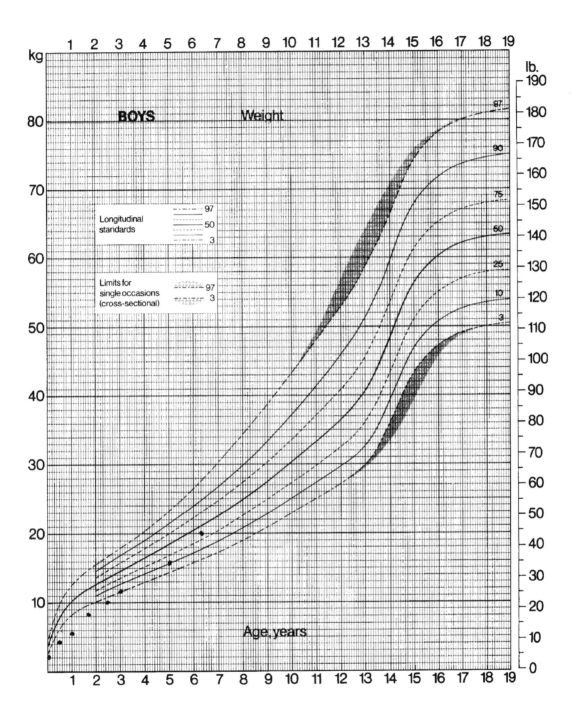

Figure 10.2c. © Castlemead Publications

Energy requirements for intrauterine growth-retarded (IUGR) infants may only be slightly increased (Tsang *et al.*, 1993), with feeding to maximum tolerance being the goal to allow catch-up to occur. Future work on the effects of catch-up growth should be carefully evaluated as there is a hypothesis that excessive catch up could predispose to adult chronic disease (Cianfarani *et al.*, 1999; Eriksson *et al.*, 1999). It is essential to ensure that catch-up length and head growth are occurring and not just the deposition of excess fat. Long-term observation often shows that VLBW infants have less success at achieving catch-up weight gain than more mature infants (Casey *et al.*, 1990). However, catch-up can occur and continue well into childhood independent of formal nutritional supplementation (Figure 10.2).

Diagnosis of Failure to Thrive

It is useful to understand patterns of growth in preterm babies before diagnosing failure to thrive. Given appropriate nutrition, well babies will grow. However, growth may have a pulsatile pattern, individual to each, which is hidden when only daily measurements are considered (Greco *et al.*, 1990). There may be a 1–2 weekly pattern irrespective of daily energy input (Gibson, 1994; Figure 10.3). A small study of preterm babies fed human milk found no relationship between energy intake and weight gain over a 3 week period during the first postnatal month (Spencer *et al.*, 1982). Likewise in a group of formula-fed babies there was a wide variability in weight gains despite comparable nutrition and environment (Spencer *et al.*, 1992). The following guidelines are a rough framework for defining when failure to thrive is occurring:

- when weight loss occurs progressively over several days (other than the early postnatal period when a diuresis is expected);

- when weight, length ± head circumference velocity decreases over 1 week;
- when weight velocity alone decreases over 2 weeks.

Causes of Failure to Thrive

There are conflicting results from studies looking at correlates with growth. Weight gain over the first 6 weeks postnatally has not been shown to be related to nutrition or illness in one study (Cooke *et al.*, 1993), whereas in another it has been found that energy intake was positively associated with weight gain over the first 56 days (Berry *et al.*, 1997). Therefore all efforts to achieve full nutritional requirements must be made. The latter study also found that short gestation was independently negatively associated with growth.

Sepsis did not appear to affect weight gain in this study, but did in another (Ehrenkranz *et al.*, 1999); nutritional input was not assessed in this study.

Dexamethasone treatment and ventilation appear to reduce growth independently (Gibson *et al.*, 1993; Leitch *et al.*, 1996; Berry *et al.*, 1997). It has been observed to take up to 30 days for catch-up length to occur after a single course of dexamethasone (Gibson *et al.*, 1993), although there are no data following several courses. If weight alone is used to assess growth, these babies are potentially at risk of overfeeding, leading to an abnormal body composition with lower lean body mass and higher body fat than controls (Leitch *et al.*, 1999). Sodium depletion is a risk factor for poor growth especially in preterm babies who have high requirements (Chance *et al.*, 1977; Haycock, 1993).

Occasionally, expressed human milk could be very low in fat, particularly if predominantly fore milk is collected. This may be deduced when an otherwise well human milk-fed baby is growing poorly with normal or

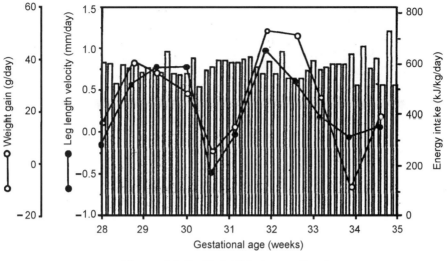

Figure 10.3   Variability in growth rate

raised serum urea levels. Milk expression technique should be evaluated and preferential feeding of hind milk or at least the stored milk with the largest fat layer (Valentine *et al.*, 1994). Estimating the fat content via the creamatocrit may be useful (Lucas *et al.*, 1978; Wang *et al.*, 1999). This is most usefully carried out on pooled samples due to the potentially high variation between expressions.

Anaemia may lead to poor weight gain (Stockman and Clarke, 1984), although this is unlikely to be a clinically important risk factor.

Increased respiratory rate indicating increased metabolic rate can be associated with cardiac disease and chronic lung disease (de Meer *et al.*, 1997) and is one of the few times an energy supplement could be considered. Maximum volumes of appropriate feed should have been trialled prior to energy supplementation. Energy supplements alone should not be added to term formula or unfortified human milk, as it may reduce energy from protein to such a level that growth is compromised, as has been demonstrated in term infants (Clarke *et al.*, 1999). Energy supplementation could theoretically exacerbate gastro-oesophageal reflux (GOR) due to delayed gastric emptying (Siegel *et al.*, 1984)

and increased osmolality (Sutphen and Dillard, 1989).

Severe intraventricular haemorrhage has been associated with poor weight gain (Ehrenkranz *et al.*, 1999). Dietetic input on the Neonatal Unit has been shown to be associated with enhanced weight gain (McDowell, 1998), reflecting the advantage of individual assessment by a trained specialist. Despite the early discrepancies in growth performance depending on the study diet in the papers of Lucas and his team, it is interesting to note that by 8 years of age these differences had disappeared (Morley and Lucas, 2000).

Treatment of Failure to Thrive

- Ensure appropriate nutritional assessment of individual babies.
- Liberalize unnecessary fluid restriction and thus increase nutrient intake.
- Ensure adequate human milk fortification.
- Evaluate the energy content of human milk using the creamatocrit technique.
- Treat sodium depletion.

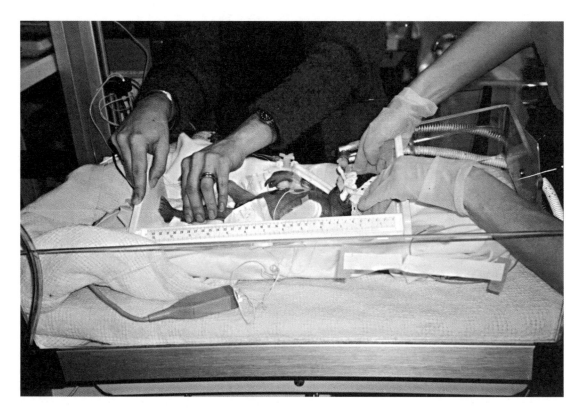

Figure 10.4 Pedobaby ruler

- Treat anaemia.
- Treat vomiting or feed refusal due to undiagnosed or inadequately treated GOR.
- Supplement with energy when there is good evidence that energy expenditure is elevated.

Growth Assessment

Weight

Weight should be plotted on the centile chart weekly, with the weight of any attachments subtracted from the total. Weight alone has several drawbacks as it often reflects fluid balance rather than tissue accretion. In addition, it is difficult to assess overall growth performance without reference to length and head growth. As the baby stabilizes and

approaches discharge, weighing should be done at a maximum of twice weekly, then once per week if possible. As discussed previously, growth rate, and therefore weight gain, will slow down and may have a more periodic pattern irrespective of short-term changes in energy input. Daily weights can add unnecessarily to parental anxiety without aiding clinical assessment.

Head circumference

This should be measured and plotted weekly, preferably by the same observer using a lasso-type tape (available from the Child Growth Foundation, Chiswick, London, UK) or a new paper tape. This measurement gives valuable information on cerebral growth with respect to

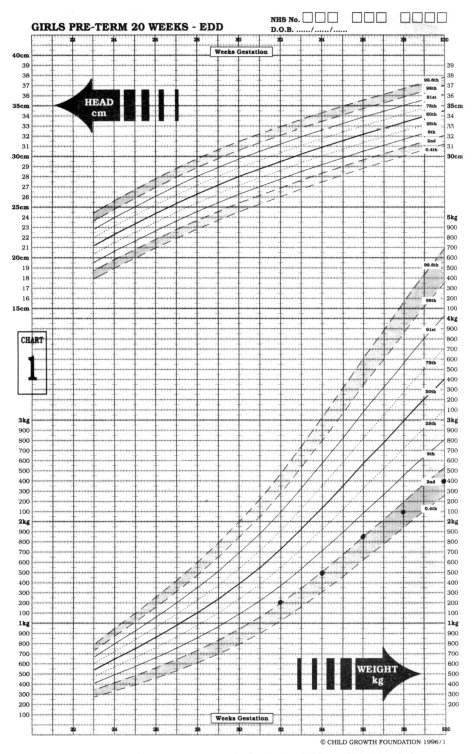

Figure 10.5 Use of appropriate growth charts. ©Child Growth Foundation 1996

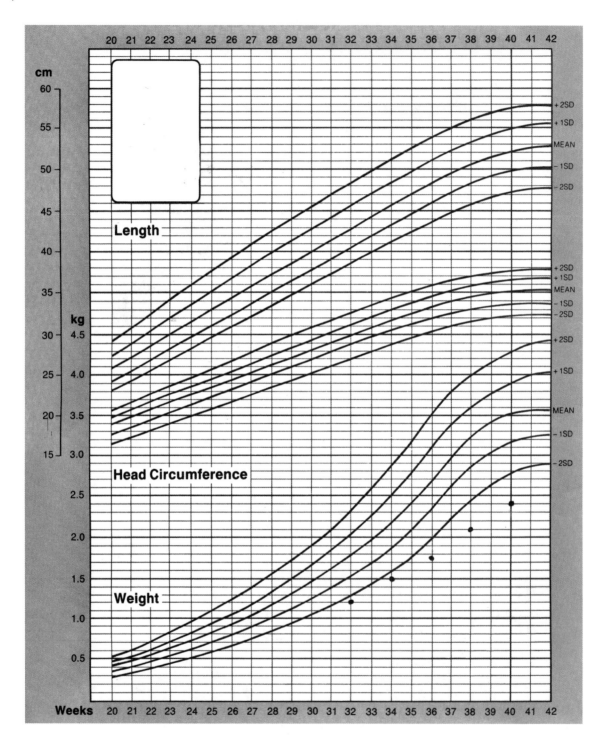

Figure 10.5b. Growth charts *continued.* © Castlemead Publications

cerebral insult as well as nutritional adequacy (Lindley *et al.*, 1999). Head growth is 'spared' in relation to length and weight in moderate undernutrition, as demonstrated quantitatively in animal studies (Weigensberg, 1990; Freedman *et al.*, 1980), but may fall off during severe illness when nutrition is compromised (Marks *et al.*, 1979).

Length

Early assessment of longitudinal growth may help give a better idea of the baby's long-term growth pattern, putting weight and head circumference changes into perspective. The measurement is essential for accurate growth assessment as it reflects both skeletal and organ growth. Length should be plotted weekly until 40 weeks postconceptual age, then every 2 weeks until discharge. Where possible the measurement should be carried out by the same two observers, or at least one consistent observer at the feet reading off the measurement, and it should follow an agreed procedure. Measurements taken by single observers and without any training can be highly unreliable (Wales *et al.*, 1997). Use of a tape measure is not recommended as it leads to large errors, even with the same observer (Rosenberg *et al.*, 1992). A simple ruler is most useful for less stable and ventilated babies; the Pedobaby is demonstrated in Figure 10.4. It measures up to 50 cm and is available from Harlow Printing Ltd (Tyne and Wear, UK).

Growth Charts

The most appropriate growth charts in the UK are the 'Four in One Growth Charts' (1996 Child Growth Foundation) based on the most recent UK growth data and including weight and head circumference centiles for preterm infants from 22 weeks (see Figure 10.5a). There

are currently insufficient data for length centiles below 32 weeks' gestation. These charts have the advantage of being included in the Personal Child Health Records held by the parents, which reduces the risk of confusion during interpretation of growth postdischarge. Other charts have length centiles below 32 weeks, but they are based on a smaller population and do not have the same centile range as the Four in One Charts, possibly leading to an erroneous diagnosis of failure to thrive compared to the recommended charts, see Figure 10.5b. Points plotted on growth charts should never be circled as this hinders interpretation of growth trends.

Conclusion

Low-birth-weight and very-low-birth-weight babies present many nutritional challenges. They are born nutritionally compromised but immaturity of the gastro-intestinal tract and endocrine homeostatic mechanisms make provision of enteral and parenteral nutrition difficult. As some feeding decisions can affect both morbidity and mortality it is essential to use the large evidence base available in conjunction with conclusions drawn from careful clinical observation.

References

Amin SB, Merle KS, Orlando MS, Dalzell LE and Guillet R (2000) Brainstem maturation in premature infants as a function of enteral feeding type. *Pediatrics* **106**, 318–322.

Anderson GH, Bryan H, Jeejeebhoy KN and Corey P (1977) Dose response relationship between amino acid intake and blood levels in newborn infants. *Am J. Clin. Nutr.* **30**, 1110–1121.

Anderson TL, Muttart CR, Bieber MA, Nicholson JF and Heird WC (1979) A controlled trial of glucose versus glucose and amino acids in premature infants. *J. Pediatr.* **94**, 947–951.

Anderson JW, Johnstone BM and Remley DT (1999) Breast-feeding and cognitive development: a meta-analysis. *Am. J. Clin. Nutr.* **70**, 525–535.

Backstrom MC, Maki R, Kuusela AL, Sievanen H, Koivisto AM, Ikonen RS, Kouri T and Maki M (1999) Randomised controlled trial of vitamin D supplementation on bone density and biochemical indices in preterm infants. *Arch. Dis. Child.* **80**, F161–F166.

Beeby PJ and Jeffrey H (1992) Risk factors for necrotising enterocolitis: the influence of gestational age. *Arch. Dis. Child.* **67**, 432–435.

Berry MA, Abrahamowicz M and Usher RH (1997) Factors associated with growth of extremely premature infants during initial hospitalization. *Pediatrics* **100**, 640–646.

Berseth CL (1992) Effect of early feeding on maturation of the preterm infants small intestine. *J. Pediatr.* **120**, 947.

Berseth CL (1996) Minimal enteral feedings. *Clin. Perinatol.*, **22**, 195–205.

Bishop NJ, King FJ and Lucas A (1993) Increased bone mineral content of preterm infants fed a nutrient enriched formula after discharge from hospital. *Arch. Dis. Child.* **68**, 573–578.

Bissett WM, Watt J, Rivers RPA and Milla PJ (1989) Post-prandial motor response of the small intestine to enteral feeds in preterm infants. *Arch. Dis. Child.* **64**, 1356–1361.

BNF (1992) *The British Nutrition Foundation. Unsaturated Fatty Acids. Nutritional and Physiological Significance*. Whitaker, London.

Boehm G, Melichar V, Senger H, Muller D and Raiha NC (1990) Effects of varying energy intakes on nitrogen retention and growth in very low birth-weight infants fed fortified human milk. *Acta Paediatr. Scand.* **79**, 228–229.

Brandt RB, Mueller DG and Schroeder JR (1978) Serum vitamin A in premature and term neonates. *J. Pediatr.* **92**, 101–104.

Brooke OG, Alvear J and Arnold M (1979) Energy retention, energy expenditure, and growth in healthy immature infants. *Pediatr. Res.* **13**, 215–220.

Byrne TA, Morrissey TB, Nattakom TV, Ziegler TR and Wilmore DW (1995) Growth hormone, glutamine, and a modified diet enhance nutrient absorption in patients with severe short bowel syndrome. *J. Parent. Enteral Nutr.* **19**, 296–302.

Cairns P and Stalker D (2000) Carnitine supplementation of parenterally fed neonates. *Cochrane Database Syst. Rev.* CD000950.

Carlson SE, Werkman SH, Peeples JM and Wilson WM (1994) Long-chain fatty acids and early visual and cognitive development of preterm infants. *Eur. J. Clin. Nutr.* **48**(Suppl. 2), 527–530.

Casey PH, Kraemer HC, Bernbaum J, Tyson JE, Sells JC, Yogman MW and Bauer CR (1990) Growth patterns of low birth weight preterm infants: a longitudinal analysis of a large, varied sample. *J. Pediatr.* **117**, 298–307.

Chance CW, Raddle IC, Willis DM and Park E (1977) Postnatal growth of infants <1.3 kg birth weight: effects of metabolic acidosis, of caloric intake and of calcium, sodium and phosphorus supplementation. *J. Pediatr.*, **91**, 787–793.

Cianfarani S, Germani D and Branca F (1999) Low birthweight and adult insulin resistance: the 'catch-up growth' hypothesis. *Arch. Dis. Child.* **81**, F71–F73.

Clarke S, MacDonald A and Booth IW (1999) Impaired growth and nitrogen deficiency in infants receiving an energy supplemented standard infant formula. *50th Study Day Paediatric Group BDA* (April), p. O1.

Connors JM, O'Callaghan MJ, Burns YR, Gray PH, Tudehope DI, Mohay H and Rogers YM (1999) The influence of growth on development outcome in extremely low birthweight infants at 2 years of age. *J. Paediatr. Child Health* **35**, 37–41.

Cooke R, Yeh YY, Gibson D, Debo D and Bell GL (1987) Soybean oil emulsion administration during parenteral nutrition in the preterm infant: effect on essential fatty acid, lipid and glucose metabolism. *J. Pediatr.* **111**, 767–773.

Cooke RJ, Zee P and Yeh YY (1985) Safflower oil emulsion administration during parenteral nutrition in the preterm infant. 1. Effect on essential fatty acid status. *J. Pediatr. Gastroenterol. Nutr.* **4**, 799–863.

Cooke RJ, Ford A and Werkmans SH (1993) Postnatal growth in infants born between 700–1500 g. *J. Pediat. Gastroenterol. Nutr.*, **16**, 130–135.

Cooke R, McCormick K, Griffin I, Embleton N, Faulkner K, Wells JC and Rawlings DC (1999) Feeding preterm infants after hospital discharge: effect of diet on body composition. *Pediatr. Res.* **46**, 461–464.

Cosgrove M, Davies DP and Jenkins HR (1996) Nucleotide supplementation and the growth of term small for gestational age infants. *Arch. Dis. Child Fetal Neonatal. Edn* **74**, F122–125.

Darlow BA and Graham PJ (2000) Vitamin A supplementation for preventing morbidity and mortality in very low birthweight infants. *Cochrane Database Syst. Rev.* **2**, CD000501.

Darlow BA, Inder TE, Graham PJ, Sluis KB, Malpas TJ, Taylor BJ and Winterbourn CC (1995) The relationship of selenium status to respiratory outcome in the very low birth weight infant. *Pediatrics* **96**, 314–319.

Darmaun D, Roig JC and Auestad NNJ (1995) Glutamine metabolism in very low birth weight (VLBW) infants. *Pediatr. Res.* **37**, 305A.

De Curtis M, Candusso M, Pieltain C and Rigo J (1999) Effect of fortification on the osmolality of human milk. *Arch. Dis. Child.* **81**, F141–F143.

de Meer K, Westerterp KR, Houwen RH, Brouwers HA, Berger R and Okken A (1997) Total energy expenditure in infants with bronchopulmonary dysplasia is associated with respiratory status. *Eur. J. Pediatr.* **156**, 299–304.

Dudrick SJ, Wilmore DW, Vars HM and Rhoads JE (1968) Long-term total parenteral nutrition with growth, development, and positive nitrogen balance. *Surgery* **64**, 134–142.

Duffy B, Gunn T, Collinge J and Pencharz P (1981) The effect of varying protein quality and energy intake on the nitrogen metabolism of parenterally fed very low birthweight (less than 1600 g) infants. *Pediatr. Res.* **15**, 1040–1044.

Dunn L, Hulman S, Weiner J and Kliegman R (1988) Beneficial effects of early hypocaloric enteral feeding on neonatal gastrointestinal function: preliminary report of a randomized trial. *J. Pediatr.* **112**, 622–629.

Ehrenkranz RA (1994) Iron requirements of preterm infants. *Nutrition* **10**, 77–78.

Ehrenkranz RA, Younes N, Lemons JA, Fanaroff AA, Donovan EF, Wright LL, Katsikiotis V, Tyson JE, Oh W, Shankaran S, Bauer CR, Korones SB, Stoll BJ, Stevenson DK and Papile LA (1999) Longitudinal growth of hospitalized very low birth weight infants. *Pediatrics*, **104**, 280–289.

el-Mohandes AE, Picard MB and Simmens SJ (1995) Human milk utilization in the ICN decreases the incidence of bacterial sepsis. *Pediatr. Res.* **37**, 306A.

el-Mohandes AE, Picard MB, Simmens SJ and Keiser JF (1997) Use of human milk in the intensive care nursery decreases the incidence of nosocomial sepsis. *J. Perinatol.* **17**, 130–134.

Eriksson JG, Forsen T, Tuomilehto J, Winter PD, Osmond C and Barker DJ (1999) Catch-up growth in childhood and death from coronary heart disease: longitudinal study. *BMJ* **318**, 427–431.

ESPGAN (1987) Nutrition and feeding of preterm infants. *Acta Paediatr. Scand.* **336**(Suppl.).

ESPGAN (1991) Comment on the content and composition of lipids in infant formula. *Acta Paediatr. Scand.* **80**, 887–896.

Evans JR, Allen AC, Stinson DA, Hamilton DC, St.John BB, Vincer MJ, Raad MA, Gundberg CM and Cole DE (1989) Effect of high-dose vitamin D supplementation on radiographically detectable bone disease of very low birth weight infants. *J. Pediatr.* **115**, 779–786.

Ewer AK and Yu VY (1996) Gastric emptying in preterm infants: the effect of breast milk fortifier. *Acta Paediatr.* **85**, 1112–1115.

Fewtrell MS, Cole TJ, Bishop NJ and Lucas A (2000a) Neonatal factors predicting childhood height in preterm infants: evidence for a persisting effect of early metabolic bone disease? *J. Pediatr.* **137**, 668–673.

Fewtrell MS, Prentice A, Cole TJ and Lucas A (2000b) Effects of growth during infancy and childhood on bone mineralization and turnover in preterm children aged 8–12 years. *Acta Paediatr.* **89**, 148–153.

Food and Agriculture Organization (1994) *Fats and Oils in Human Nutrition*, pp. 6–7. Food and Agriculture Organization, Rome.

Foote KD, MacKinnon MJ and Innis SM (1991) Effect of early introduction of formula vs fat free parenteral nutrition on essential fatty acid status of preterm infants. *Am. J. Clin. Nutr.* **54**, 93–97.

Forget P, Van den Neucker A, Degraeuwe P, van Aalst K, Sprinkel G, van Kreel B and Kester A (1995) Steatorrhea in premature infants is linked with functional pancreatic immaturity. *Pediatr. Res.* **37**, 307A.

Freedman LS, Samuels S, Fish I, Schwartz SA, Lange B, Katz M and Morgano L (1980) Sparing of the brain in neonatal undernutrition: amino acid transport and incorporation into brain and muscle. *Science*, **207**, 902–904.

Friel JK and Andrews WL (1994) Zinc requirement of premature infants. *Nutrition* **10**, 63–65.

Friel JK, Andrews WL, Matthew JD, McKim E, French S and Long D (1993) Improved growth of very low birthweight infants. *Nutr. Res.* **13**, 611–620.

Gaziano JM, Johnson EJ, Russell RM, Manson JE, Stampfer MJ, Ridker PM, Frei B, Hennekens CH and Krinsky NI (1995) Discrimination in absorption or transport of beta-carotene isomers after oral supplementation with either all-trans- or 9-cis-beta-carotene. *Am. J. Clin. Nutr.* **61**, 1248–1252.

Georgieff MK, Hoffman JS, Pereira GR, Bernbaum J and Hoffman Williamson M (1985) Effect of neonatal caloric deprivation on head growth and 1-year developmental status in preterm infants. *J. Pediatr.* **107**, 581–587.

Gibson AT (1994) Early postnatal growth – what should we measure? Why should we bother? Abstract from: *Controversies in Nutrition: Feeding the Preterm Infant*, Hammersmith Hospital, London.

Gibson AT, Pearse RG and Wales JKH (1993) Growth retardation after dexamethasone administrating assessment by knemometry. *Arch. Dis. Child.* **69**, 505–509.

Goldman HI, Goldman JS, Kaufman I and Liebman OB (1974) Late effects of early dietary protein intakes on low birth weight infants. *J. Pediatr.* **85**, 764–796.

Goldman SL and Hirata T (1980) Attenuated response to insulin in very low birth weight infants. *Pediatr. Res.* **14**, 50–53.

Greco L, Capasso A, De Fusco C and Paludetto R (1990) Pulsatile weight increases in very low birth-weight babies appropriate for gestational age. *Arch. Dis. Child.* **65**, 373–376.

Greene HL, Hambidge KM, Schanler R and Tsang RC (1988) Guidelines for the use of vitamins, trace elements, calcium, magnesium, and phosphorus in infants and children receiving total parenteral nutrition: report of the Subcommittee on Pediatric Parenteral Nutrient Requirements from the Committee on Clinical Practice Issues of the American Society for Clinical Nutrition. *Am. J. Clin. Nutr.* **48**, 1324–1342. [Published errata appear in *Am. J. Clin. Nutr.* (1989) **49**, 1332 and (1989) **50**, 560.]

Greer FR, McCormick A and Loker J (1984) Changes in fat concentration of human milk during delivery by intermittent bolus and continuous mechanical pump infusion. *J. Pediatr.* **105**, 745–749.

Griffin IJ, Cooke RJ, Reid MM, McCormick KPB and Smith JS (1999) Iron nutritional status in preterm infants fed formulas fortified with iron. *Arch. Dis. Child.* **81**, F45–F49.

Hall RT, Wheeler RE, Benson J, Harris G and Rippetoe L (1993) Feeding iron-fortified premature formula during initial hospitalization to infants less than 1800 grams birth weight. *Pediatrics* **92**, 409–414.

Hamosh M (1987) Lipid metabolism in premature infants. *Biol. Neonate* **52**(Suppl. 1), 50–64.

Hamosh M, Mehta NR, Fink CS, Coleman J and

Hamosh P (1991) Fat absorption in premature infants: medium-chain triglycerides and long-chain triglycerides are absorbed from formula at similar rates. *J. Pediatr. Gastroenterol. Nutr.* **13**, 143–149.

Hay WW, Lucas A, Heird WC, Ziegler E, Levin E, Grave GD, Catz CS and Yaffe SJ (1999) Workshop summary: nutrition of the extremely low birth weight infant. *Pediatrics* **104**, 1360–1368.

Haycock GB (1993) The influence of sodium on growth in infancy. *Pediatr. Nephrol.* **7**, 871–875.

Heimler R, Doumas BT, Jendrzejczak BM, Nemeth PB, Hoffman RG and Nelin LD (1993) Relationship between nutrition, weight change, and fluid compartments in preterm infants during the first week of life. *J. Pediatr.* **122**, 110–114.

Hibberd CM, Brooke O and Carter ND (1982) Variations in the composition of breast milk during the first five weeks lactation: implications for the feeding of preterm infants, *Arch. Dis. Child.* **57**, 658–662.

Holland P, Wilkinson A, Diez J and Lindsell D (1990) Prenatal deficiency of phosphate, phosphate supplementation and rickets in very low birth weight infants. *Lancet* **335**, 697–701.

Horwood L, Darlow B and Mogridge N (2001) Breast milk feeding and cognitive ability at 7–8 years. *Arch. Dis. Child. Fetal Neonatal Edn* **1**, 7.

Howlett A and Ohlsson A (2000) Inositol in preterm infants with RDS. (Cochrane Review.) *Cochrane Database Syst. Rev.* CD000366.

Huston R, Jelen BJ, Ray LK and Borschel MW (1996) Parenteral and enteral selenium supplementation in low birthweight preterm infants. *Pediatr. Res.* **39**, 311A.

Jacobson SW, Chiodo LM and Jacobson JL (1999) Breastfeeding effects on intelligence quotient in 4- and 11-year-old children. *Pediatrics* **103**, e71.

Jocson MA, Mason EO and Schanler RJ (1997) The effects of nutrient fortification and varying storage conditions on host defense properties of human milk. *Pediatrics*, **100**, 240–243.

Johnson L, Bowen FW and Abbasi S (1985) Relationship of prolonged pharmacological serum levels of vitamin E to incidence of sepsis and necrotising enterocolitis in infants with birth weight 1500 g or less. *Pediatrics* **75**, 619–638.

Johnson L, Quinn GE, Abbasi S, Gerdes J, Bowen FW and Bhutani V (1995) Severe retinopathy of prematurity in infants with birth weights less than 1250 grams: incidence and outcome of treatment with pharmacologic serum levels of vitamin E in addition to cryotherapy from 1985 to 1991. [See comments.] *J. Pediatr.* **127**, 632–639.

Kashyap S and Heird WC (1994) Protein metabolism during infancy. *Nestle Nutr. Serv.* **6**, 139a.

Kennedy KA, Tyson JE and Chamnanvanikij S (2000) Early versus delayed initiation of progressive enteral feedings for parenterally fed low birth weight or preterm infants. *Cochrane Database Syst. Rev.* **2**, CD001970.

Keshen TH, Miller R, Jahoor F, Jaksic T, Reeds PJ (1997) Glucose production and gluconeogenesis are negatively related to body weight in mechanically ventilated, very low birth weight neonates. *Pediatr. Res.* **41**, 132–138.

King C (1998) *Neonatal Unit Parenteral Nutrition Policy*. Dietetics Department, Hammersmith Hospital, London.

King C (1999) *Neonatal Unit Enteral Feeding Policy*. Nutrition and Dietetic Department, Hammersmith Hospital, London.

King C (2001) *Neonatal Unit Short Bowel Policy*. Nutrition and Dietetic Department, Hammersmith Hospital, London.

Koletzko B, Thiel I and Abiodun PO (1992) The fatty acid composition of human milk in Europe and Africa. *J. Pediatr.* **120**, S62–S70.

Kuschel CA and Harding JE (2000a) Multicomponent fortified human milk for promoting growth in preterm infants. *Cochrane Database Syst. Rev.* **2**, CD000343.

Kuschel CA and Harding JE (2000b) Protein supplementation of human milk for promoting growth in preterm infants. *Cochrane Database Syst. Rev.* **2**, CD000433.

Lacey JM, Crouch JB, Benfell K, Ringer SA, Wilmore CK, Maguire D and Wilmore DW (1996) The effects of glutamine-supplemented parenteral nutrition in premature infants. *J. Parent. Enteral Nutr.* **20**, 74–80.

Landman J, Sive A, De V, Hesse H, Van der Elst C and Sacks R (1992) Comparison of enteral and intramuscular vitamin A supplementation in preterm infants. *Early Hum. Devl.* **30**, 163–170.

Leach JL, Baxter JH, Molitor BE, Ramstack MB and Masor ML (1995) Total potentially available nucleosides of human milk by stage of lactation. *Am. J. Clin. Nutr.* **61**, 1224–1230.

Leitch CA, Antriches JA, Karn CA and Denne SC (1996) Growth reduction during dexamethasone therapy is not caused by increased energy expenditure. *Pediatr. Res.* **39**, 314A.

Leitch CA, Ahlrichs J, Karn C and Denne SC (1999) Energy expenditure and energy intake during dexamethasone therapy for chronic lung disease. *Pediatr. Res.* **46**, 109–113.

Lindley AA, Benson JE, Grimes C, Cole TM and Herman AA (1999) The relationship in neonates between clinically measured head circumference and brain volume estimated from head CT-scans. *Early Hum. Dev.* **56**, 17–29.

Lockitch G, Jacobson B, Quigley G, Dison P and Pendray M (1989) Selenium deficiency in low birth weight neonates: an unrecognized problem. [See comments.] *J. Pediatr.* **114**, 865–870.

Lucas A (1994) Role of nutritional programming in determining adult morbidity. *Arch. Dis. Child.* **71**, 288–290.

Lucas A and Cole TJ (1990) Breast milk and neonatal necrotising enterocolitis. *Lancet* **336**, 1519–1523.

Lucas A and Hudson GJ (1984) Preterm milk as a source of protein for low birth weight infants. *Arch. Dis. Child.* **59**, 831–836.

Lucas A, Gibbs JA, Lyster RL and Baum JD (1978) Creamatocrit: simple clinical technique for estimating fat concentration and energy value of human milk. *Br. Med. J.* **1**, 1018–1020.

Lucas A, Gore SM, Cole TJ, Bamford MF, Dossetor JF, Barr I, Dicarlo L, Cork S and Lucas PJ (1984) Multicentre trial on feeding low birthweight infants: effects of diet on early growth. *Arch. Dis. Child.* **59**, 722–730.

Lucas A, Bloom SR and Aynsley Green A (1986) Gut hormones and 'minimal enteral feeding'. *Acta Paediatr. Scand.* **75**, 719–723.

Lucas A, Brooke OG, Morley R, Cole TJ and Bamford MF (1990) Early diet of preterm infants and development of allergic or atopic disease: randomised prospective study. *Br. Med. J.* **300**, 837–840.

Lucas A, King F and Bishop NB (1992a) Post discharge formula consumption in infants born preterm. *Arch. Dis. Child.* **67**, 691–692.

Lucas A, Morley R and Cole TJ (1992b) Breast milk and subsequent intelligence quotient in children born preterm. *Lancet* **339**, 261–264.

Lucas A, Bishop NJ, King FJ and Cole TJ (1992c) Randomised trial of nutrition for preterm infants after discharge. *Arch. Dis. Child.* **67**, 322–327.

Lucas A, Morley R, Cole TJ and Gore (1994) A randomised multicentred study of human milk vs formula and later development in preterm infants. *Arch. Dis. Child.* **70**, F141–F146.

Lucas A, Quinlan P, Abrams S, Ryan S, Meah S and Lucas PJ (1997) Randomised controlled trial of a synthetic triglyceride milk formula for preterm infants. *Arch. Dis. Child Fetal Neonatal Edn* **77**, F178–F184.

Lucas A, Morley R and Cole T (1998) Randomised trial of early diet in preterm babies and later intelligence quotient. *Br. Med. J.* **317**, 1481–1487.

MacFie J, Holmfield JHM, King RFG and Hill GL (1983) Effect of the energy source on changes in energy expenditure and respiratory quotient during total parenteral nutrition. *J. Parent. Enteral Nutr.* **7**, 1–5.

Marks KH, Maisels MJ, Moore E, Gifford K and Friedman Z (1979) Head growth in sick premature infants: a longitudinal study. *J. Pediatr.* **94**, 282–285.

McClure RJ and Newell SJ (1999) Randomised controlled trial of trophic feeding and gut motility. *Arch. Dis. Child Fetal Neonatal Edn* **80**, F54–F58.

McClure RJ and Newell SJ (2000) Randomised controlled study of clinical outcome following trophic feeding. *Arch. Dis. Child Fetal Neonatal Edn* **82**, F29–F33.

McDowell S (1998) An audit of growth rate for infants on the neonatal unit, Childrens Hospital, Leicester Royal Infirmary NHS Trust. *BAPEN* 8–10 December, p. PC54.

McKiernan J and Hull D (1982) The constituents of neonatal milk. *Pediatr. Res.* **16**, 60–64.

Meetze WH, Valentine C and McGuigan JE (1992) Gastrointestinal priming prior to full enteral nutrition in very low birth weight infants. *J. Pediatr. Gastroenterol. Nutr.* **15**, 163–170.

Melnick G, Crouch JB, Caksackkas HL and Churella HR (1988) Iron status of low birth weight infants fed formulas containing high or low iron content. *Pediatr. Res.* **23**, 488A.

Michie CA and Raffles A (1990) Iron supplementation in the preterm or low birthweight infant [letter; comment]. *Arch. Dis. Child.* **65**, 559.

Moody GJ, Schanler RJ, Lau C and Shulman RJ (2000) Feeding tolerance in premature infants fed fortified human milk. *J. Pediatr. Gastroenterol. Nutr.* **30**, 408–412.

Morley R and Lucas A (2000) Randomized diet in the neonatal period and growth performance until 7.5–8 y of age in preterm children. *Am. J. Clin. Nutr.* **71**, 822–828.

Mupanemunda RH, Lee DS, Fraher LJ, Koura IR and Chance GW (1994) Postnatal changes in serum retinol status in very low birth weight infants. *Early Hum. Dev.* **38**, 45–54.

Narayanan I, Singh B and Harvey D (1984) Fat loss

during feeding of human milk. *Arch. Dis. Child.* **59**, 475–477.

Neu J, Shenoy V and Chakrabarti R (1996) Glutamine nutrition and metabolism: where do we go from here? *FASEB J.* **10**, 829–837.

Neu J, Roig JC, Meetze WH, Veerman M, Carter C, Millsaps M, Bowling D, Dallas MJ, Sleasman J, Knight T and Auestad N (1997) Enteral glutamine supplementation for very low birth weight infants decreases morbidity. *J. Pediatr.* **131**, 691–699.

Neville MC (1989) Regulation of milk fat synthesis. *J. Pediatr. Gastroenterol. Nutr.* **8**, 426–429.

Ojeda F, Carver JD, Torres BA, Minervini G, Norkus E and Barness L (1994) Retinyl palmitate [RP] absorption in preterm [PT] infants. *Pediatr. Res.* **35**, 317A.

Olivares M, Llaguno S, Marin V, Hertrampf E, Mena P and Milad M (1992) Iron status in low-birth-weight infants, small and appropriate for gestational age. A follow-up study. *Acta Paediatr.* **81**, 824–828.

Olson AL, Nelson SE and Rebouche CJ (1989) Low carnitine intake and altered lipid metabolism in infants. *Am. J. Clin. Nutr.* **40**, 624–628.

Ong TJ, Mehta A, Ogston S and Mukhopadhyay S (1998) Prediction of lung function in the inadequately nourished. *Arch. Dis. Child.* **79**, 18–21.

Patton S, Canfield LM, Huston GE, Ferris AM and Jensen RG (1990) Carotenoids of human colostrum. *Lipids* **25**, 159–165.

Penn D, Schmidt-Somerfield E and Wolf H (1980) Carnitine deficiency in premature infants receiving total parenteral nutrition. *Early Hum. Dev.* **4**, 23–34.

Pickering L, Masor M, Granoff D, Erickson J, Paule C and Hilty M (1996) Human milk [HM] levels of nucleotides in infant formula reduce incidence of diarrhea. *FASB J.* **10**, A554.

Polberger SK, Axelsson IA and Raiha NC (1989) Growth of very low birth weight infants on varying amounts of human milk protein. *Pediatr. Res.* **25**, 414–419.

Polberger SKT, Axelsson IE and Raitia NCR (1990) Urinary and serum urea as indicators of protein metabolism in very low birth weight infants fed varying human milk protein intakes. *Acta Paediatr. Scand.* **79**, 737–742.

Polberger S, Raiha NC, Juvonen P, Moro GE, Minoli I and Warm A (1999) Individualized protein fortification of human milk for preterm infants: comparison of ultrafiltrated human milk protein and a bovine whey fortifier. *J. Pediatr. Gastroenterol. Nutr.* **29**, 332–338.

Powell-Tuck J (1993) Glutamine, parenteral feeding, and intestinal nutrition. *Lancet* **342**, 451–452.

Powls A, Botting N, Cooke RW, Pilling D and Marlow N (1996) Growth impairment in very low birthweight children at 12 years: correlation with perinatal and outcome variables. *Arch. Dis. Child Fetal Neonatal. Edn* **75**, F152–F157.

Premji S and Chessell L (2001) Continuous nasogastric milk feeding versus intermittent bolus milk feeding for premature infants less than 1500 grams. (Cochrane Review.). *Cochrane Database Syst. Rev.* CD001819.

Puntis JW, Holden CE, Smallman S, Finkel Y, George RH and Booth IW (1991) Staff training: a key factor in reducing intravascular catheter sepsis. *Arch. Dis. Child.* **66**, 335–337.

Putet G, Senterre J, Rigo J and Salle B (1984) Nutrient balance, energy utilization, and composition of weight gain in very-low-birth-weight infants fed pooled human milk or a preterm formula. *J. Pediatr.* **105**, 79–85.

Quan R, Barness LA and Uauy R (1990) Do infants need nucleotide supplemented formula for optimum nutrition? *J. Pediatr. Gastroenterol. Nutr.* **11**, 429–437.

Quan R, Yang C, Rubinstein S, Lewiston NJ, Stevenson DK and Kerner-JA J (1994) The effect of nutritional additives on anti-infective factors in human milk. *Clin. Pediatr. Phil.* **33**, 325–328.

Raju T, Langenberg P, Bhutani V and Quinn GE (1997) Vitamin E prophylaxis to reduce retinopathy of prematurity: A reappraisal of published trials. *J. Pediatr.* **131**, 844–850.

Reichman B, Chessex P, Putet G, Verellen G, Smith JM, Heim T and Swyer PR (1981) Diet, fat accretion, and growth in premature infants. *New Engl. J. Med.* **305**, 1495–1500.

Reichman B, Chessex P, Verellen G, Putet G, Smith JM, Heim T and Swyer PR (1983) Dietary composition and macronutrient storage in preterm infants. *Pediatrics* **72**, 322–328.

Rosenberg SN, Verzo B, Engstrom JL, Kavanaugh K and Meier PP (1992) Reliability of length measurements for preterm infants. *Neonatal Netw.* **11**, 23–27.

Ross G, Krauss AN and Auld PA (1983) Growth achievement in low-birth-weight premature infants: relationship to neurobehavioral outcome at one year. *J. Pediatr.* **103**, 105–108.

Rowe PM (1996) Beta-carotene takes a collective beating. [News; see comments.] *Lancet* **347**, 249.

Rudolph FB (1994) Symposium: dietary nucleotides: a recently demonstrated requirement for cellular development and immune function. *J. Nutr.* **124**(Suppl), 1431S–1432S.

Rudolph N, Allen L, Colindres J, Christie E, Wong S, Gulrajani M and Braithwaite A (1994) Early iron supplementation in prematures: an advantage or not? *Pediatr. Res.* **35**, 319A.

Saini J, MacMahon P, Morgan JB and Kovar IZ (1989) Early parenteral feeding of amino acids. *Arch. Dis. Child.* **64**, 1362–1366.

Sanchez Pozo A, Ramirez M, Gil A, Maldonado J, Van Biervliet JP and Rosseneu M (1995) Dietary nucleotides enhance plasma lecithin cholesterol acyl transferase activity and apolipoprotein A-IV concentration in preterm newborn infants. *Pediatr. Res.* **37**, 328–333.

Schanler RJ, Hurst NM and Lau C (1999a) The use of human milk and breastfeeding in premature infants. *Clin. Perinatol.* **26**, 379–398, vii.

Schanler RJ, Shulman RJ and Lau C (1999b) Feeding strategies for premature infants: beneficial outcomes of feeding fortified human milk versus preterm formula. *Pediatrics* **103**, 1150–1157.

Schanler RJ, Shulman RJ, Lau C, Smith EO and Heitkemper MM (1999c) Feeding strategies for premature infants: randomized trial of gastrointestinal priming and tube-feeding method. [See comments.] *Pediatrics* **103**, 434–439.

Schlesinger L, Arevalo M, Arredondo S, Lonnerdal B and Stekel A (1993) Zinc supplementation impairs monocyte function. *Acta Paediatr.* **82**, 734–738.

Shaw JCL (1982) Iron absorption by the premature infant. The effect of transfusion and iron supplements on the serum ferritin levels. *Acta Paediatr. Scand.* (Suppl. 299), 83–89.

Shenai JP (1999) Vitamin A supplementation in very low birth weight neonates: rationale and evidence. *Pediatrics* **104**, 1369–1374.

Shenai JP, Rush MG, Stahlman MT and Chytil F (1990) Plasma retinol-binding protein response to vitamin A administration in infants susceptible to bronchopulmonary dysplasia. *J. Pediatr.* **116**, 607–614.

Siegel M, Lebenthal E and Krantz B (1984) Effect of caloric density on gastric emptying in premature infants. *J. Pediatr.* **104**, 118–122.

Signer E, Murphy GM, Edkins S and Anderson CM (1974) Role of bile salts in fat malabsorption of premature infants. *Arch. Dis. Child.* **49**, 174–180.

Simmer K (2000) Longchain polyunsaturated fatty acid supplementation in preterm infants. *Cochrane Database Syst. Rev.* **2**, CD000375.

Singhal A, Cole TJ and Lucas A (2001) Early nutrition in preterm infants and later blood pressure: two cohorts after randomised trials. *Lancet* **357**, 413–419.

Spencer SA, Hendrickse W, Roberton D and Hull D (1982) Energy intake and weight gain of very low birthweight babies fed raw expressed breast milk. *Br. Med. J. Clin. Res. Edn* **285**, 924–926.

Spencer SA, McKenna S, Stammers J and Hull D (1992) Two different low birth weight formulae compared. *Early Hum. Dev.* **30**, 21–31.

Stockman JA and Clarke DA (1984) Weight gain: a response to transfusion in selected preterm infants. *Am. J. Dis. Child.* **138**, 828–830.

Sulkers EJ, von Goudoever JB, Leunisse C, Wattimena JL and Sauer PJ (1992) Comparison of two preterm formulas with or without addition of medium-chain triglycerides (MCTs). I: Effects on nitrogen and fat balance and body composition changes. *J. Pediatr. Gastroenterol. Nutr.* **15**, 34–41.

Suskind R, Edelman R, Kulapongs P, Pariyanonda A and Sirisinha S (1976) Complement activity in children with protein-calorie malnutrition. *Am. J. Clin. Nutr.* **29**, 1089–1092.

Sutphen JL and Dillard VL (1989) Dietary caloric density and osmolality influence gastroesophageal reflux in infants. *Gastroenterology* **97**, 601–604.

Tsang RC, Lucas A, Uauy R and Zlotkin S (1993) *Nutritional Needs of the Preterm Infant: Scientific Basis and Practical Guidelines*. Caduceus Medical, New York.

Tubman TR and Thompson SW (2000) Glutamine supplementation for preventing morbidity in preterm infants. *Cochrane Database Syst. Rev.* **2**, CD001457.

Tyson JE, Wright LL, Oh WOM, Kennedy KA, Mele L, Ehrenkranz RA, Stoll BJ, Lemons JA, Stevenson DK, Bauer CR, Korones SB and Fanaroff AA (1999) Vitamin A supplementation for extremely-low-birth-weight infants. *New Engl. J. Med.* **340**, 1962–1968.

UKAMB (1999) *Guidelines for the Establishment and Operation of Human Milk Banks in the UK*, 2nd edn. Royal College of Paediatrics and Child Health, London.

Uraizee F and Gross SJ (1989) Improved feeding tolerance and reduced incidence of sepsis in sick very low birth weight (VLBW) infants fed maternal milk. *Pediatr. Res.* **25**, 298A.

Valentine C, Hurst NM and Schanler RJ (1994) Hind milk improves weight gain in low birth weight infants fed human milk. *J. Pediatr. Gastroenterol. Nutr.* **18**, 474–477.

Van-Aerde JEE, Saver PJJ and Pencharz PB (1989) Effect of replacing glucose with lipid on the energy metabolism of newborn infants. *Clin. Sci.* **6**, 581–588.

van-Lingen RA, van-Goudoever JB, Luijendijk IH, Wattimena JL and Sauer PJ (1992) Effects of early amino acid administration during total parenteral nutrition on protein metabolism in pre-term infants. *Clin. Sci. Colch.* **82**, 199–203.

Wales JK, Carney S and Gibson AT (1997) The measurement of neonates. *Horm. Res.* **48**(Suppl. 12-10), 10.

Wang CD, Chu PS, Mellen BG and Shenai JP (1999) Creamatocrit and the nutrient composition of human milk. *J. Perinatol.* **19**, 343–346.

Wardle SP, Hughes A, Chen S and Shaw NJ (2001) Randomised controlled trial of oral vitamin A supplementation in preterm infants to prevent chronic lung disease. *Arch. Dis. Child Fetal Neonatal Edn* **84**, F9–F13.

Warner JT, Linton HR, Dunstan FD and Cartlidge PH (1998) Growth and metabolic responses in preterm infants fed fortified human milk or a preterm formula. *Int. J. Clin. Pract.* **52**, 236–240.

Weigensberg M (1990) Brain growth is preserved in malnourished neonatal rats. *Pediatr. Res.* **27**, 293A.

Weismann K and Hoyer H (1985) Serum alkaline phosphatase and serum zinc levels in the diagnosis and exclusion of zinc deficiency in man. *Am. J. Clin. Nutr.* **41**, 1214–1219.

Williamson S, Finucane E and Ellis H (1978) Effect of heat treatment of human milk absorption of nitrogen, fat, sodium, calcium and phosphorus by preterm infants. *Arch. Dis. Child.* **53**, 553–563.

Winick M and Rosso P (1969) Head circumference and cellular growth of the brain in normal and marasmic children. *J. Pediatr.* **74**, 774–778.

Woolfson AMJ, Heatley RV and Allison SP (1979) Insulin to inhibit protein catabolism after injury. *New Engl. J. Med.* **300**, 14–17.

Ziegler EE, O'Donnell AM, Nelson SE and Komon SJ (1976) Body composition of the reference fetus growth. *Growth* **40**, 329–341.

Zlotkin SH, Bryan MH and Anderson GH (1981) Intravenous nitrogen and energy intakes required to duplicate in-utero nitrogen accretion in prematurely born human infants. *J. Pediatr.* **99**, 115–120.

11

NUTRITION IN CHILDHOOD

Elizabeth Poskitt

LEARNING OUTCOMES

- The impact of physical growth on nutrient needs.

- The impact of pubertal development on lifestyle and nutritional needs.

- The impact of deficient nutrition (for both macro- and micronutrients) on growth and health at different stages in childhood.

- The role of developing skills and intellect on dietary habits and nutritional needs.

- The interaction of families and society on the diets and nutrition of children at different stages in childhood.

Introduction

Childhood can be understood as the whole period from birth to maturity in late teens or early twenties. Infancy has been dealt with elsewhere in this book (Chapters 8 and 9), so this chapter discusses issues of nutrition and development particularly relevant to the age group 2–20 years. However, we shall overlap into younger and older age groups from time to time. Growth and development, as markers of good nutrition, are continuous processes which cannot easily be divided into specific sections or ages.

Age-related Changes in Body Composition Relevant to Nutrition

If we look at development and growth, there are enormous differences between children of 2 years (mean weight: boys, 12.3 kg; girls,

11.8 kg) and those in late adolescence (mean weight at 16 years: boys, 62.1 kg; girls, 56.0 kg) (Needman, 2000). The former are virtually totally dependent on parents (or other carers) for nutrition and for many other aspects of nurture. The latter are still immature in mental reactions and limited in experience, but physiologically capable of reproduction and, even if they have ceased linear growth, continuing to acquire both fat and lean body mass (LBM). Adolescents may or may not be good at composing and cooking meals for themselves, but almost certainly they have the ability, and sometimes sufficient money, with which to live very satisfactory independent existences – in total contrast to 2-year-old children.

It is not only in size and developmental abilities that young children differ from adolescents. Body composition is also different. Nutritional requirements and nutritional problems must be assessed taking children's age and maturity into account as well as their absolute size. Further, whilst gender-related differences in physical features and nutritional requirements are small in young children, by adolescence the differences are considerable (Table 11.1).

Growth is not a steady process occurring gradually over years. Rates are very rapid *in utero*, but slow from birth until about 2 years of age when they 'flatten out' and remain at fairly constant levels until the growth spurt (period of accelerated growth) that takes place in both sexes with puberty (Tanner and Kelnar, 1992). Thus growth velocity curves have the particular shape indicated in Figure 11.1. However the tissues deposited over the time in which growth rates change are not constant either. In fact there is a cyclic process of fattening and slimming that repeats itself in childhood (Table 11.1). Human infants are only modestly fat at birth but accrue fat at an extremely rapid rate in early infancy so they treble the amount of fat in their bodies in the time it takes them to double body weight (around 4–5 months of life; Fomon, 1974). From about 1 year of age, there is a period when children 'slim' naturally, in that fat forms a smaller part of newly deposited tissues and the percentage of body weight that is fat declines. These changes in body composition also reflect changes in energy balance at weaning, when nutrient intakes may be barely adequate because of difficulties often experienced moving children from totally fluid diets to weaning diets of mixed solids. Fat stores may be mobilized to help meet energy needs.

Increasing energy expenditure in weight-bearing activity is also relevant in the proportionately greater deposition of lean mass after the first 6 months of life and particularly after 1 year of age. Children less than 6 months old

Table 11.1 Variation in body composition with age in childhood

Age	Mean weight (kg)	Whole body: water, percentage of body weight	Whole body: fat, percentage of body weight	Fat-free mass: water, percentage of lean body mass	Fat-free mass: protein, percentage of lean body mass
Birth	3.5	72	14	84	14
4 months	7	60	26	82	15
12 months	10	59	24	78	19
2 years	12	60	21	78	18
5 years	18	60	21	74	20
10 years	32	60	17	72	20
25 years, men	70	60	12	72	21
25 years, women	60	55	25	72	21

Data derived from Fomon (1974); Lentner (1981); Widdowson (1981); WHO (1983).

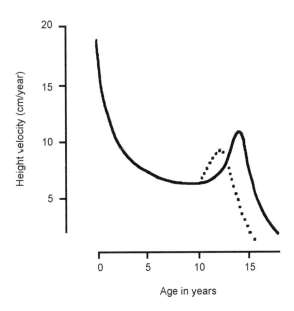

Figure 11.1 Height velocity curves (cm/year) for boys and girls related to age. Velocities for both sexes similar until 10 years so the curve for girls (·····) is superimposed on the boys' curve (———) under 10 years (from Tanner, 1989)

spend their days lying or sitting supported. Crying, kicking, rolling over and bouncing are the heights of their activity. Children of 1 year are usually 'cruising' around the furniture with great enthusiasm even if they are not yet walking unaided (Day, 1992). Weight-bearing activities increase further as new motor skills are acquired. Energy consumed in physical activity increases and may stimulate muscular development affecting the content of whole body mass. Certainly, by the age of 5, many children look slimmer than they have ever done before – or possibly will ever do so in the future. This can lead to parental concerns about children 'losing weight' or getting 'too thin' when in fact the children are gaining weight very satisfactorily but showing the change from rotund infants to trim young children.

Around 5 years of age, but often beginning earlier in children with relatively greater height for age, a further fattening trend begins. This is the so-called 'adiposity rebound' (Rolland-Cachera *et al.*, 1984). Children developing adiposity rebound before the age of 5 seem more likely to develop obesity that will persist into adult life. This may be a particular characteristic of fattening at this age. It is more likely, however, to reflect the fact that children who are fattening when the physiological trend encourages slimming have either greater genetic or unusually strong environmental pressures to lay down fat. Presuming that the pressures continue to exert effects when fat deposition is more vigorous, these children could be expected to remain at great risk of obesity.

Girls show a very brief period of relative slimming with rapid growth early in the pubertal process, prior to further increase in height and significant increase in the percentage of body weight that is fat as puberty advances. Fat deposition, particularly around breasts and hips, results in the typical adult female figure. Teleologically this fattening can be interpreted as laying down reserves for the nutritional demands of reproduction.

The male growth spurt occurs later in puberty, continues longer, and is associated with massive deposition of lean tissue in comparison with the female growth spurt (Tanner and Kelnar, 1992). The process of development of lean body mass may utilize some of the fat component of the body. Boys who were quite plump prior to the onset of puberty often become relatively slim, tall adolescents.

Material in chapters 1 and 12 should be read in relation to this chapter.

Puberty

The age of onset of puberty and – as a specific marker of maturation – the age of menarche, fell quite dramatically over the twentieth century in many countries. However recent data suggest that in the UK (Whincup *et al.*,

2001), the Netherlands (Mul *et al.*, 2001) and possibly other parts of Western Europe, the age of menarche has stabilized. Data on change in the age at onset of puberty are less consistent in the USA (Lee *et al.*, 2001; Herman-Giddens *et al.*, 2001). In many developing societies, the age at onset of puberty is probably still falling, particularly amongst young people in the poorest communities. These changes in maturation have been attributed to improved childhood nutrition with accelerated growth and accelerated physical development as accompaniment. Other factors, such as greater luminescence due to electric lighting, may also have influenced cerebrally initiated hormonal controls of puberty.

It is difficult to know what nutritional factors, if any, contribute to early puberty since many of the countries where the changes have been greatest also show falls in mean energy intakes of children over at least the latter part of the same period. Energy balance must nevertheless be positive in these communities since the populations are, in general, fatter. Nutritionally, is it greater energy intakes, higher protein intakes, or improved micronutrient nutrition which drives the age of puberty downwards? We do not know.

The association between nutrition and timing of growth and maturation is interesting and still unexplained, although studies of leptin are beginning to suggest ways in which physiological processes might take place.

Over 30 years ago Frisch and Revelle (1970) suggested that a certain body weight and proportion of fat to lean mass was the trigger for menarche, reproductive maturity and fertility. The amenorrhoea that occurs with starvation, with intense exercise and dieting such as practised by ballerinas, and in anorexia nervosa develops below the critical weight of 48 kg. Frisch (1987) has suggested that 17 per cent fat mass is necessary for onset of menstruation, and fertility is attained at approximately 22 per cent fat mass. Not all data support this hypothesis. Obese children below

the age of puberty may have more than the critical fat mass and critical body weight and yet show no evidence of puberty (Crawford and Osler, 1975). Early puberty is not uncommon in obese girls, but precocious puberty is not. Nevertheless, the concept that changing body composition may be one of the triggering factors for menarche is an interesting one. Since leptin levels are higher in females than in males at all ages, and since leptin levels reflect the size of body fat stores, leptin may be the link between nutritional status and the hormonal changes of physiological maturation (Roemmich and Rogol, 1999; Mauras, 2001).

Children do reflect, to a greater or lesser extent, the growth pattern of their parents (Tanner *et al.*, 1975). Thus children of very tall parents are likely to be tall (and usually also heavy) for age. Small parents tend to have small children, although a small parent with small children could suffer from an inherited growth-restricting condition.

Assessment of Nutritional Status

Nutritional status in children is assessed clinically, anthropometrically and biochemically. Anthropometric assessment is the procedure most frequently performed (and most affected by age and development). Weight, because it is so susceptible to illness-induced change, is widely used clinically as a general assessment of a child's state of health rather than as a specific *nutritional* assessment. Weight and height and other measurements must be related to tables or charts of expected values for age (Tanner *et al.*, 1966).

Most countries with maternal and child health services have reference weight-for-age charts for children covering at least the first 5 years of life (Freeman *et al.*, 1995; Needman, 2000). The charts have usually been derived from national or other child cohorts measured cross-sectionally. Health workers in many countries are accustomed to measuring the weights of children attending 'well baby' clinics, school assessments or their doctors. Weight can be plotted on charts against age. It can also be related to reference growth centiles, as percentage of expected weight for age (widely used where undernutrition is common), weight for height (often used if age is unlikely to be known accurately), or standard deviation score (SDS) compared with mean weight for age (Cole, 1994, 1997). Other anthropometric measurements can be related similarly to mean values for age. Weight for age depends to a significant degree on height for age and, particularly in Westernized societies where malnutrition is not a major concern, weight and height should be considered together in the nutritional assessment of children.

The current British reference standards for weight and height for age are divided into centiles with average weight as the 50th centile for age (Freeman et al., 1995; Cole, 1997). Children below average weight (or height) are on lower centiles and children above average weight are on higher centiles. For practical purposes, children below the third or above the 97th centile have been regarded as out of the normal range, although by definition 3 per cent of normal children should fall into these ranges. More extreme centiles, such as the 0.4 and 99.6 centiles on the most recent growth charts developed by Cole (1997), might be more suitable cut-off points for screening. Being outside the 'normal' range indicates a child probably needs growth review, particularly if this centile position is not part of a lifelong pattern of growth but the result of 'growth faltering'.

Assessing children anthropometrically against age-related standards can be useful for plotting growth in relation to age and change in growth over time. Charts which present not only means but also the standard deviations (s.d.) of the measurements have been developed (Tanner et al., 1966; WHO,

1983; Freeman et al., 1995). The weight for age standard deviations score (SDS) also known as Z-score is:

$$\text{Actual weight} - \text{Mean weight for age}$$
$$\div \text{SD of mean weight for age}$$

For children below average weight, SDS will be minus numbers. For practical purposes, $-2\,\text{SD}$ approximates to the third centile and $+2\,\text{SD}$ to the 97th centile for age. SDS of -3 (or $+3$) are sufficiently far from average values to suggest abnormality, although there is no absolute score at which abnormality can be diagnosed (or excluded) with absolute certainty.

Normal growth can be expected to show weight and height increasing with age along similar centiles or with similar and persistent SDS (Rudolf et al., 2000). After infancy (when there is often adjustment across growth centiles) and until the onset of puberty, weight and height usually follow particular centiles remarkably consistently, although they are not necessarily on identical centiles. Thus a 'stocky' child may have a relatively higher weight than height score but this difference in centile position presents the pattern of growth which is followed at least until puberty. Weights and heights for age which drift downwards across the centiles before puberty suggest abnormal growth (Figure 11.2).

The onset of the pubertal growth spurt can lead to temporary deviation of growth from the prepubertal centile position, particularly for centiles developed from cross-sectional rather than longitudinal data. Cross-sectional data have the effect of 'flattening' the steep rise of the individual pubertal growth acceleration (Tanner and Whitehouse, 1976). Children with early puberty and early growth spurts may appear predestined for tall stature since their early growth acceleration takes them upwards across the weight and, particularly, height centiles. However these children's growth normally ceases early. The stature attained, although above average for age when growth

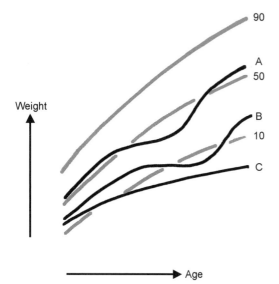

Figure 11.2 Figurative growth curves of three children with failure to thrive plotted against 10th, 50th and 90th weight centiles for age. Children A and B show growth faltering (although child A's weight remains within 'normal' centiles), but complete catch-up growth and return to previous weight centiles. Child C shows persistent growth faltering (abnormal weight velocity)

onset of puberty. 'Bone age' estimations (from hand and wrist X-rays) are thus widely used in clinical assessment of children with growth problems.

One of the problems of evaluating normality from weight and height centiles is the increasing obesity found in children as well as adults in westernized populations (Flegal, 1999; Chinn and Rona, 2001). How much do, or should, growth standards eliminate the asymmetry produced by increasing overweight and obesity in most European and North American societies (Cole *et al.*, 2000)? Obesity will be discussed further later in this chapter.

Issues Relevant to Development and Dietary Needs

Nutritional requirements and growth rates

ceases, is rapidly overtaken by that of later maturing children. Children with late onset of puberty, particularly boys since they have greater increments in height, weight and lean body mass at puberty than girls, may suffer socially and psychologically as they appear (usually wrongly) abnormally small for their age before maturation finally begins. As these boys have been growing steadily whilst 'waiting' for growth to accelerate, they often begin their growth spurt at a greater height than did earlier maturing peers, allowing them very adequate 'catch-up' growth. Ultimate height is then within the normal range and even above average.

Bone maturation, indicated by the appearance, development and fusion of epiphyses, is a better indication of the individual's stage of maturation than height alone and can be helpful in predicting future growth and the

Rates of growth are important determinants of nutrient needs. Any individual undergoing catch-up growth (accelerated growth velocity following a period of growth faltering) needs increased nutrient intakes, particularly for energy and micronutrients/kg body weight. These needs also apply to preschool children and those in early school years who are still growing rapidly and prone to infections. Intakes may be reduced by infection-induced anorexia and growth may be temporarily halted during infection and other illnesses. Pyrexia may also have more specific effects on nutritional utilization since it raises metabolic rate and is associated with reduced gastro-intestinal absorption of iron (Beresford *et al.*, 1971) and possibly other micronutrients. Thus young children need energy-dense diets and these may be difficult to achieve without high proportions of total energy from fat. High-fibre diets are not recommended for young children since they result in bulky, low-energy-density diets which are often rather 'filling'. The aims of good nutrition in young children include developing a nutritionally sound and sustainable dietary progression from breast-feeding and weaning towards the recommendations for adult diets.

At what age should children consume diets equivalent in quality to those recommended for adults? Five years is the age at which children in UK commence school and seems, arbitrarily, the age at which more adult concerns for the quality of the diet begin to replace the concerns for quantity which predominate with very young children. It is also the age at which the consumption of school dinners (or nowadays often 'packed lunches') begins. School dinners have been a cause of nutritional concern since, in the interests of keeping down costs and encouraging children to eat, they have frequently failed to meet dietary recommendations. This issue is discussed further in Chapter 12.

Direction of desirable dietary change

Breast-fed infants consume diets with more than 50 per cent of the total energy derived from fat. The diet is wholly liquid and devoid of dietary fibre but a source of all essential nutrients. The fats include high levels of monounsaturated and polyunsaturated fatty acids (PUFA) including long chain PUFA. The only sugar in breast milk is lactose, which does not occur naturally in foods other than milk, although nowadays it is added as bulk to many foods (and medicines). Today most dietary recommendations for adults suggest no more than 35 per cent total energy from fat, a proportion of PUFAs to SFA of about 1; a total dietary fibre of around 30 g/day, of which approximately 18 g is non-starch polysaccharide, and satisfactory micronutrient intakes. In

food-based dietary guidelines, this latter has been suggested as at least 7 per cent of energy coming from vegetables (excluding potatoes; WHO, 1982; Department of Health and Social Security, 1984; World Cancer Research Fund, 1997). This has been interpreted as 400 g vegetables (excluding potatoes), 30 g of pulses (beans/peas/lentils etc.) and fruit each day (James and Ralph, 2000) or, in simpler terms, at least five portions of fruit or vegetables daily (Department of Health and Social Security, 1984). Table 11.2 outlines how developmental skills are involved in the process of moving from sucked milk diets to mixed diets of liquids and solids where the solids are varied in texture and may require substantial chewing. If children are to adapt to the dietary recommendations developed for adults in many Westernized countries, it is vital that they grow up familiar with meals containing wholemeal cereals, fruit and vegetables and that they are at ease with chewable foods.

In progression from 50 per cent dietary energy from fat to less than 35 per cent dietary energy from fat as older children and adults, toddlers may go through phases of consuming diets of less than 30 per cent total energy from fat – levels which may put the children at risk of undernutrition. UK children aged $1\frac{1}{2}$–$4\frac{1}{2}$ years consumed diets with, on average, 36 per cent total energy from fat, but 15 per cent of children consumed diets with less than 30 per cent total energy from fat (Gregory et al., 1995a). Twenty-one per cent of the same cohort of children were still consuming diets with more than 40 per cent total energy from fat. On average 16 per cent of the total energy intake was from saturated fats. Dietary modification needs to develop more balanced mixtures of foods and, as a consequence, nutrients. Dietary fibre intake should increase only gradually through childhood so adult recommendations may not be achieved until adolescence or later. Cereals, fruit and vegetables should form major components of the diet after weaning.

Table 11.2   Age and development of feeding/nutrition skills

Age	Feeding skills
Birth	Integrated sucking and swallowing reflexes
3 months	Conveys bolus of food from front of mouth to back of mouth
5 months	Conveys objects placed in hand to mouth
	Drinks from hand-held cup with biting movements
$5\frac{1}{2}$ months	Reaches out for objects and conveys to mouth
$6\frac{1}{2}$ months	Begins to make chewing movements
	Feeds self with biscuit, rusk or other small item
	Transfers objects from one hand to the other
7 months	Learns to shut mouth, shake head and indicate 'No'
9 months	Picks up raisin-sized object with thumb and forefinger
	Throws food to ground with great enthusiasm – and expects someone else to pick it up
10 months	Holds beaker of liquid but drops it when finished
12 months	Tries to spoon feed but unable to stop rotation of spoon (and loss of food) before it reaches mouth
15 months	Manipulates spoon and food on spoon to mouth
18 months	Determined to be independent at mealtimes
2 years	Expresses own self and independence in – often irrational – food refusal. This spell may last some years
5 years	Eating in company with peers may lead to eating a greater variety of foods than previously accepted
	May also lead to strong preferences for 'popular' foods

Food choices

We have already indicated that childhood is not just a period of changing size but also a period of developing skills – mental and physical. Skills and understanding impact on nutrition through influencing children's ability to select and consume food, to access extra foods and to exert choice (Table 11.2). In young children, choice may seem well developed since food refusal is common. However expressions of choice by very young children may not be so much conscious decisions on preference but, instead, tests of parental response. After having adamantly refused food, the children may suddenly appear to forget this and eat up happily. By contrast, school-age children's choices are heavily influenced by the diets and attitudes of their peers, who may themselves be influenced by the media, particularly by food advertising on the television. Adolescent eating habits are like-

wise very sensitive to peer pressures and may seem at times to be returning to the dietary perversity of young children, although with much more self awareness (Truswell and Darnton-Hill, 1981; Jeffrey et al., 1982). Adolescents' decisions about what and when they will eat are notoriously inconsistent and frequently bizarre. Diets vary from day to day and meal to meal. Since the nutrient demands of growth are high, nutritional deficiencies, particularly for energy and micronutrients such as iron, are common in adolescence.

Adolescents are also beginning to move away from the shelter of families and often consume large amounts of cheap, ready to eat, food outside the home. This means their diets are frequently high in saturated fats, sugar and carbonated drinks (Truswell and Darnton-Hill, 1981). They may commence alcohol consumption, tobacco smoking and even taking recreational/non-prescribed drugs. These latter are not exactly nutritional matters but tobacco smoking does affect energy partitioning in the body both by reducing appetite and increasing BMR. Thus smoking can impact on nutritional status even without production of ill health. These habits conflict with the need to develop healthy lifestyles in adolescence in order to reduce the risks of non-communicable diseases in adult life. Diets and activities followed at this age may continue as adult lifestyles and even as the lifestyles followed in the adolescents' future families.

Milk in children's diets

In the UK, perhaps more than in other EU countries, milk and milk products have traditionally made a considerable contribution to energy, protein and micronutrient intakes throughout childhood. The National Diet and Nutrition Survey (Gregory *et al.*, 1995b) data for British children aged 1.5–4.5 years showed an average consumption of 26 per cent dietary energy from milk and milk products amongst the age group 1.5–2.5 years and a mean consumption of 16 per cent energy from milk and milk products in the 3.5–4.5-year-old age group. Nineteen per cent of food energy came from cow's milk in the younger age group and 12% from cow's milk in the older age group.

Today there are choices in the 'milk' available to children. Under 1 year, cow's milk, other than that modified as infant and follow-on formulas, is not recommended (Department of Health, 1994). Since milk may be making an important contribution to meeting the requirements of energy and fat-soluble vitamins in the diets of young children, recommendations are that skimmed and semi-skimmed milk (because of their reduced energy and fat-soluble vitamin concentration) are not given to children as drinks under 2 years. Small amounts of these milks used in cooking are likely to be mixed with other nutrients and are probably safe. Skimmed and semi-skimmed milks are also not recommended for children under 5 except that semi-skimmed milk is viewed as safe for children over 2 years to drink *provided* they are consuming otherwise 'balanced' diets (Department of Health, 1994). From 5 years on, there are no UK recommendations on the form of milk given to children. It seems appropriate, assuming children are thriving, that semi-skimmed or skimmed milks are gradually introduced into the diets of children over 5, so as to reduce the percentage of total energy from dietary fat. As a source of calcium, vitamin A, riboflavin and high-quality dietary protein, as well as many other nutrients, milk remains a useful component of children's diets. Whole milk can be particularly useful complementing micronutrient deficiencies in the diets of non-vegan (i.e. those accepting dairy products in their diets) vegetarian children (Poskitt, 1988).

Nutritional Problems in Young Children

Young children's intakes can be increased through more frequent meals. This is particularly relevant for vegetarian diets where low-energy-density diets may mean young children have difficulty consuming sufficient volumes of food to meet their nutritional needs (Poskitt, 1988). Usual recommendations for young children are that they should have three main meals each day (early morning, midday and late afternoon/evening) with two snacks in between the meals. The meals should have a substantial helping (half the plateful) of bread, pasta or other cereals or potatoes, with a protein source (meat, fish or pulses), calcium source (which might be as milk rather than solid food) and always some fruit and vegetables to provide micronutrients (Department of Health, 1994). Each meal should have a source of vitamin C since, through its reducing properties, ascorbic acid enhances absorptio·

of some micronutrients, especially iron. The amounts of fat recommended depend on whether the diets are for well-nourished children (modest fat intake) or for children who may be showing growth faltering (encourage addition of fats or oils to meal). Plant-derived fats and oils should predominate.

There is a tendency for children who have not been encouraged to chew to be habituated to foods which do not require chewing. Learning skills are acquired most easily when practised at the earliest age at which the ability to perform the skill occurs. Learning to manipulate and chew solid foods, as with other skills, is usually more successful if encouraged at the age at which the skill naturally develops, rather than trying to introduce that skill at a later stage in development. This is sometimes the cause of problems of poor weight gain, failure to thrive and micronutrient deficiencies, when transfer from bottle to cup is delayed.

Fussy eaters

It is not unusual for young children to cause concern because they will only eat a limited number of foods. Occasionally this faddism is sufficiently severe for children to develop micronutrient inadequacy. If the foods consumed are low in fat as well as micronutrients, energy intakes may also be inadequate.

Failure to 'wean' from bottle to cup can interfere with the progressive weaning process whereby initially soft mushy foods and then lumpy foods and hand-held, chewable foods gradually take over from a liquid milk diet. Sucking from a bottle can offer solace and comfort to children. Thus some children who continue bottle-feeding long beyond infancy consume excessive volumes of milk or juice (Shane and Rolles, 1995). Energy intakes vary from low to high, depending on the energy density of the fluids in the bottle. In a study of 105 children between 2 and 7

years in the UK, 15 per cent of the children consumed almost 50 per cent of their recommended daily energy intake in drinks, largely fruit squash (Petter et al., 1995).

Some carers worry excessively about inadequate nutrition because their children refuse certain foods simply because the foods are unfamiliar. They offer favourite foods so the children do at least 'eat something'. Food refusal appears rewarded. Thus mealtimes become battlegrounds between innately determined young children and their frustrated, anxious mothers. Children rarely starve themselves and, whilst it is inappropriate to present children with situations where, for an indefinite period they get no other food until they have 'eaten up', they need to learn that food refusal does not automatically lead to more attractive but potentially nutritionally less appropriate foods.

A firm approach can be difficult at times. The concept of food as an outward sign of love and care is so fundamental to parenting. Further, it is unwise to take too firm an approach when children are already tired or significantly hungry, such as before bed. The slight risk of hypoglycaemia makes it undesirable for children to go to bed with 'empty' stomachs. Several small energy-dense meals which contain sources of micronutrients should be offered regularly rather than only when hunger or tiredness make children uncooperative (see Table 12.8 for examples of snack meals). As children grow older the pattern of three substantial meals a day with two (perhaps three in adolescence) modest snacks should develop.

Macronutrient Deficiency and Excess

Failure to thrive

This is failure to gain weight and height at the expected rate (the expected rate being weight gain as shown on standard growth charts). Although often associated with psycho-social deprivation (see below) there are a number of well-recognized nutritional and medical causes. Some of these are categorized and listed in Table 11.3.

Failure to thrive is of concern in development since, if it continues, poor nutrition can affect brain development, learning and cognitive abilities. It is most frequently a problem in children under 2 years so we are not discussing it at length in this chapter except to outline the broad categories of causes and some examples for failure to thrive with pathological cause. 'Emotional deprivation' or 'psychomotor growth retardation' can be a problem in older children and is discussed further here.

Emotional deprivation

Some children from socially deprived environments where parent–child interaction is poor, fail to grow, perhaps despite apparently adequate nutritional intakes. These children have particular characteristics in that they are usually both short and underweight with passive affect, quiet and still with the so-called 'radar gaze' (observant but still and silent) and cool peripheries (McCarthy, 1974). Occasionally these children are aggressive, disruptive and uncontrollable. They may have bizarre appetites, stealing food from others at school or even from dustbins. Poor muscle tone and sometimes delayed motor development can cause them to resemble children with coeliac syndrome.

It is not entirely clear why these children with 'emotional deprivation' do not grow. Within one family, some children seem more readily affected than others. There may be a genetic predisposition to react to adverse circumstances in this way or perhaps one child in a family is picked out for emotional abuse or deprivation. Are these children, despite appearances, not actually consuming

Table 11.3 Classification of symptomatic factors contributing to failure to thrive in young children

Basic cause	Clinical situation

Too little in	Inadequate food
	  poverty
	  famine
	Diet not sufficiently energy dense:
	  carers too 'health conscious'
	  strict vegetarianism
	Excessive vomiting
	Illness, medical causes of vomiting
	Anorexia
	Infection and other illnesses

Too much out	Energy losses in urine:
	  diabetes mellitus
	Energy losses through skin:
	  exfoliative dermatitis
	Energy losses in gastro-intestinal tract:
	  protein-losing enteropathy
	  blood/protein loss: hookworm

Failure to absorb	Malabsorption syndromes:
	  cystic fibrosis
	  coeliac syndrome

Failure to utilize	Chronic illness, chronic infection,
	  cystic fibrosis
	  urinary tract infection
	Lack of another nutrient essential for metabolism
	Anoxia
	Cyanotic congenital heart disease

Increased requirements	Elevated BMR:
	  thyrotoxicosis
	  congenital L to R cardiac shunts
	Increased growth rates:
	  catch-up growth
	Increased respiratory rates:
	  cystic fibrosis
	  congenital heart disease

expected requirements for normal nutrition? Could it be that the stress experienced by the children is such that they have increased requirements – perhaps due to more or less permanently elevated stress hormones – which their diets do not meet? Metabolically, emotionally deprived children are difficult to study since the hormonal and biochemical abnormalities disappear rapidly when the children's immediate environments change. Early investigations suggested rapidly reversible increased cortisol and lowered growth hormone levels in psycho-socially deprived children (Powell *et al.*, 1973; Rayner and Rudd, 1973).

Diagnosis, which can be difficult if the failure in family dynamics is well hidden, may be established by the sudden change in affect, behaviour and growth when children are removed from depriving environments into warm caring environments.

Intellectually these children may fare poorly. However there is no evidence to make poor nutrition the *cause* of the low achievement since lack of a warm caring environment can hamper learning as much as lack of food.

Nutritional stunting

Stunting is defined as height for age < 90% expected value on reference charts. Weight for age is usually equally below expected so weight for height and BMI for age are often within the normal range. Stunting, particularly in deprived and disadvantaged environments, is often viewed as a nutritional condition and a consequence of inadequate diet. However it is usually extremely resistant to resolution through dietary means (Hoare *et al.*, 1996; Poskitt *et al.*, 1999) and reduction of stunting in a population seems dependent on major changes in the social environment (Esray, 1996; Rousham and Gracey, 1997). Thus the role of inadequate nutrition as a cause of stunting is unclear. If children are eating recommended allowances and yet not gaining weight and height as expected, it could be concluded that these children need more food than average in order to achieve the same gain in weight and linear growth. This may be the case (Donnet *et al.*, 1982; Hoare *et al.*, 1996), but why this is so still demands explanation.

Stunting, although usually discussed in the context of countries with low GDP, may be manifest, to a lesser degree, in the relatively shorter stature of children from disadvantaged areas and socio-economically deprived families in Westernized richer countries. Habicht *et al.* (1974) showed that the differences in height for children under 5 from upper and lower social classes within a racial group were greater than the differences in height between children from the upper social classes of different racial groups. The prevalence of stunting in a child population may be a very significant indicator of the social development of a country.

Stunting in young children is associated with poor later outcomes in terms of small adult height and weight, reduced muscular fitness and possibilities of poor pregnancy outcome in increased incidence of low birth-weight (Darboe and Poskitt, 2001). Evidence suggests that stunted children are also more likely to have poor educational outcomes (see below), but again it is not clear whether this is directly due to nutritional factors or to the influence of the environment of disadvantage. Economically, stunting in childhood may have an enormous impact on adult productivity, although this is a statistic that is difficult to determine.

Role of protein-energy deficiency in problems of growth and development, especially in relation to neurological impairment

Across the world, protein-energy malnutrition – marasmus, kwashiorkor, nutritional stunting – remains one of the major nutritional problems of young children. The profound and often prolonged energy deficiencies that contribute to these problems have been thought to lead to the arrest of brain growth and development and long-term consequences.

The impact of protein-energy malnutrition (PEM) on any individual is heavily influenced by factors such as age of onset, duration of poor nutrition, speed with which normal nutrition is restored, extent of changes in the home environment following nutritional rehabilitation, and presence or absence of associated illnesses and micronutrient deficiencies. Thus, if adverse socio-environmental factors in the environment can be removed, even if the nutritional problems are not immediately corrected, there may be less long-term physical and intellectual damage. Children who are too weak or too miserable through malnutrition will miss out on the normal interactions and experiences of childhood. Acquisition of motor and intellectual skills will be delayed, thus affecting children's capacity to react appropriately for age to their environment after recovery. The recovery process must stimulate psychomotor as well as anthropometric catch up (McKay *et al.*, 1978; Walker *et al.*, 2000).

Whilst it is possible that PEM does specifically affect brain functioning, there is little good evidence that preventive nutritional supplementation can improve psychomotor outcomes for children in areas where PEM is common. There is no clear mechanism for a direct effect of PEM on cerebral function (Grantham-McGregor *et al.*, 2000). There is, however, some evidence that nutritional supplementation *per se* can improve development in children after severe PEM, but the effects of nutritional supplementation are usually enhanced by associated programmes for psychomotor stimulation (Grantham-McGregor *et al.*, 1991; Husaini *et al.*, 1991). Modern programmes for the management of PEM in children include, along with nutritional rehabilitation, training for carers in carer–child interaction, communication and child stimulation through play. These procedures not only seem to improve nutritional outcomes but intellectual outcomes for the children as well (Grantham-McGregor *et al.*, 1997; Gardner *et al.*, 1999).

The growth outcome of severe childhood malnutrition is unpredictable. Most evidence suggests that the ultimate height of children severely malnourished in early childhood is less than expected by comparison with better nourished siblings or with the distribution of height within the population. The almost universal nature of poor nutrition within some societies can make it difficult to compare individual outcomes with general outcomes. It is relatively unusual for children who have been severely malnourished to go back to greatly improved local circumstances. Thus the depriving environment may continue despite better nutrition.

Obesity

Obesity in childhood is increasing in prevalence in virtually all Westernized countries and amongst affluent families in countries in the process of westernization (Wang, 2001). The reasons for the epidemic of obesity (which is occurring in adults as well as children) are not entirely clear. Certainly children are healthier and therefore less likely to suffer the growth-retarding effects of infection. Surprisingly, however, most assessments of children's nutritional intakes over the years have suggested quite significant falls in mean daily energy intakes, although the quality of dietary intakes and the situations under which food is consumed have changed a lot over the years. More food is eaten out of the home today. More food is also consumed outside specific meals. Snack foods are largely 'ready to eat' commercially produced items ranging from sweets, biscuits, crisps, icecream and sweetened, carbonated drinks, to hamburgers, Chinese take-away and pizza.

Many families cook little at home but buy ready-made meals which require heating in the microwave but little other preparation. Such meals are often energy dense and contain high levels of saturated fats. Widdowson (1947), referring to her study of 10 years earlier, remarked that the change in children's beverages was perhaps the greatest indicator of how diets had changed over the previous 200 years. 'Small beer' had been replaced by tea and milk (Widdowson, 1947). The same may be true for the period since. Fruit squashes, commercially produced undiluted fruit juices (which are quite energy dense), and the sugary Coca Cola and Pepsi of today have replaced the tea, home-diluted fruit squash and tap water of 50 years ago (Petter *et al.*, 1995). The variety, even within the same brand, of snack items and the innovative concepts behind marketing, produce almost irresistible pressures on children today to eat for excitement and experience, rather than for need.

Important also, to the epidemic of obesity, is the decline in *activity* of children and in particular the increase in *inactivity*. Children walk, play outside the house, and use stairs much less than 20–30 years ago. Television seems particularly relevant to the obesity epidemic. In the USA relative fatness for age in pre-adolescent boys seems to increase with the hours spent watching television each week (Klesges *et al.*, 1993).

Although obesity in its more severe form can be diagnosed 'by eye', the definition of obesity which can distinguish between the obese/overweight and the higher levels of 'normal' fatness is an area of interest and controversy (Cole *et al.*, 2000). Childhood definitions of obesity need to take into account differing fatness in children of differing ages. In adult life the BMI [body mass index: weight in kg/(height in m)^2] is widely used in community studies as a simple indicator of excessive weight which is most commonly due to excessive fat. Relating BMI values to mortality rates has shown that mortality and morbidity rates begin to rise for adults with BMI greater than $25 \, \text{kg/m}^2$ and rates increase considerably with BMI $> 30 \, \text{kg/m}^2$. However, in childhood mean BMI values vary with age and follow a sinuous course making the provision of one set of cut-off points for all ages impractical. There are no data relating particular levels of BMI in childhood to adverse health outcomes either in childhood or adult life. Cole *et al.* (2000) have suggested that the age-related cut-off points for overweight and obesity should be the childhood centile values equivalent to those which equate with morbidity data in adult life, namely BMIs of 25 and $30 \, \text{kg/m}^2$ at the age of 18 years.

BMI is only an indirect indicator of fatness. Theoretically, diagnosing obesity from BMI centile levels should lead to constant prevalence of approximately 9 per cent overweight and 0.5 per cent obesity at whatever age in childhood. This seems unrealistic. Thus the method, although very practical, will have to be evaluated in different populations to see how children diagnosed as overweight or obese on other grounds relate to this definition (Poskitt, 2000). Ideally it would also be valuable to relate centile position to childhood as well as to adult morbidity. Although the very obese are likely to remain very obese, a significant proportion of children who are obese slim to normal BMI in later childhood or adolescence. Only about one-third of obese adults were obese as children, so the centile cut-off points may not prove very useful in anticipating adult obesity. However, as obesity becomes commoner in childhood, so it is likely that the proportion of adult obese who were fat children will increase, since it is unlikely that there is a totally reversed relationship between obesity in childhood and obesity in adult life (Chinn and Rona, 2001).

In recent years, a lot of stress has been put on the importance of obesity in early life for later obesity. This may be overdone (Parsons *et al.*, 1999). We have already referred to the spontaneous changes in the rates of fat deposition that take place throughout childhood. It was established some years ago that most obese infants slim down in the first years of life and do not remain fat (Poskitt and Cole, 1977). The prognosis for the obese child after infancy,

Table 11.4   Some approaches to prevention/management of childhood obesity

Policy	Possible approach
Reduce energy intake without reducing volume of food	Low-energy versions of margarine, yoghurts etc. Semi-skimmed or skimmed milks Grill, boil, bake without added fats instead of frying 'Oven' chips
Increase time required to consume foods/increase satiety by 'wholefood' versions	Whole fruits rather than juices or purees Wholemeal breads and pastas
Organize mealtimes and snacks so eating confined to recognized episodes rather than continuous process	Three main meals a day and two or three snacks. Snacks preferably whole fruit/raw vegetables rather than sweets and biscuits Family meals so slower eating process may encourage satiety
Reduce intake of 'empty' calories and unnecessary very energy-dense foods	Limit intakes of sweets, biscuits, sweetened juices and carbonated drinks
Discourage inactivity	Encourage active lifestyle through using stairs, walking whenever possible, running errands around the house for others, helping with housework, etc. Develop hobbies so other interests than television-watching and computer games
Encourage activity	Play games and go for walks and outings as a family. Look for opportunities for safe physical activity outside the home

particularly for the severely obese, is less optimistic.

It is generally agreed, although without strong evidence, that it is easier – and more effective – to prevent childhood obesity than to treat it once it is established. Unfortunately there are few studies on the prevention of obesity in childhood from which to glean advice. Table 11.4 lists possible approaches to developing a childhood lifestyle which might diminish the risk of developing obesity or which might reduce moderate obesity. The similarity between these approaches and the recommendations for healthy living for all outlined at the end of the chapter are significant. The prevention of obesity does not demand very different approaches to the prevention of other non-communicable disease of adult life. Action is, however, needed since

the rising prevalence of childhood obesity in Westernized countries (Chinn and Rona, 2001) and some industrializing countries is beginning to pose major problems for health services, as well as for public services, which have to consider the large size of many of their clients when planning public transport, theatres, access to public areas etc. Practical measures for weight management in childhood can be found in Chapter 12.

Micronutrient Deficiencies

Micronutrients are usually defined as those nutrients required in quantities less than 1 g/ day. Calcium is borderline in this respect since some recommendations indicate just over 1 g/

Table 11.5 UK dietary reference values for some micronutrients in childhood

Age (years)	Thiamin (mg)	Vitamin A (μg)	Vitamin C (mg)	Calcium (mmol)	Zinc (μmol)	Iodine (μmol)
1–3	0.5	400	30	8.8	75	0.6
4–6	0.7	500	30	11.3	100	0.8
7–10	0.9	600	30	13.8	110	0.9
Males						
11–14	0.9	600	35	25	140	1.0
15–18	1.1	700	40	25	145	1.0
Females						
11–14	0.7	600	35	20	140	1.0
15–18	0.8	600	40	20	110	1.1

Department of Health (1991).

day at some ages. Nevertheless calcium is usually classed as a micronutrient, although perhaps rather unique in view of the weight of skeletal calcium in the body.

Table 11.5 outlines dietary reference values (DRVs) for several micronutrients of importance in childhood nutrition (Department of Health, 1991). Reference values for iron are given later in the chapter. It will be apparent that micronutrient requirements do not relate directly to weight in young children. Requirements of young children are much higher, in proportion to weight, than the requirements for adults.

The concept of a DRV (or recommended dietary allowance, RDA) for a nutrient involves the understanding that all other nutrients in the diet are sufficient. This is an unnatural situation since malnutrition rarely occurs for a single nutrient. It is now recognized that internutrient interactions and the interdependence of micronutrients are critical to many metabolic processes (Munoz *et al.*, 2000). Thus recommendations, if we only knew what to recommend, might be more suitably presented as combined micronutrient needs rather than DRVs for individual micronutrients.

Interaction between micronutrients may take the form of enhancement or interference at the level of gastro-intestinal absorption.

Sometimes there is mutual interaction in metabolic processes (Powers *et al.*, 1983; Munoz *et al.*, 2000; Zimmermann *et al.*, 2000b). Thus disappointing responses to well-designed micronutrient supplementation trials could be explained by the interdependency of micronutrient metabolism (Allen *et al.*, 2000). Rivera *et al.* (2001) demonstrated improved growth in Mexican infants receiving multiple micronutrient supplementation when compared with single nutrient supplementation.

Micronutrients are involved in building new tissues as catalysts for enzymes, as part of enzymes involved in tissue formation (zinc, copper, B vitamins, vitamin D), and as substantive parts of tissues (calcium and iron particularly). Many micronutrients are involved in maintenance of normal immunological resistance to infection (especially vitamin A, iron and vitamin C). Young children are particularly vulnerable to infection due to their lack of previous experience, unhygienic habits, low natural resistance through immature immunological reactions and close contact with other groups of infected persons such as other young members of the family and playmates. Table 11.6 lists some of the varied factors contributing to micronutrient deficiencies in children. The micronutrient

Table 11.6 Factors contributing to micronutrient deficiencies

Basic cause	General condition	Specific condition
Too little in	Inadequate variety of foods	Poverty; single staple
	Consumption of foods low in micronutrients	Single staple
	Removal or destruction of nutrients in processing/cooking	Loss of B vitamins in polished rice Loss of vitamin C in cooking
	Non-bioavailability of micronutrients	Inhibition of iron absorption by calcium Zinc binding by phytates
Too much out	Losses from gastro-intestinal tract	Zinc in intestinal secretions
	Losses via kidney	Phosphates in congenital and chronic kidney disease
	Losses via skin	Zinc, folates, iron in exfoliative conditions
	Losses in other tissues	Haemorrhage leading to loss of iron
Failure to absorb	Genetic conditions: acrodermatitis enteropathica	Zinc
	Acquired conditions: cystic fibrosis	Fat-soluble vitamins
	Gluten-sensitive enteropathy	Iron, folic acid
	Reduced iron absorption in pyrexia	Iron
	Reduced calcium absorption in vitamin D deficiency	Calcium
	Binding of micronutrients to phytates	Iron, calcium
Failure to utilize	Chronic illness	Poor incorporation of iron into haem
	Inhibitors in food	Inhibition of iodine utilization by thiocyanates
Increased requirements	Catch-up growth	All growth requires extra nutrients and high levels of micronutrients, accelerated catch-up growth requires even more
	Inadequate summer sunshine	Vitamin D in pigmented individuals and those in northern climes where vitamin D levels may be low

problems discussed in detail in this chapter are those where deficiencies have significant impact throughout childhood and which are not discussed elsewhere in the book.

Iron deficiency anaemia

Worldwide, iron deficiency is probably the most common micronutrient deficiency. Iron is low in many diets and bioavailability is affected by the form in which the iron occurs in the food, other constituents of the food, and the health and nutritional status of the con-sumer (Hunt, 2001), as shown in Table 11.7. Iron acts as an important component of many enzymes and of cytochromes, which have mediating roles in energy transport within cells (Table 11.8). However the major role of iron in the body is as an essential component for the transport of oxygen in haemoglobin and for energy transport by myoglobin in muscles. Immune responsiveness is impaired in iron deficiency with reduced DNA activity leading to reduced T cell production and function. Neutrophils show lowered myeloper-oxidase and lowered overall phagocytic activ-ity. Iron is also an important cofactor in the

Table 11.7 Factors influencing iron absorption

Positive factors	Negative factors
Iron in diet as haem	Iron associated with high phytate diet
Food includes meat	Foods with phytates, phenols
Iron in ferrous form	Iron in ferric form
Diet contains ascorbic acid or other reducing agent	Calcium or other inhibitors in diet
Iron deficiency	Tissues saturated with iron
	Chronic illness/infection
	Pyrexia

Table 11.8 Role of iron in metabolism

Iron requirement	Biochemical process
As component of haem in haemoglobin molecule	Responsible for oxygen-carrying capacity of blood
As component of myoglobin	Metabolic action leading to contraction of muscle
As component of cytochromes	Intracellular transport of energy
As component of other enzymes	Many metabolic processes

metabolism of neurotransmitters such as dopamine and it may be required for myelin production in the developing brain. Certainly the iron content of the brain increases with age. Seventy per cent of the iron in the maturing brain is in the myelin fraction and 15 per cent in mitochondrial, 5 per cent in microsomal and 5–10 per cent in the soluble fractions of the brain. Development of the dendritic trees and myelinization account for increase in brain iron until about 10 years of age. It is not clear how much the presence of adequate iron is necessary for these processes to take place (Youdin, 1990). Haemoglobin is one of the main sites for iron in the body. Haemoglobin levels may be preserved initially in iron deficiency, whilst iron stores in bone marrow and reticulo-endothelial system are depleted. However, in its most severe form iron deficiency leads to iron-deficiency anaemia (IDA) and the clinical problems which arise from the reduced oxygen-carrying capacity of the blood.

Newborn infants have relatively high haemoglobin levels to cope with the low intrauterine oxygen tension and the need to increase oxygen capture by haemoglobin. Even when mothers are iron-deficient, haemoglobin levels in the newborn may be satisfactory, although extreme iron deficiency in the mother is reflected in very poor iron nutrition in the infant.

The relatively high oxygen concentration in the extrauterine environment probably explains the quiescent bone marrow in the first few weeks of postnatal life. Haemoglobin levels fall and, as infants grow, the bone marrow responds once more to meet the needs of expanding blood volumes. However, rates of growth seem to outstrip young children's ability to produce red cells and haemoglobin. Thus haemoglobin levels of young children are, on average, lower than those of older children and adults even when they are not iron-deficient (Table 11.9). Because milk diets are not particularly good sources of iron (although the small quantities of iron in breast milk are very well absorbed), and because weaning foods are frequently low in iron, IDA is very

Table 11.9 Minimum acceptable levels of haemoglobin according to age[a]

Age (years)	Haemoglobin level g/l
0.5–6.0	110
>6.0–14	120
>14 boys	130
>14 girls	120
Adult men	130
Adult women	120
Pregnant women	110

[a]WHO (1973).

Table 11.10 Iron requirements in childhood according to age and sex[a]

Age (years)	LRNI (mg/day)	EAR (mg/day)	RNI (mg/day)
0–0.33	0.9	1.3	1.7
0.33–0.5	2.3	3.3	4.3
0.5–1.0	4.2	6.0	7.8
2	3.7	5.3	6.9
5	3.3	4.7	6.1
10	4.7	6.7	8.7
15 boys	6.1	8.7	11.3
girls	8.0	11.4	14.8
25 men	4.7	6.7	8.7
women	8.0	11.4	14.8

[a]Department of Health (1991).

common in young infants. Severe anaemia in infants and young children in Europe may be less common than in the past because the addition of iron and vitamin supplements to formula milks, including to the follow-on formulas intended for infants postweaning, has increased the iron intake of many young children. Once children move on to neat cow's milk, the very low iron content of cow's milk plus, in some children, the risk of blood loss as a manifestation of cow's milk protein allergy, contribute further to iron deficiency.

Adolescents are another group where iron nutrition may be poor. The adolescent diet is likely to be poor in bioavailable iron. Growth places huge demands – in both sexes – on iron as the blood volume expands, muscle size increases dramatically in boys, and, in girls, the onset of menstruation increases iron requirements. Table 11.10 lists UK recommendations for iron intake (Department of Health, 1991) according to age and sex in childhood.

Iron-deficiency anaemia is characterized by falling haemoglobin levels and increasing problems of breathlessness with, ultimately, high output cardiac failure. Iron-deficiency anaemia is a microcytic, hypochromic anaemia. Plasma iron is low and plasma transferrin level is high. The body adapts to low haemoglobin levels if these develop gradually. Children with IDA which is primarily dietary in origin and which can develop very slowly may reach extremely low levels of haemoglobin (e.g. 30 g/l) before any problem is recognized.

Clinically, iron-deficient children are often miserable and apathetic, with poor appetites and negative behaviours. Apathy may be replaced by irritability and poor attention span. The children may present with bizarre eating habits (pica), often with a particular penchant for soil.

A number of studies suggests that iron deficiency *per se* is associated with impaired learning and cognition (Bruner *et al.*, 1996; Aukett *et al.*, 1986). Logan *et al.* (2001), in a very critical evaluation of studies on the effects of iron therapy in children under 3 years with IDA, concluded that the evidence that psychomotor progress and cognition could be improved by iron treatment was not good. However, they concluded that the number of children involved in the studies they accepted for consideration was small and results could be compatible with 'substantial beneficial effect in children with iron-deficiency anaemia'. They concluded that there was 'urgent need for large scale randomized controlled trials of iron therapy in young infants with iron-deficiency anaemia'. Despite these uncertain conclusions there remains a significant literature purporting to show improved mental functioning in iron-deficient children of all ages, even when not anaemic, following iron supplementation (Grantham-McGregor and Ani, 2001). The NHANES III study, involving children aged 6–16 years, found lower maths scores in children with biochemical evidence of iron deficiency even when not anaemic, compared with children with normal iron-related biochemistry (Halterman *et al.*, 2001). Bruner *et al.* (1996) found improved verbal learning and verbal memory following iron supplementation of non-anaemic USA schoolchildren. Otero *et al.* (1999) demonstrated not only lower WISC (Wechsler Intelligence Scale for Children) scores in information, comprehension and verbal performance and full-scale IQ, but more theta and delta activity on EEG in iron-deficient, when compared with non-iron-deficient, Mexican schoolchildren. Whether these problems lead on to permanently impaired intellectual ability is questionable (Pollitt, 2000).

It is difficult to distinguish the clinical effects of iron deficiency from those of poor home environments and/or the IDA that so often accompanies deficiency. Despite the involvement of iron in many immune reactions, few studies show conclusively that iron deficiency, *per se*, leads to increased infection or worse outcomes from infection. This may be because, in most cases, there is a strong socio-economic pattern to iron deficiency with greater prevalence in the more disadvantaged groups who are usually more prone to infection anyway (Grantham-McGregor *et al.*, 2000). Moreover any effect may be through positive effects on vitamin A nutrition. Munoz *et al.* (2000) showed that supplementation of children between 18 and 36 months with vitamin A, zinc and iron was more effective in raising plasma retinol levels than either supplementation with vitamin A alone or with vitamin A and zinc.

Iron deficiency causes a microcytic, hypochromic anaemia. Serum iron is low and transferrin levels are high. Iron absorption is 'controlled' at the level of the gastro-intestinal mucosa by the availability of unsaturated transferrin to bind and transport iron into and across mucosal cells. Iron circulates in the plasma bound to transferrin. Thus transferrin saturation can give an indication of need for iron, but transferrin levels may be reduced by low protein states. Ferritin, synthesized in cells from the reticulo-endothelial system, provides a better indicator of iron stores in the body. Plasma levels of ferritin fall in parallel with falls in stainable bone marrow iron and rise as stores return to normal. However, ferritin is an acute phase reactant and can also be an uncertain indicator of iron stores in situations where infection and inflammation accompany possible deficiency.

Although widespread in foods, iron bioavailability is variable. Iron in the haem molecule is absorbed intact as haem. Table 11.7 indicates some of the factors influencing iron bioavailability and intestinal absorption. Phytates and zinc can inhibit iron absorption. Iron absorption is facilitated by iron in the ferrous form rather than the ferric form. Dietary vitamin C facilitates reduction of dietary iron from ferric to ferrous forms and can improve iron absorption, although under normal (rather than experimental) conditions this effect may be quite small (Cook and Reddy, 2001). The traditional administration of iron therapy or supplemental iron has been on a daily basis. Iron is an unpleasant nutrient to take therapeutically. It is reassuring that recent studies suggest iron therapy/supplements once or twice a week are as effective in supplementing low-iron diets as daily supplements, although possibly less effective in restoring iron status to normal in severe iron deficiency, as the same dose of iron administered on a daily basis (Angeles-Agdeppa *et al.*, 1997; Thu *et al.*, 1999). Where poor micronutrient nutrition is rife, iron therapy should be administered with vitamin C to facilitate absorption and vitamin A and riboflavin to improve incorporation of iron into haemoglobin.

Iron is a micronutrient where therapeutic and toxic doses are relatively close to one another. Further, when circulating transferrin levels are low, as in severe malnutrition, adverse effects of iron may be facilitated by the presence of free, unbound, iron in the plasma which excites free radical activity and inhibits immune responsiveness. The gastro-intestinal barrier restricts iron absorption in the presence of infection and when circulating transferrin levels are low. Parenteral iron bipasses these controls, thus risking iron over-load. This is particularly dangerous in malnu-trition and it is advisable to avoid giving iron therapy until children with malnutrition are beginning to show signs of recovery, for fear of precipitating overwhelming infection (WHO, 1998). Parenteral iron, now rarely given in childhood, is contraindicated in malnutrition since low iron-binding protein in the blood may cause dangerous levels of free iron to circulate and encourage oxidative reactions. Further information on practical measures to maintain optimal iron status and to treat IDA can be found in Tables 12.7–12.9.

Zinc deficiency

The most severe manifestations of zinc defi-ciency are found in infants with acrodermatitis enteropathica where there is congenital absence of a ligand facilitating zinc absorption in the intestine. If untreated, these children die of intractable diarrhoea, severe failure to thrive, eczema and often overwhelming infec-tion. The earliest suggestions that dietary zinc deficiency had consequences for genetically normal children came from findings of short stature and delayed puberty responding to zinc supplementation in Egyptian adolescent boys (Prasad et al., 1963; Sandstead et al., 1967). In the USA growth retardation in weanlings has also been shown to respond to zinc supple-mentation (Walravens et al., 1983; Hambidge,

1986). Clinical signs of zinc deficiency, except in extreme cases, are non-specific. Ageusia (loss of sense of taste), poor growth, dry skin, diarrhoea and lowered resistance to infection are all associated with many other conditions. Weeping flexural eczema and blistering skin lesions are only features of severe zinc defi-ciency and again may be imitated by a number of conditions. Moreoever plasma zinc levels are not good indicators of overall body zinc status. Thus interpreting the effect of low zinc intakes can be very difficult. The hormone thymulin, involved in T cell differentiation is zinc-dependent and may be responsible for reduced cell-mediated immunity in the pre-sence of low zinc nutrition (Prasad, 1998). Recent work also suggests that zinc may be involved in cognitive processes. Bhatnagar and Taneja (2001) concluded that evidence sup-ported improved mental development and func-tional activity in zinc-supplemented young children, although data for older children were less clear-cut. However zinc supplementation in one study in Bangladesh showed that infants given zinc ended up with marginally lower developmental indices than those who did not receive supplemental zinc – possibly because of the general micronutrient imbalance caused by offering only one nutritional supplement (Hamadani et al., 2001). Zinc is also involved in vitamin A metabolism (Munoz et al., 2000) and may exert some immune effects through the action of vitamin A – demonstrating once again the mutual interdependence of micro-nutrients in many physiological processes.

Zinc levels in plasma are not very helpful as indicators of zinc deficiency. This may explain the varied responses to zinc supplementation despite apparently low zinc intakes. In the Gambia for example, zinc supplementation studies produced no improvement in growth, nor evidence of reduced infection, nor reduced morbidity from infection in schoolchildren in an area with high prevalence of nutritional stunting and diets low in zinc (Powers et al., 1983; Bates et al., 1993).

Significant food sources of zinc are animal products. Bioavailability is strongly influenced by the physical and chemical nature of the zinc in the food. Absorption of zinc is inversely proportional to the concentration of zinc in the intestine, perhaps because of the ready saturation of zinc receptors involved in uptake and transport of zinc. A further complicating factor is the prevalence of zinc antagonists in diets with a phytate to zinc ratio of >15.

Diets can thus be divided into (WHO, 1996):

High zinc availability	Diets low in cereal fibre and phytic acid
	Phytate/zinc ratio <5
	Adequate animal or fish protein
Moderate zinc availability	Mixed diets containing animal and fish and cereal proteins
	Lacto-ovo, ovovegetarian or vegan diets not containing unrefined grains or flour
	Phytate/zinc ratio 5–15 (<10 if fortified with calcium)
Low zinc availability	Unrefined, unfermented cereals, especially if fortified with calcium >50% energy from high phytate foods
	Phytate/zinc ratio >15
	High intake of soya high phytate products
	High calcium intakes (>1 g/day)

Zinc is found in all body fluids, including gastro-intestinal secretions. Requirements depend on, or are affected by, losses in intestinal secretions and through sweat and/or skin epithelial cell loss particularly. Most zinc in the body is present as a component of lean body mass – muscle and bone. Thus requirements are affected by:

- body surface area (which increases *in toto* with growth although decreasing in proportion to body weight);
- intestinal length, which increases with increased body size and weight;
- energy intakes;
- lean body mass as a proportion of total body mass.

Since catch-up growth following periods of malnutrition or growth faltering (often secondary to diarrhoea with loss of zinc) involves rapid deposition of new tissue, zinc requirements are greatly increased during recovery from malnutrition. Further, zinc is an important component of lean body mass so requirements also increase during periods of accelerated growth.

Iodine deficiency

Worldwide iodine deficiency and iodine deficiency disorders (IDD) affect millions of people (Maberly, 1994). The economic consequences are enormous. 'Ending iodine deficiency forever' has been a major programme of international agencies for the past 10 years and has been reasonably effective. UNICEF (2001) estimates 90 million newborns each year are now protected from significant loss of learning ability by national programmes to iodize salt.

Iodine deficiency is classically manifest in the development of visible thyroid enlargement (goitre). The prevalence of goitre in a community is used as an indication of the severity of iodine deficiency in the area. However it is clear that, where there is iodine deficiency, even those who do not show classical signs may nevertheless be affected by the consequences of long-standing iodine deficiency, for example by reduced perinatal survival, or by impaired learning in later childhood. Recognition of subclinical risk has led to programmes for universal iodine supplementation wherever there is potential risk of deficiency rather than programmes to reach only the obviously at-risk individuals. It is, however, interesting that areas of Europe (such as Derbyshire, UK) where goitre used to be fairly common seem to have overcome iodine deficiency without

Table 11.11   Long-standing effects of iodine deficiency in fetal and later life

Time of main iodine deficit	Consequences	Clinical details
In utero	Neurological cretinism	Hypertonic/ataxic cerebral palsy
		Low IQ
		Deaf mutism
		Growth retardation
	Myxoedematous cretinism	Growth retardation
		Low IQ
		Hypothyroid
		Myxodematous facies:
		coarse features
		prominent tongue
		Dry skin
		Hoarse voice
	Increased risk of low birth-weight	
	Increased risk of perinatal mortality	
In utero/postnatal	Impaired psychomotor development	Increased risk of low IQ:
		impaired learning
		impaired cognition
Infancy/childhood	Hypothyroidism	Goitre
	Growth retardation	Short stature
	Psychomotor damage	Low IQ
		Reduced learning ability
		Reduced physical strength
	Hyperthyroidism (especially with iodine supplementation)	

specific dietary supplementation. Presumably greater variety in the diet and the inclusion of foods produced in non-iodine-deficient areas have resolved the problem. Thus a general improvement in diets and consumption of a greater variety of foods, including non-locally produced foods, together with the reduction of poverty and food insecurity, should be the long-term aim in combatting IDD.

Table 11.11 lists the main complications of iodine deficiency in childhood. The neurological cretin with deafness and profound irreversible neurological impairment is the worst outcome of severe maternal deficiency throughout pregnancy. Indeed it is possible that the developing inner ear is the one system, apart from the thyroid gland, which requires iodine as such since the damage occurs very

early in gestation, before the infant's thyroid gland is functional. The typical hypothyroid cretin, who may gain some growth and intellectual benefit from iodine or thyroid hormone supplementation, may be the result of milder damage taking place later in pregnancy when suboptimal levels of maternal or foetal thyroid hormone cease to be adequate for normal development.

More important, because much larger numbers of children are involved than those presenting with obvious IDD, is the greater risk of lower IQ, impaired learning and reduced cognition amongst children born to unsupplemented mothers compared with iodine-supplemented mothers in deficient areas. Deficient iodine intakes may contribute to apathy and/or problems with decision-making amongst some of the older children and adults in iodine deficient areas.

Reduced iodine intakes lead to reduced tetra-iodotyrosine (thyroxine: T_4) production by the thyroid gland. This stimulates increased release of thyroid-stimulating hormone (TSH) from the anterior pituitary gland in the brain and this in turn stimulates increased thyroid iodine capture. The brain is dependent on circulating T_4 levels for maintenance of intracerebral levels of the more active component of thyroid hormone: triiodotyrosine (T_3; Delange, 2000). It is of interest that one of the enzymes involved in conversion of T_4 to T_3 is selenium dependent and thus micronutrient deficiency other than for iodine may be involved in some of the problems of low iodine levels. Both selenium deficiency and iodine deficiency arise in mountainous areas where minerals have been leached out of the soil and washed away by heavy rain, or in areas affected by repeated flooding. Iodine supplementation alone may not resolve goitre in areas where there is selenium as well as iodine deficiency (Zimmermann *et al.*, 2000a). The same authors (Zimmermann *et al.*, 2000b) have found poor response in goitre size with iodine supplementation given to iron-deficient subjects.

Iodine uptake by the thyroid gland is affected by thiocyanates in some foodstuffs. The cyanogenic glycosides, present in many widely consumed staples although, apart from cassava, in insignificant amounts, are digested and converted into thiocyanates in the body. Vegetables of the *Brassica* family likewise give rise to thiocyanates. For most of these foods, the quantities consumed are only likely to be important if iodine intakes are already at critically low levels. Where these foods are commonly eaten, daily dietary recommendations for iodine should be doubled.

Because iodine is well absorbed and any iodine not utilized in thyroid hormone synthesis is excreted in the urine, 24 h urinary iodine excretion can be a useful way of estimating the level of iodine nutrition within populations. Since complete 24 h urinary collections are often difficult to obtain, urinary iodine/creatinine ratio may be used as a proxy for 24 h iodine excretion. Twenty-four-hour excretion of iodine is not very reliable for assessment of iodine nutrition in individuals. The distribution and mean values of iodine concentration in spot specimens from groups of over 40 individuals can be more informative for population studies than 24 h collections of uncertain completeness.

Where practical, blood levels of T_4 or TSH are used to screen children for thyroid deficiency and could be used to detect children with iodine deficiency. However the countries where these tests are usually available are commonly those of the Westernized world where iodine deficiency is no longer, or never has been, a problem. Thyroid screening of the newborn in these countries anticipates sporadic congenital thyroid deficiency and inborn errors in thyroid metabolism rather than infants affected by iodine deficiency.

Whatever the cause, treatment for perinatal thyroid deficiency needs to be rapid and effective if the neurological consequences are to be kept to a minimum.

Calcium nutrition

The main component of bone mineral is calcium apatite. Needs for calcium are greatly affected by rates of bone deposition. The calcium content of the body and bone mineral density (BMD) increase with growth. Bone mineral density may be influenced particularly by the hormonal changes at puberty. Nutritionally, however, the interaction of vitamin D and calcium for the deposition of bone mineral remains a critical issue in the development of BMD and, as discussed in the section on vitamin D, subclinical vitamin D deficiency may be more common in adolescence than currently recognized.

Bone mineral continues to accrue throughout childhood and early adult life, reaching a peak bone mass (PBM) between the ages of 16 and 30 years. A high PBM guards against the effects of calcium loss after middle age. Concern to optimize PBM through nutrition should centre attention on nutrients such as protein, vitamins D, A and K as well as calcium. The acquisition of high PBM is of particular relevance to adolescent girls in whom pregnancy and lactation may make demands on their calcium nutrition and in whom bone loss in late middle age will be proportionately greater than for boys.

From 40 years onwards, there is gradual bone loss in both sexes but accelerated bone loss in women at menarche as oestrogen levels fall. Loss of bone mineral and the consequences in terms of osteoporosis manifest as bone fractures, pain and disability are major problems for the elderly in many Westernized societies. Calcium intakes in the bone accretion phase of growth are thought to be relevant to PBM with high calcium intakes in adult life slowing bone mineral loss with age. Of the many other micronutrients involved in bone formation, vitamin D as its chief active metabolite 1-25-di-hydroxy vitamin D is essential for calcium absorption in the gastro-intestinal tract, retention of phosphate by the kidney, and remodelling (through absorption and rediposition of calcium apatite) of bones and bone mineral to allow bone growth.

Work from The Gambia suggests that, even where calcium intakes are very low, the bone mineral content of adolescents and adults is appropriate for their overall size when compared with that of individuals in societies where traditional intakes of calcium are much higher (Dibba et al., 2000). Bone loss at middle age follows the same pattern as in Western Europe, and yet complications from osteoporosis are almost non existent (Aspray et al., 1996). The difference between the Gambian and the Westernized populations seems to reside in the amount of heavy manual work

and physical exercise undertaken. In societies where calcium intakes are low, but physical activity levels high, calcium retention in bone may be facilitated and, because of activity, be deposited and aligned where it provides the bone with most strength. Thus it is possibly not the amount of calcium in the diet (within limits), but the distribution of the calcium forming the supportive matrix in the bone which determines the risk of fracture as bone mineral loss occurs. It is, however, possible that the protective factors lie not in the bones but in the good muscular and ligamentous strength guarding the bones during falls and unusual stresses.

A study from The Gambia indicates that, when calcium in the diet is very low and growth stunting common, long-term (over 1 year) supplementation of the diet with calcium can lead to increased BMD in preadolescent children (Dibba et al., 2000).

It is of interest that some of the studies of calcium absorption and bone mineralization suggest differences in the effect of calcium as supplementary calcium salts and calcium as a component of milk (Merrilees et al., 2000). If bone mineralization is more effective when the calcium is supplied in milk, is this indicative of better calcium absorption or indicative of the role of proteins or other components of milk in bone growth and development? Calcium absorption is readily affected by other dietary components such as phytates and other minerals.

Vitamin D deficiency and rickets

Vitamin D deficiency rickets used to be very common in Western Europe and particularly the UK, where industrial smog and the cloudy climate hindered adequate exposure to ultraviolet sunlight of around 300 nm (only reaching the northerly latitude of Britain between mid-February and late October). The Clean Air Act of the mid-1950s probably did much to remove the risk of rickets in healthy Caucasian children, although increased vitamin D supplementation of diets was also instrumental, as was increasing affluence and the chance for more children to have summer holidays (Poskitt et al., 1979). The influx of immigrants from the West Indies and particularly from the Indian subcontinent to UK in the second half of the twentieth century demonstrated that rickets and osteomalacia could still be risks in Britain for those in whom skin synthesis of vitamin D is limited by increased skin pigmentation, extensive skin covering by clothes and limited exposure to sunshine. The relatively low calcium absorption from many Asian diets because of high-phytate flours may also mean that requirements for vitamin D are relatively higher than for those with higher calcium bioavailability from the diet. A review of the practical measures that can be adapted to maintain vitamin D status (and other vitamins) can be found in Chapter 12.

Vitamin D can be obtained from foods (fatty fish, offal, cream, cheese and supplemented margarine and some canned milks and milk powders), but the main source for most people, even in high-latitude countries, is synthesis in the skin from the impact of ultraviolet light of 300 nm on 7-de-hydrocholesterol in the skin. The extent of skin pigmentation is of little importance in vitamin D synthesis except in situations where the amount of sunshine exposure is restricted.

Cholecalciferol synthesized in the skin is converted to 25-hydroxy vitamin D in the liver and this is the main circulating component of vitamin D in the blood. The active component of vitamin D is 1-25-di-hydroxy vitamin D, which is synthesized in the kidney. Where active vitamin D production is adequate, other metabolites of 25-hydroxy vitamin D, such as 24-25-di-hydroxy vitamin D, are synthesized. These have much less activity and are excreted in bile and urine.

The stimuli for the production of 1-25-di-hydroxy vitamin D are parathyroid hormone, low serum calcium and low serum phosphate. 1-25-di-hydroxy vitamin D stimulates calcium absorption from the intestine by increasing the calcium-binding proteins in the intestinal mucosal cells and by direct effects on calcium absorption as well. In the bones, bone mineral resorption is increased, allowing, together with parathyroid hormone activity, high calcium and phosphate concentrations in the vicinity of osteoblastic activity, further deposition of bone mineral and reorganization and growth of bone.

Rickets – clinical vitamin D deficiency – is a disease of growing children. The most obvious effects are in the bones, which are poorly ossified, soft and malleable so the children have painful bowed legs (or arms if they are not yet walking and thus still weight bearing on their arms). The ribs are also soft and tend to be pulled in at the attachment of the diaphragm causing 'Harrison's sulcus' around the lower ribs with pigeon chest appearance above. Accumulation of uncalcified cartilage and osteoid at the end of the metaphyses leads to swelling just above the epiphyseal plates at wrists, knees and the ends of the bony ribs (leading to the characteristic 'rickety rosary'). Bossing of the skull due to still open cranial fontanelles and soft skull bones distorted by the brain growing underneath them are other features in young children. In older children the changes may be present but less dramatic. The clinical signs are exacerbated by the muscular weakness which accompanies the bony problem. In very young children, the effect of vitamin D deficiency may be to produce hypocalcaemia and/or hypocalcaemic convulsions. In older children, secondary hyperparathyroidism stimulates calcium resorption from bone, and serum calcium levels usually rise into the low normal range. However, secondary hyperparathyroidism leads to low phosphate levels which, with elevated alkaline phosphatase levels (normal range 100–800 U/l), provide biochemical support for the diagnosis of rickets.

There are a number of congenital (e.g. familial vitamin D-dependent rickets; X-linked dominant hypophosphataemic rickets) and acquired (e.g. bone disease secondary to chronic renal failure and to malabsorption syndromes) conditions which can give rise to the clinical appearance of vitamin D deficiency rickets. Usually, if serum vitamin D levels are normal, muscular weakness is not a significant feature. Biochemical findings are variable depending on the nature of the causative problem. True vitamin D deficiency usually responds rapidly to administration of vitamin D, whereas these other conditions are largely 'vitamin D resistant rickets', that is they are unresponsive to oral vitamin D except in doses many times higher than the DRV.

Vitamin D deficiency is a potential problem in adolescents as well as young children. Rapid rates of growth coupled with diets low not only in vitamin D but calcium as well, may contribute to 'subclinical' rickets with some bone pain and radiological evidence of rickets. It can be quite difficult to be sure of evidence of rickets on some limb X-rays and vague bone and muscle pains are not uncommon in rapidly growing teenagers. Classical findings should include serum calcium which is below or at the lower end of the normal range, low serum phosphate and high alkaline phosphatase with clinical response to oral vitamin D. Alkaline phosphatase levels may be elevated as a response to growth in normal adolescent boys and are not diagnostic in the absence of other supportive biochemistry. Evidence of circulating levels of 25-hydroxyvitamin D below the accepted normal level ($> 25\,nmol/l$) thus remain the diagnostic test for deficiency and potential rickets or osteomalacia.

Of recent years inadequate vitamin D nutrition in Caucasian British children after infancy had not been seen as a significant nutritional problem. However there is growing evidence that low levels of 25-hydroxy vitamin D are not uncommon in adolescents living in more northerly countries (Du et al., 2001). Data from Finland (Outila et al., 2001) suggest that low levels of 25-hydroxy vitamin D in the winter months are associated with reduced BMD in the lower forearm, suggesting that low levels of the circulating vitamin may be having negative effects on calcium deposition in the skeleton. This is concerning since O'Hare et al. (1984) in Scotland found quite widespread low levels of 25-hydroxy vitamin D in children admitted to hospital. Six per cent of Asian girls, and some Caucasian girls, between 13 and 15 years had biochemical evidence of rickets.

Although the changes of vitamin D deficiency may be very dramatic at the time of presentation, given time and normal nutrition, growth in the bones usually resolves all the deformity. This is perhaps less true for adolescents close to the end of their growth period than for younger children with many years of bone growth and remodelling ahead of them.

Conclusion

Nutrition in childhood, as stated at the beginning of this chapter, is a dynamic process. Table 11.12 outlines some of the changes which need to be encompassed to achieve healthy diets in adult life. Table 11.13 outlines important principles underlying strategies for good nutrition in childhood. Further practical measures can be found in Chapter 12, in the section 'School-age children' (pp. 365–6) and in Table 12.24 where school meal guidelines are reviewed. The main achievement of these principles should be to recognize that nutrition and the overall lifestyle in childhood can have significant bearing on an individual's predisposition to some of the non-infective diseases of adult life. Simple dietary changes can alter this predisposition. Problems such as obesity, whilst not, as sometimes thought, merely the

Table 11.12   Nutritional issues that should be considered for child to progress from infant diet to that of adult

Age	Diet	Nutritional issues
Young infant	Wholly breast-fed	Entirely liquid diet Quite low energy food All essential nutrients in one food No fibre in diet >50% total energy from fat
Weaning diet	Milk: formula or breast plus some 'solid' foods as purées and porridges	Diet low energy density, ~1 kcal/g Very little or no fibre May be low in fat – some weaning diets even in developed countries may have fat content <30% total energy Often high refined sugar content to diet
Young child	Mixed diet. May be quite limited in variety Little unprocessed meat Children often not keen to chew and whole fruit largely absent. Vegetables usually eaten only with reluctance	Varies according to food offered and children's pickiness. Fat content may range from 25 to >40% total energy Iron content may be very low Fibre intake largely from breakfast cereals
Schoolchild	Diet may be influenced by school meal. School dinners whether provided from home or canteen often high in total energy, energy from fat and refined sugar and low in vegetable fibre. Micronutrient intake in school dinners commonly low	School dinners may achieve >45% energy from fat Saturated fat may be majority of fat Sugar and sweetened drinks very popular Maybe high salt intake Fibre predominantly from breakfast cereals
Adolescent	May be a balanced adult diet or a thoroughly irregular diet Diet eaten away from home without supervision. May be excessive soft drink consumption	Important that diet is encouraged to follow recommendations for adults whenever possible Other aspects of 'healthy living' important as well as diet

consequence of greed and overindulgence, can be managed even if not totally cured with appropriate dietary and lifestyle changes. Likewise, environmental factors which induce diet can interact with the genetic make-up to reduce or prevent predisposition to certain diseases. Furthermore, the ability to eat 'healthily' can, contrary to some popular opinion, be thoroughly enjoyable. A varied healthy lifestyle should leave opportunity for enjoyable indulgence as well. Our outline recommendations for sensible healthy eating in later childhood with the aim of healthy adult life are described below. Chapter 12 (Table 12.23 and the section 'Healthy eating recommendations for pre-

schoolchildren', p. 364) provides details for younger children.

1. Nutrition in the form of dietary intake is only one aspect of healthy living. Activity levels, and avoiding high levels of inactivity, as well as more nebulous aspects, such as the development of self-esteem and avoiding smoking, are important as well.
2. Some degree of organization of eating into meals and snacks makes it easier to consume 'balanced' diets in appropriate quantities.
3. Consumption of fluids is important, but water is often the most appropriate drink.

Table 11.13 Outline of principles for good nutrition in childhood and adolescence

Age group	Nutritional principles
Children <3 y: weaning diets	Should include three main meals and two smaller meals
	Diets should be energy dense and varied to provide micronutrients: good sources of iron and vitamin C with each meal to encourage micronutrient absorption
	Whole milk rather than skimmed or semi-skimmed at least until 2 years
	High fibre diets should be avoided but fibre in diets gradually increased
Pre-school children 3–5 y	Three meals, two snacks, but other food in between meals discouraged. Increasing foods with fibre content
	Perhaps some semi-skimmed milk if children taking an otherwise balanced diet
	Careful modification of diet if child getting progressively fatter rather than slimming down from 'puppy' fat
	Encourage active lifestyle and discourage periods of inactivity in front of television
	Discourage eating between meals and outside recognized snack periods
	Fresh fruit as snacks. Water as beverage. Low energy fruit squash rather than carbonated drinks
	Vegetarian diets need careful attention for energy adequacy and micronutrient bioavailability
Schoolchildren 5–10 y	Control of high energy snack foods
	Maintain active lifestyle both at home and in school – encourage walking to school etc., or at least using bus rather than car
	Encourage hobbies, interests and activities other than television watching and computer games. Restrict television viewing
	Create nutritionally adequate and healthy school meals which are palatable and acceptable
	Watch for obesity and develop lifestyle management to cope with this
	Guard for dieting obsessions which might suggest early anorexia nervosa/bulimia
	Educate to understand advertising pressures in food and nutrition
Adolescents	Encourage adolescents to look after themselves and eat healthily despite peer pressures
	Encourage activity. Discourage inactivity
	Encourage high micronutrient intake
	Source of vitamin C with every meal
	Approximately 1 pint of reduced-fat milk/day
	Give supportive constructive advice to those becoming obese
	Recognize the stresses of adolescence and the need for adolescents to show independence and to develop their own lifestyles
	Maintaining 'contact' with children at this critical point in life may ultimately be more important than an ideal dietary intake

Carbonated drinks are not desirable since their acidity and sugariness can be very damaging to teeth. They are of little nutrient value (empty calories: sugar but without other macro- or micronutrient content) and can put children off eating other foods by gaseous distension in the stomach.

4. Current aims are that, for children over 5 years, no more than 35 per cent of the total energy should be derived from fat energy and no more than 10 per cent of dietary energy should be derived from saturated fats. In view of the importance of the long-chain PUFA for brain development in infancy, older children should be advised also to optimize intakes of n-6 and n-3 PUFA. Linoleic acid should provide at least 1 per cent total energy and α-linolenic acid

at least 0.2 per cent total energy, but total PUFA intake should not exceed 10 per cent total energy. Thus monounsaturated fatty acids (chiefly as oleic acid) should, as 10–15 per cent total energy, form the largest fraction of dietary fat.

5. Carbohydrates in the form of unrefined high-fibre versions should provide at least 50 per cent of total energy.

6. Drinking water should be fluoridated at the level of 1 ppm (1 mg/l) if it contains less than 0.7 ppm fluoride naturally. Alternatively children should take fluoride tablets (0.5 mg/day 2–4 years and 1 mg/day more than 4 years) daily.

7. It is desirable that each meal includes a source of vitamin C since this facilitates absorption of iron and other micronutrients.

8. Tea and coffee should preferably not be consumed with meals since they may inhibit some micronutrient absorption.

9. Milk at 500 ml (1 pint) per day – skimmed or semi-skimmed – is a useful contribution to calcium needs.

10. Wholemeal cereals are preferable to refined cereals. Recommendations for fibre intake are in the region of 18 g/day for adults. This amount is probably not appropriate for children. For children from 5 years upwards, a graded proportion of this amount is indicated.

References

Allen LH, Rosado JL, Casterline JE, Lopez P, Munoz E, Garcia OP and Martinez H (2000) Lack of hemoglobin response to iron supplementation in anemic Mexican pre-schoolers with multiple micronutrient deficiencies. *Am. J. Clin. Nutr.* **71**, 1485–1494.

Angeles-Agdeppa I, Schultink W, Sastroamidjojo S, Gross R and Karyadi D (1997) Weekly micronutrient supplementation to build iron stores in female Indonesian adolescents. *Am. J. Clin. Nutr.* **66**, 177–183.

Aspray TJ, Prentice A, Cole TJ, Sawo Y, Reeve J and Francis RM (1996) Low bone mineral content is common but osteoporotic fractures are rare in elderly rural Gambian women. *J. Bone Miner. Res.* **11**, 1019–1025.

Aukett MA, Parks YA, Scott PH and Wharton BA (1986) Treatment with iron increases weight gain and psychomotor development. *Arch. Dis. Child.* **61**, 849–857.

Bates CJ, Evans PH, Dardenne M, Prentice A, Lunn PG, Northrop-Clewes CA, Hoare S, Cole TJ, Horan SJ, Longman SC *et al.* (1993) A trial of zinc supplementation in young rural Gambian children. *Br. J. Nutr.* **69**, 243–255.

Beresford CH, Neale RJ and Brooke OG (1971) Iron absorption and pyrexia. *Lancet* **i**, 568–572.

Bhatnagar S and Taneja S (2001) Zinc and cognitive development. *Br. J. Nutr.* **85**(Suppl. 2), S139–145.

Bruner AB, Joffe AQ, Duggan AK, Casella JF and Brandt J (1996) Randomised study of cognitive effects of iron supplementation in non-anaemic iron deficient adolescent girls. *Lancet* **348**, 992–996.

Chinn S and Rona RJ (2001) Prevalence and trends in overweight and obesity in three cross sectional studies of British children 1974–94. *Br. Med. J.* **322**, 24–26.

Cole TJ (1994) Do growth centile charts need a face-lift? *Br. Med. J.* **308**, 641–642.

Cole TJ (1997) Growth monitoring with the British 1990 growth reference. *Arch. Dis. Child.* **76**, 47–49.

Cole TJ, Bellizzi MC, Flegal KM and Dietz WH (2000) Establishing a standard definition for childhood overweight and obesity: international survey. *Br. Med. J.* **320**, 1240–1243.

Cook JD and Reddy MB (2001) Effect of ascorbic acid intake on nonheme-iron absorption from a complete diet. *Am. J. Clin. Nutr.* **73**, 93–98.

Crawford JD and Osler DC (1975) Body composition at menarche: the Frisch–Revelle hypothesis revisited. *Pediatrics* **56**, 449–458.

Darboe MK and Poskitt EME (2001) Nutritional stunting: a family continuum. *Proc. Nutr. Soc.* **60 (OCA)**, 19A.

Day RE (1992) Psychosocial and intellectual development. In: *Forfar and Arneil's Textbook of Paediatrics*, 4th edn, ed. Campbell AGM and McIntosh N, pp. 449–467. Churchill Livingstone, Edinburgh.

Delange F (2000) The role of iodine in brain development. *Proc. Nutr. Soc.* **59**, 75–80.

Department of Health (1991) *Dietary Reference Values*

of Food Energy and Nutrients in the United Kingdom. Report on Health and Social Subjects no. 41. HMSO, London.

Department of Health (1994) Weaning and the Weaning Process. HMSO, London.

Department of Health and Social Security (1984) Diet and Cardiovascular Disease. Report on Health and Social Subjects no. 28. HMSO, London.

Dibba B, Prentice A, Ceesay M, Stirling DM, Cole TJ and Poskitt EME (2000) Effect of calcium supplementation on bone mineral accretion in Gambian children accustomed to a low calcium diet. Am. J. Clin. Nutr. 71, 544–549.

Donnet ML, Cole TJ, Scott TM and Stanfield JP (1982) Diet, growth and health of infants in a disadvantaged inner city environment in Glasgow. In: Nutrition and Health, ed. Turner MR, pp. 183–195. MTP Press, Lancaster.

Du X, Greenfield H, Fraser DR, Ge K, Trube A and Wang Y (2001) Vitamin D deficiency and associated factors in adolescent girls in Beijing. Am. J. Clin. Nutr. 74, 494–500.

Esray SA (1996) Water, waste and well being: a multi-country study. Am. J. Epidemiol. 143, 608–623.

Flegal KM (1999) The obesity epidemic in children and adults: current evidence and research issues. Med. Sci. Sports Exercise 31, S509–514.

Fomon SJ (1974) Infant Nutrition, 2nd edn, p. 34–94. WB Saunders, Philadelphia, PA.

Freeman JV, Cole TJ, Chinn S, Jones PR, White EM and Preece MA (1995) Cross sectional stature and weight reference curves for the UK 1990. Arch. Dis. Child. 73, 17–24.

Frisch RE (1987) Body fat, menarche, fitness and fertility. Hum. Reprod. 2, 521–533.

Frisch RE and Revelle R (1970) Height and weight at menarche and a hypothesis of critical body weight and adolescent events. Science 169, 397–399.

Gardner JM, Grantham-McGregor SM, Himes J and Chang S (1999) Behaviour and development of stunted and non stunted Jamaican children. J. Child Psychol. Psychiat. 40, 819–827.

Grantham-McGregor S and Ani C (2001) A review of studies on the effect of iron deficiency on cognitive development in children. J. Nutr. 131, 649S–666S.

Grantham-McGregor SM, Powell CA, Walker SP and Himes JH (1991) Nutritional supplementation, psychosocial stimulation, and mental development of stunted children: the Jamaican Study. Lancet 338, 1–5.

Grantham-McGregor SM, Walker SP, Chang SM and Powell CA (1997) Effects of early childhood supplementation with and without stimulation on later development in stunted Jamaican children. Am. J. Clin. Nutr. 66, 247–253.

Grantham-McGregor SM, Walker SP and Chang S (2000) Nutritional deficiencies and later behavioural development. Proc. Nutr. Soc. 59, 47–54.

Gregory JR, Collins DL, Davies PSW, Hughes JM and Clarke PC (1995a) National Diet and Nutrition Survey: Children Aged 1½ to 4½ Years, Vol. 1 Report of the Diet and Nutrition Survey, pp. 94–128. HMSO, London.

Gregory JR, Collins DL, Davies PSW, Hughes JM and Clarke PC (1995b) National Diet and Nutrition Survey: Children Aged 1½ to 4½ years, Vol. 1 Report of the Diet and Nutrition Survey, pp. 27–48. HMSO, London.

Habicht JP, Martorell R, Yarborough C, Malina RM and Klein RE (1974) Height and weight standards for preschool children. Lancet 1, 611–615.

Halterman JS, Kaczorowski JM, Aligne A, Auigner P and Szilagyi PG (2001) Iron deficiency and cognitive achievement among school age children and adolescents in the United States. Pediatr. 107, 1381–1386.

Hamadani JD, Fuchs GJ, Osendarp SJM, Khatun F, Huda SN and Grantham-McGregor SM (2001) Randomized controlled trial of the effects of zinc supplementation on the mental development of Bangladeshi infants. Am. J. Clin. Nutr. 74, 381–386.

Hambidge KM (1986) Zinc deficiency in the weanling. Acta Paediatr. Scand. 323 (Suppl.), 52–58.

Herman-Giddens ME, Wang L and Koch G (2001) Secondary sexual characteristics in boys: estimates from the national health and nutrition examination survey III, 1984–1994. Arch. Pediatr. Adolescent Med., 155, 1022–1028.

Hoare S, Poppitt SD, Prentice AM and Weaver LT (1996) Dietary supplementation and rapid catch-up growth after acute diarrhoea in childhood. Br. J. Nutr. 76, 479–490.

Hourihane JO and Rolles CJ (1995) Morbidity from excessive intake of high-energy fluids: the 'squash drinking syndrome'. Arch. Dis. Child. 73, 277.

Hunt JR (2001) How important is dietary iron bioavailability? Am. J. Clin. Nutr. 73, 3–4.

Husaini MA, Karyadi L, Husaini YK, Sandjaja Karyadi D and Pollitt E (1991) Developmental effects of short-term supplementary feeding in nutritionally at risk Indonesian infants. Am. J. Clin. Nutr. 54, 799–804.

James WPT and Ralph A (2000) Policy and a prudent diet. In: Human Nutrition and Dietetics, 10th edn, ed. Garrow JS, James WPT and Ralph A, pp. 837–845. Churchill Livingstone, Edinburgh.

Jeffrey DB, McLellarn RW and Fox DT (1982) The development of children's eating habits: the role of television commercials. *Health Educ. Q.* **9**, 174–189.

Klesges RC, Shelton ML and Klesges LM (1993) Effects of television on metabolic rate: potential implications for childhood obesity. *Pediatrics* **91**, 281–286.

Lee PA, Guo SS and Kulin HE (2001) Age of puberty: data from the United States of America. *APMIS* **2**, 81–88.

Lentner C (ed.) (1981) *Geigy Scientific Tables, 8th edition, Vol. I, Units of Measurement, Body Fluids, Composition of the Body, Nutrition.* Ciba-Geigy, Basel.

Logan S, Martins S and Gilbert R (2001) Iron therapy for improving psychomotor development and cognitive function in children under the age of 3 with iron deficiency. In: *Cochrane Library Issue*, Vol. 3. Oxford Update Software, Oxford.

Maberly GF (1994) Iodine deficiency disorders: contemporary scientific issues. *J. Nutr.* **124**(Suppl.), 1473S–1478S.

Mauras N (2001) Growth hormone and sex steroids. Interactions in puberty. *Endocrinol. Metab. Clin. N. Am.* **30**, 529–544.

McCarthy D (1974) Effects of emotional disturbance and deprivation (maternal rejection) on somatic growth. In: *Scientific Foundations of Paediatrics*, ed. Davis J and Dobbing J, pp. 56–67. William Heinemann Medical Press, London.

McKay H, Sinisterra L, McKay A, Gomez H and Lloreda P (1978) Improving cognitive ability in chronically deprived children. *Science* **200**, 270–278.

Merrilees MJ, Smart EJ, Gilchrist NL, Frampton C, Turner JG, Hooke E, March RL and Maguire P (2000) Effects of food supplements on bone mineral density in teenage girls. *Eur. J. Nutr.* **39**, 256–262.

Mul D, Fredriks AM, van Buuren S, Oostdijk W, Verloove-Vanhorick SP and Wit JM (2001) Pubertal development in the Netherlands 1965–1997. *Pediatr. Res.* **50**, 479–486.

Munoz EC, Rosado JL, Lopez P, Furr HC and Allen LH (2000) Iron and zinc supplementation improves indicators of vitamin A status of Mexican preschoolers. *Am. J. Clin. Nutr.* **71**, 789–794.

Needman RD (2000) Pre-school years. In: *Nelson Textbook of Pediatrics*, 16th edn, ed. Behrman RE, Kliegman RM and Jenson HB, pp. 43–50. WB Saunders, Philadelphia, PA.

O'Hare AE, Uttley WS, Belton NR, Westwood A, Levin SD and Anderson F (1984) Persisting vitamin D deficiency in the Asian adolescent. *Arch. Dis. Child.* **59**, 766–770.

Otero GA, Aguirre DM, Porcayo R and Fernandez T (1999) Psychological and electroencephalographic study in school children with iron deficiency. *Int. J. Neurosci.* **99**, 113–121.

Outila TA, Kärkkäinen MUM and Lamberg-Allardt CJE (2001) Vitamin D status affects serum parathyroid hormone concentrations during winter in female adolescents: associations with forearm bone mineral density. *Am. J. Clin. Nutr.* **74**, 206–210.

Parsons TJ, Power C, Logan S and Summerbell CD (1999) Childhood predictors of adult obesity. *Int. J. Obes.* **23**(Suppl 8), S1–S107.

Petter LP, Hourihane JO and Rolles CJ (1995) Is water out of vogue? A survey of the drinking habits of 2–7 year olds. *Arch. Dis. Child.* **72**, 137–140.

Pollitt E (2000) Developmental sequel from early nutritional deficiencies: conclusive and probability judgements. *J. Nutr.* **130**(Suppl.), 350S–353S.

Poskitt EME (1988) Vegetarian weaning. *Arch. Dis. Child.* **63**, 470–478.

Poskitt EME (2000) Body mass index and child obesity: are we nearing a definition? *Acta Paediatr. Scand.* **89** 507–509.

Poskitt EME and Cole TJ (1977) Do fat babies stay fat? *Br. Med. J.* **1**, 7–9.

Poskitt EME, Cole TJ and Lawson DEM (1979) Diet sunlight and 25-hydroxy vitamin D in healthy children and adults. *Br. Med. J.* **1** 221–223.

Poskitt EME, Cole TJ and Whitehead RG (1999) Less diarrhoea but no change in growth: 15 years' data from three Gambian villages. *Arch. Dis. Child.* **80**, 115–120.

Powell GF, Hopwood NJ and Barratt ES (1973) Growth hormone studies before and during catch-up growth in a child with emotional deprivation and short stature. *J. Clin. Endocrinol. Metab.* **37**, 674–679.

Powers HJ, Bates CJ, Prentice AM, Lamb WH, Jepson M and Bowman H (1983) The relative effectiveness of iron and iron with riboflavin in correcting microcytic anemia in men and children in rural Gambia. *Hum. Nutr. Clin. Nutr.* **37C**, 413–425.

Prasad AS (1998) Zinc and immunity. *Mol. Cell. Biol.* **188**, 63–69.

Prasad AS, Miale A, Farid Z, Schulert A and Sandstead HH (1963) Zinc metabolism in patients with iron deficiency anaemia, hypogonadism and dwarfism. *J. Lab. Clin. Med.* **61**, 557–549.

Rayner PH and Rudd BT (1973) Emotional deprivation in three siblings associated with functional pituitary growth hormone deficiency. *Aust. Paediatr. J.* **9**, 79–84.

Rivera JA, Gonzaalez-Cossio T, Flores M, Romero M, Rivera M, Tellez-Rojo MM, Rosado JL and Brown KH (2001) Multiple micronutrient supplementation increases the growth of Mexican infants. *Am. J. Clin. Nutr.* **74**, 657–663.

Roemmich JN and Rogol AD (1999) Hormonal changes during puberty and their relationship to fat distribution. *Am. J. Hum. Biol.* **11**, 209–224.

Rolland-Cachera M-F, Deheeger M, Guilloud-Bataille M, Avons P, Patois E and Sempe M (1984) Adiposity rebound in children: a simple indicator for predicting obesity. *Am. J. Clin. Nutr.* **39**, 129–135.

Rousham EK and Gracey M (1997) Persistent growth faltering among aboriginal infants and young children in North West Australia: a retrospective study from 1969–93. *Acta Paediatr.* **86**, 46–50.

Rudolf MCJ, Cole TJ, Krom AJ, Sahota P and Walker J (2000) Growth of primary school children: a validation of the 1990 references and their use in growth monitoring. *Arch. Dis. Child.* **83**, 298–301.

Sandstead HH, Prasad AS, Schulert AR, Farid Z, Miale A Jr, Bassilly S and Darby WJ (1967) Human zinc deficiency, endocrine manifestations and response to treatment. *Am. J. Clin. Nutr.* **20**, 422–442.

Tanner JM (1989) *Foetus into Man*, 2nd edn, p. 14. Castlemead, Hertford.

Tanner JM and Kelnar CJH (1992) Physical growth development and puberty. In: *Forfar & Arneil's Textbook of Paediatrics*, 4th edn, ed. Campbell AGM and McIntosh N, pp. 389–445.

Tanner JM and Whitehouse RH (1976) Clinical longitudinal standards for height, weight, height velocity, weight velocity and stages of puberty. *Arch. Dis. Child.* **51**, 170–179.

Tanner JM, Whitehouse RH and Takaishi M (1966) Standards from birth to maturity for height, weight, height velocity and weight velocity for British children in 1965. *Arch. Dis. Child.* **41**, 454–471.

Tanner JM, Whitehouse RH, Marshall WA and Carter BS (1975) Prediction of adult height from height bone age and occurrence of menarche at ages 4 to 16 with allowance for mid parent height. *Arch. Dis. Child.* **50**, 14–26.

Thu BD, Schultink W, Dillon D, Gross R, Leswara ND and Khoi HH (1999) Effect of daily and weekly micronutrient supplementation on micronutrient deficiencies and growth in young Vietnamese children. *Am. J. Clin. Nutr.* **69**, 80–86.

Truswell AS and Darnton-Hill I (1981) Food habits of adolescents. *Nutr. Rev.* **39**, 73–88.

UNICEF (2001) *The State of the World's Children 2002*. UNICEF, New York.

Walker SP, Grantham-McGregor SM, Powell CA and Chang SM (2000) Effects of growth restriction in early childhood on growth, IQ, and cognition at age 11 to 12 years and the benefits of nutritional supplementation and psychosocial stimulation. *J. Pediatr.* **137**, 36–41.

Walravens PA, Krebs NF and Hambidge KM (1983) Linear growth of low income preschool children receiving zinc supplement. *Am. J. Clin. Nutr.* **38**, 195–201.

Wang Y (2001) Cross-national comparison of childhood obesity: the epidemic and the relationship between obesity and socioeconomic status. *Int. J. Epidemiol.* **30**, 1129–1136.

Whincup PH, Gilg JA, Odoki K, Taylor SJC and Cook DG (2001) Age at menarche in contemporary British teenagers. A survey of girls born between 1982 and 1986. *Br. Med. J.* **322**, 1095–1096.

WHO (1973) *Nutritional Anemia*. WHO Technical Report Series no. 3. WHO, Geneva.

WHO (1982) *Prevention of Coronary Heart Disease*. Technical Report Series no. 678. WHO, Geneva.

WHO (1983) *Measuring Change in Nutritional Status*. WHO, Geneva.

WHO (1996) *Trace Elements in Human Nutrition and Health*, pp. 72–104. WHO, Geneva.

WHO (1998) *Management of the Child with Severe Malnutrition in Hospital*. WHO, Geneva.

Widdowson EM (1947) *A Study of Individual Children's Diets*. MRC Special Report series no. 257, p. 56. HMSO, London.

Widdowson EM (1981) Changes in body proportions and composition during growth. In: *Scientific Foundations of Paediatrics*, 2nd edn, ed. Davis J and Dobbing J, pp. 330–342. William Heinemann Medical Books, London.

World Cancer Research Fund (1997) *Food Nutrition and the Prevention of Cancer: a Global Perspective*. WCRF, London.

Youdin MBH (1990) Neuropharmacological and neurobiochemical aspect of iron deficiency. In: *Brain Behaviour and Iron in the Infant Diet*, ed. Dobbing J, pp. 83–106. Springer, London.

Zimmermann M, Adou P, Torresani T, Zeder C and Hurrell R (2000a) Effect of iodized oil on thyroid size and thyroid hormone metabolism in children with concurrent selenium and iodine deficiency. *Eur. J. Clin. Nutr.* **54**, 209–213.

Zimmermann M, Adou P, Torresani T, Zeder C and Hurrell R (2000b) Persistence of goiter despite oral iodine supplementation in goitrous children with iron deficiency anaemia in Côte d'Ivoire. *Am. J. Clin. Nutr.* **71**, 88–93.

12

PRACTICAL ADVICE ON FOOD AND NUTRITION FOR THE MOTHER, INFANT AND CHILD

Margaret Lawson

LEARNING OUTCOMES

- National and local nutrition policies should include practical information on foods and feeding during pregnancy, lactation for the infant and during childhood and should highlight the scientific evidence underpinning the advice. A policy should enable health-care workers to evaluate evidence and to translate it into relevant practice.

- It is important for infant health that women begin pregnancy with an adequate nutritional status, and maintain good nutritional health throughout pregnancy and lactation. In particular Department of Health advice on folic acid supplementation should be followed.

- The optimum method of feeding infants for the first 4–6 months of life is by exclusive breast-feeding. Women who choose not to breast-feed should be supported by advice on suitable infant formulas. Appropriate weaning foods can be introduced after the age of 4–6 months.

- Pre-school-aged children have high nutrient requirements and they may be influenced by psycho-social issues affecting food intake. It is important that pre-schoolchildren receive a flexible feeding regimen that is not 'adult' in content and is not too low in fat or too high in dietary fibre.

- School-age, pre-adolescent children have fewer nutritional problems than other age groups, and it is important that they receive both education about and practical examples of a healthy lifestyle, including a healthy diet.

- Adolescence is a time of rapid growth and high nutrient requirements; it is also a time when independence from parental influences and peer pressure may lead to a poor nutrient intake. It is a challenge to provide nutrition advice in the context of a holistic health message that is acceptable to teenagers.

- A number of nutritional and feeding problems may arise throughout childhood. These include gastro-intestinal disorders, food allergy, failure to thrive and obesity. Relevant and consistent advice on all of these topics needs to be formulated for carers and older children in order to maintain nutritional health.

Introduction

One of the roles of the health-care professional is to translate nutritional information generated from research and audit or from national guidelines or legislation into practical food-based advice that can be understood and followed by members of the larger population. To optimize health messages, coherent information and education should be given to the public by all members of the health-care team. In order for this to happen it is important that the team members are not left to make their own interpretation of research findings or legislation, with the risk that misleading and sometimes inaccurate messages are being conveyed. The drawing up and implementation of local food and nutrition policies for such aspects of health as pregnancy, infants and children is essential for the delivery of effective education. Audit of the impact of local food and nutrition policies will advise policy-makers of areas which remain sub-optimal and where further research or resources are required.

National nutrition policies and other policies which impact on nutrition have been in place for many years, but these are general policies for the population as a whole and historically in the UK have been more concerned with agriculture, food production and food safety than with health (Helsing, 1997).

Nutritional policies relating to health have been slow to develop in the UK (James *et al.*, 1997). Policies intended for mothers, infants and children are sparse compared with those in countries such as the USA, although the school meals scheme was introduced in England and Wales in 1906 and the Welfare Food Scheme throughout the UK in 1946. Policies such as the Food Stamp Scheme, the Special Supplemental Nutrition Program for Women, Infants and Children (WIC), the School Breakfast Program and the Summer Food Service Program have been in place in the USA for a number of years and have been shown to be effective in terms of delivery (Kennedy and Cooney, 2001) and in improving the nutritional status of vulnerable groups (Yip *et al.*, 1987).

An outline of examples of local food and nutrient initiatives is given in Figure 12.1. A Food and Nutrition Group is formed under the aegis of local health or local government agencies. In order for policies and guidelines to be successfully implemented, the support of such bodies that have statutory powers is vital. The Food and Nutrition Group has responsibility for developing strategies and policies to

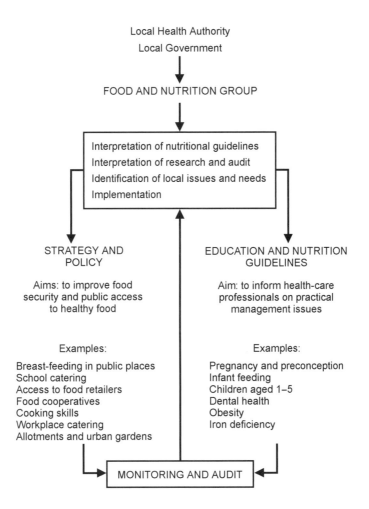

Local Health Authority
Local Government

FOOD AND NUTRITION GROUP

Interpretation of nutritional guidelines
Interpretation of research and audit
Identification of local issues and needs
Implementation

STRATEGY AND POLICY

Aims: to improve food security and public access to healthy food

Examples:

Breast-feeding in public places
School catering
Access to food retailers
Food cooperatives
Cooking skills
Workplace catering
Allotments and urban gardens

EDUCATION AND NUTRITION GUIDELINES

Aim: to inform health-care professionals on practical management issues

Examples:

Pregnancy and preconception
Infant feeding
Children aged 1–5
Dental health
Obesity
Iron deficiency

MONITORING AND AUDIT

Figure 12.1 Local nutrition policies

improve food security and access to healthy food for the population. This will involve liaising with statutory bodies (e.g. the local authority), schools, adult education institutions and private sector industry. Although it is vital to identify future directions at a corporate level, it is important that a document dealing with these matters is kept separate from documents dealing entirely with education and nutrition guidelines. Practical nutrition information should be easily accessible and understandable for health-care professionals imparting advice to the public. A detailed discussion on strategy and social policy is

outside the remit of this book – for a review see Grossman and Webb (1991).

A local nutrition policy is likely to form part of a more widely based local health policy that addresses a number of health issues, including nutrition. The membership of a Nutrition Education Group should be drawn from as wide a range of health professionals as possible. Key members of a group preparing a policy for infants and young children would comprise paediatric dietitians, community dietitians and nutritionists, paediatricians, health visitors, midwives, practice nurses, school nurses, clinical psychologists, speech and language therapists, dentists and health promotion personnel. Consultation with all target groups should be sought before the policy is launched.

The overall objectives of such a group might be: to encourage consistent health messages given by health professionals; to make available to health professionals a scientifically based and current document on which to base advice; to provide advice and information to the population. This chapter gives examples of recommendations that might be contained in a local nutrition policy aimed at educating health-care professionals. It translates the scientific evidence contained in the preceding chapters into food-based practical advice. In general the practical advice given here as an illustration is designed for the UK, but the interpretation and translation of evidence contained in the book may differ according to the environment and local conditions. Material in Chapters 1, 3, 5 and 7–12 should be read in relation to this chapter.

Preconception, Pregnancy and Lactation

Rationale for policy

Nutrition before conception and during pregnancy and lactation have been discussed in Chapters 2 and 3, which give details of the scientific evidence which underpins a preconception, pregnancy and lactation nutrition policy.

In well-nourished Western societies the demands of pregnancy and lactation are generally met by a balanced healthy diet. Women are receptive to advice at this time and advice and counselling should be available to all women both before conception and throughout pregnancy. Local policies should take into account the proportion of the population that is at particular risk of starting pregnancies with

Table 12.1 Women at risk of sub-optimum pregnancy outcome

History of previous obstetric difficulties
History of previous neural tube defect
*Body mass index <20 or >30
Adolescents
Women who smoke
Women with alcohol or recreational drug problems
Low income
Ethnic minority groups with English as second language
Women on restricted diets, e.g. vegan, macrobiotic
Short interval since last birth (<2 years between births)
Families with history of atopic disease

*Body mass index $= wt(kg)/ht(m)^2$.

a nutritional deficit or who may become deficient during their pregnancy. Table 12.1 gives examples of such groups, and these should be targeted for health education.

The recommended dietary intake for many nutrients is not increased during pregnancy and lactation (see Tables 5.1 and 5.2). Recommendations for supplemental folic acid (Department of Health, 1991, 2000) have been published. Guidance on alcohol consumption has been made (Department of Health, 1995) and guidance for food hygiene has been given (Department of Health, 1996). There is no universally agreed optimum weight gain during pregnancy; the recommendations used here are based on those made by Feig and Naylor (1998), although other recommendations are discussed in Chapters 3 and 5.

Practical measures

Preconception

Women should be encouraged to adopt a healthy lifestyle 3–6 months before they plan to conceive. They should also check that they are immune to *Rubella* well before conception.

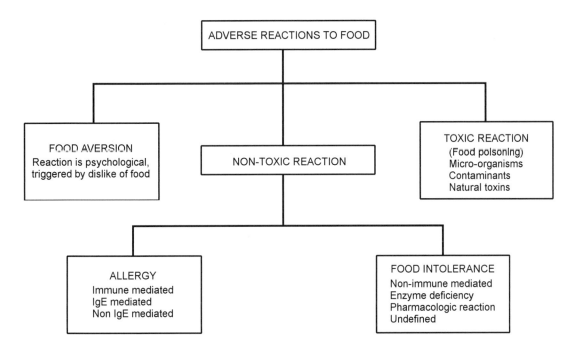

Figure 12.2 Adverse reactions to food

Table 12.2 Dietary sources of some minerals and trace elements

Mineral	Food source
Calcium	Nuts, pulses, wheat flour and wheat products, spinach[a] Milk, cheese, fish eaten with bones
Phosphorus	Wholegrain, cereals and wholewheat products, nuts, pulses, soft drinks[a] Fish eaten with bones
Magnesium	Green vegetables, wholegrain cereals, nuts[a]
Iron	Wholegrain cereals, fortified breakfast cereals, pulses, dark green vegetables[a] Liver, meat, egg yolk
Zinc	Wholegrain cereals, nuts[a] Shellfish, meat
Copper	Green vegetables, pulses, nuts[a] Liver, fish, shellfish
Selenium	Wholegrain cereals[a] Liver, meat, fish
Iodine	Vegetables[a] Milk, egg, fish, shellfish, meat
Chromium	Yeast, wholegrain cereals, pulses, nuts[a] Meat

[a]Non-animal sources.

Table 12.3 Dietary sources of essential fatty acids

Omega 3 – α-linolenic acid
Fatty fish
Seed oils – rapeseed
Marine oils
Meat
Cereal
Green leafy vegetables

Omega 6 – linoleic acid
Plant oils – soya
              corn
              sunflower
              safflower
Nuts
Vegetables
Cereals

Preconceptionally women should stop smoking, avoid alcohol (or maximum 1 unit per day), stop the use of recreational drugs and review usage of over-the-counter and prescribed medicines (for drugs which potentially harm the fetus see Table 5.3). The contraceptive pill should be stopped 4–8 weeks prior to the planned conception and barrier contraceptive methods substituted.

A healthy diet based on cereals and starchy foods (see Figure 9.9) should be followed. It is particularly important that women begin pregnancy with adequate iron stores (see Table 12.2 for dietary sources of iron) and adequate intakes of essential fatty acids (Table 12.3).

Body mass index (BMI) ideally should be $23–24\,kg/m^2$ at conception. Women with a

Table 12.4 Dietary sources of vitamins

Vitamin	Food source
Vitamin A	*Carotene*: dark green vegetables, carrots, yellow/orange fruit[a]
	Added to margarine
	Retinol: liver, fish oils, milk, butter, egg
Vitamin D	Added to margarine
	Egg, oily fish
Vitamin E	Vegetable oils, whole grain cereals[a]
	Butter, egg
Vitamin K	Dark green vegetables[a]
	Liver
Thiamine, vitamin B_1	Wholegrain cereals, yeast, nuts, pulses[a]
	Liver, meat
Riboflavin, vitamin B_2	Yeast[a]
	Milk, egg
Niacin	Yeast, wholegrain cereals, peanuts[a]
	Meat, fish, liver
Biotin	Wholegrain cereals[a]
	Milk, egg, meat, fish
Pyrodoxine, vitamin B_6	Wholegrain cereals, peanuts, bananas[a]
	Egg, liver, meat, fish
Cobalamin, vitamin B_{12}	Egg, milk, liver, meat, fish
Pantothenic acid	Wholegrain cereals, vegetables[a]
	Egg, milk, meat, fish
Ascorbic acid, vitamin C	Citrus fruits, berry fruits, green vegetables, potatoes[a]
Folic acid	Green vegetables, fruit, nuts, pulses, yeast extract[a]
	Egg, liver

[a]Non-animal sources.

Table 12.5 Folic acid content of foods

More than 50 µg per average serving		20–50 µg per average serving	
Food	Quantity of folic acid/serving (µg)	Food	Quantity of folic acid/serving (µg)
Brussels sprouts	100	Cauliflower	45
Spinach	80	Peas	40
Broccoli	60	Potatoes	
Green beans	50	old	45
Orange (peeled)	60	new	35
Black-eyed beans	130	Carrot	25
Yeast or malt extract	95	Spring greens	25
e.g. Marmite (1 teaspoon)		Chick peas	30
Fortified breakfast cereal	100	Baked beans	30
		Milk (500 ml)	35
		Yoghurt (1 carton)	25
		Bread (two slices[a])	
		wholemeal/granary	30
		white	20
		Chapatti (two medium)	20

[a]Some bread is fortified with folic acid, and will provide larger quantities.

BMI <20 prior to conception need to gain weight, since they are at increased risk of a preterm or low-birth-weight baby. Very overweight women should allow a longer time scale and should aim to reduce their BMI to <30 2–3 months prior to conception. This will enable them to adopt a more nutrient-dense diet before they become pregnant.

A folic acid supplement of 400 µg per day is recommended for 3–6 months prior to conception and should be continued up until the 12th week of pregnancy. In cases where a previous pregnancy has resulted in a child with a neural tube defect, women should take a prescribed supplement of 5 mg folate daily. In addition 200 µg folic acid should be consumed in the diet (see Tables 12.4 and 12.5 for sources).

Pregnancy

No alcohol should be consumed for the first 12 weeks of pregnancy; thereafter up to one unit per day is not thought to cause any adverse outcome. The use of substitution therapy should be considered for pregnant women who have a chronic drug abuse habit.

Since infection by *Toxoplasma*, *Listeria*, *Campylobacter* and *Salmonella* can damage the unborn child, particular care must be taken with food hygiene. Specifically, pregnant women should not consume raw or lightly cooked eggs, undercooked poultry or shellfish, unpasteurized milk or products made from these, mould-ripened cheeses (Brie, Camembert), blue-veined cheeses, liver or meat patés.

From the 12th week of pregnancy the diet should provide 300 µg folate per day (see Tables 12.4 and 12.5). To avoid large intakes of vitamin A, pregnant women should avoid liver, liver paté, liver sausage and fish liver oils.

A balanced diet providing foods from all food groups should be followed during pregnancy (Figure 9.9). Women from some cultural groups restrict some foods during pregnancy and consume other foods preferentially as they believe foods may have an effect on pregnancy outcome. There is no harm in these practices,

Table 12.6   Diets for cow's milk protein allergy and lactose intolerance

Food	Cow's milk protein free	Low lactose
Milks	Cow's milk not suitable Goat or sheep milk may be tolerated	None suitable
Cheese/yoghurt/ice cream/cream	Cow's milk products not suitable Goat and sheep products may be tolerated	Yoghurt and ice cream not suitable Hard cheese and double cream have < 1 g lactose/100 g and may be tolerated
Butter and margarine	Butter not suitable Check margarine ingredients	Butter usually tolerated Check margarine ingredients
Special infant formulas	Low lactose milks not suitable Hydrolysed and soya formulas usually tolerated	Low-lactose milk, hydrolysed and soya formulas all suitable
Eggs	Suitable	Suitable
Soya products	Soya milk, cheese and desserts usually tolerated	Soya milk, cheese and desserts all suitable
Unprocessed meat, fish, poultry	Suitable	Suitable
Unprocessed fruit, vegetables and pulses	Suitable	Suitable
Proprietary infant weaning foods and infant cereals	May contain milk – check ingredients	May contain milk – check ingredients
Breakfast cereals	May contain milk – check ingredients	Most adult varieties suitable
Breads, flour, rice, oats, dry pasta	Suitable	Suitable
Cakes, biscuits and pastry	May contain milk – check ingredients	May contain milk – check ingredients
Sugar, soft and fizzy drinks	Suitable	Suitable
All processed foods	May contain milk – check ingredients	May contain milk – check ingredients

Milk substitutes – see Table 12.14 for details of milks suitable for infants and prescribability.
Infants and children with lactose intolerance – low-lactose infant formula or infant soya formula.
Infants and children with milk protein intolerance – infant soya formula or extensively hydrolysed infant formula.
Children >2 years and adults – calcium-fortified adult soya milk.

provided a varied and balanced diet is taken, but there is no evidence to support these beliefs.

Fluid intake should be 1.5–21 per day throughout pregnancy. Women who consume large quantities of caffeine should restrict their intake to a maximum of 4 cups of tea/coffee or cola drinks per day. Ground coffee is particularly high in caffeine.

Women with a family history of atopic disease may sensitize their infant *in utero* and may wish to avoid peanuts throughout pregnancy. Evidence to support the restriction of cow's milk and milk products during the last trimester of pregnancy is inconclusive. If milk is avoided it is important to ensure that the rest of the diet contains sufficient calcium and riboflavin and supplements may be needed. See Table 12.6 for details of a milk-free diet.

Nausea and vomiting during the early weeks of pregnancy can be alleviated by the consumption of frequent small starchy snacks. It is important to maintain an adequate fluid intake even when feeling nauseous.

The optimum weight gain during pregnancy is 6.8–11.4 kg. There should be little or no weight gain for the first 20 weeks. Energy requirements are increased by approximately 200 kcal/day for the last trimester.

Women who begin pregnancy overweight or obese should not follow a very restricted diet

Table 12.7 Foods which supply iron in the diet

Contains easily absorbed iron	Containing less easily absorbed iron – always eat with a source of vitamin C
Breast milk	Fortified baby milks
	Bread (white/brown/wholemeal)
Meat – lamb, beef, corned beef, pork, ham, bacon, sausages, burgers, liver, liver paté, liver sausage, kidney, chicken, turkey	Flour, pastry, chappatti
	Malt bread, dried fruit cake, ginger cake
	Digestive and ginger biscuits
	Wholemeal spaghetti and pasta
Oily fish – tuna, sardines, mackerel, pilchards, trout, kippers, salmon, fish paste, taramasalata, white fish, fish fingers	Breakfast cereal/rusks with extra iron
	Beans – kidney, haricot, mung, chick peas, baked beans, peas
	Lentils and dhal
	Nuts (no whole nuts under 5 years)
	Peanut butter, tahini, humus, tofu
	Curry powder and pastes, spices
	Egg yolk
	Dark green vegetables – broccoli, spinach, Brussels sprouts, green cabbage, watercress
	Mushrooms, sweet potato, tomato, avocado
	Prunes, raisins, sultanas, dried apricots, dates
	Chocolate, cocoa powder, liquorice

during their pregnancy as this increases the risk of a preterm or low-birth-weight infant. Weight gain should be the minimum recommended (6.8 kg).

An adequate intake of iron is important, although iron requirements are not increased. Iron supplements are commonly prescribed but these should be in response to haematological signs of deficiency. It should be possible to obtain sufficient iron from the diet (see Tables 12.7 and 12.8). Women following a meat-free diet are particularly vulnerable to iron deficiency. Table 12.9 gives suggestions for increasing iron in non-meat diets.

A supplement of 10 μg per day of vitamin D is recommended if the mother is not obtaining sufficient from the diet (see Table 12.4) and from exposure to sunlight. Asian women who customarily cover their body in public are particularly prone to vitamin D deficiency (with sequelae for both the infant and the mother's health) and they should be encouraged to take a supplement of 10 μg, particularly during the last trimester.

Although no additional intake of calcium, magnesium and zinc is recommended during pregnancy, the usual intake of these minerals in women in the UK is low, and women

Table 12.8   Snacks which are high in iron

Liver paté sandwich or on toast	Cornflakes/iron-fortified cereal and milk with $\frac{1}{2}$ glass grapefruit juice
Fish or meat paste sandwich or on toast	
Bacon sandwich	Drinking chocolate and iron-fortified toddler/junior milk
Hot dog sausage in bread roll	Baby rusk, butter and banana
Taramasalata and pitta bread	Dried apricots
Peanut butter sandwich or on toast with $\frac{1}{2}$ glass fresh orange juice	Slice of fruit cake or dark ginger cake with 1 glass apple juice
Humus and tortilla chips with two small tomatoes	Two chocolate digestive biscuits with six strawberries
Small packet of Twiglets with $\frac{1}{2}$ glass fruit cordial	Two slices of malt bread and butter/margarine with $\frac{1}{2}$ glass pineapple juice
Baked beans on toast with small green salad	
Portion of dhal and chappatti with slice of mango	Small packet of mixed nuts with 1 orange
	Small packet of nuts and raisins with kiwi fruit

Table 12.9   Increasing the iron in non-meat/vegetarian diets

- Use peas, beans and lentils to add to vegetable stews (canned beans are just as good as dried ones and take less time to prepare)
- Use baked beans as the basis of a meal
- Make your own 'veggieburgers' using lentils, potato and egg
- Wholemeal pasta with a tomato sauce will give both iron and vitamin C
- Add tahini or peanut butter to vegetable dishes
- Curry powder, pastes and curry spices are rich in iron (mild curries can be given to children)
- Use dhal to accompany curries
- Add ground almonds or other ground nuts to desserts such as yoghurt or milk puddings
- Use dried raisins, sultanas, apricots and dates in desserts and cakes
- Cow's milk is low in iron. Adults and children over the age of 2 years can use a liquid soya milk, which is higher in iron. For children between the ages of 1 and 2 years continued use of a fortified infant formula or follow-on milk should be considered
- Do not drink tea with meals

should be encouraged to choose foods that are rich sources (Tables 12.2 and 12.10). Additional intake of the B vitamins, thiamine and riboflavin and of vitamins C and A is recommended, in addition to folate (see above). Food sources of these are listed in Table 12.4.

If there is concern over the micronutrient content of the diet a multivitamin/mineral supplement may be useful. A number are marketed as being suitable for pregnancy. No more than 100 per cent of the Reference Nutrient Intake (RNI) should be taken as a daily supplement. In particular, supplements

containing more than 1250 µg vitamin A are contraindicated during pregnancy.

Long-chain polyunsaturated fatty acids, synthesized in the body from essential fatty acids, are particularly important during pregnancy and women who do not consume many green vegetables or wholegrain cereals may be at risk of deficiency of the omega 6 series (see Table 12.3 for food sources).

Women who follow a restricted diet – vegan, macrobiotic or fruitarian – are at particular risk of nutrient deficiency, and a vitamin/mineral supplement containing vitamin B_{12} may be important.

Table 12.10 Calcium content of foods

> 500 mg per serving		250–500 mg per serving		100–250 mg per serving	
Food	Quantity of calcium/serving (mg)	Food	Quantity of calcium/serving (mg)	Food	Quantity of calcium/serving (mg)
Milk – whole or low fat (500 ml)	680	Hard (Cheddar) cheese	250	Bread (two slices) brown or white	100
Soya milk – fortified (500 ml)	680	Yoghurt (1 carton)	250	Fish – salmon (canned) or prawns	100
Fish –		Fish – Pilchards (canned)	300		
whitebait	860	Almonds	250	Broccoli	100
sardines (canned)	550			Watercress	100
Tofu	510			Dried apricots	100
Spinach	600			Dried figs	140
				Stewed rhubarb	100
				Brazil nuts	180
				Milk chocolate	110

Lactation

A balanced healthy diet should be followed during lactation, with particular emphasis on dairy foods and those that supply calcium (Figure 9.9 and Tables 12.2 and 12.10). An adequate fluid intake of at least 2 l per day should be consumed throughout lactation. Despite a number of myths and beliefs, there is no evidence that particular foods are 'good' or 'bad' during lactation, nor that some foods encourage or inhibit milk production.

Alcohol consumption during lactation is permitted in moderation (1–2 units/day), although alcohol is secreted into the breast milk and is likely to make the infant sleepy. Spicy and strongly flavoured foods such as chilli and onions may cause loose stools in the infant. There is no particular reason to avoid such foods, unless the infant has diarrhoea, although many mothers choose to do so.

Since food antigens can pass into breast milk, some infants may experience colic or become sensitized to proteins such as milk. Where there is a strong family history of atopy or where siblings have had food allergic symptoms in early life there may be some advantage to keeping the consumption of milk and milk products to a minimum during lactation. It is extremely important that a milk-free diet (see Table 12.6) during lactation contains alternative sources of calcium, riboflavin and protein.

A supplement of vitamins A, D and C or a multivitamin supplement for pregnancy is advisable for women whose diet is poor.

Feeding the Infant

Rationale for policy

Nutrition during infancy is particularly important for a number of reasons. During infancy the need for energy and nutrients on a per kilogram weight basis is higher than at any other time of life and compromised growth during the early months of life may be associated with long-term physical and cognitive problems. Recommendations for nutrient intake for infants are given in Tables 8.7 and 11.5.

The topic of breast-feeding has been fully discussed in Chapter 8 and will not be repeated here. The advantages of breast-feeding should be summarized at the beginning of a written infant feeding policy so that health-care professionals give a consistent message when advising parents.

Although breast-feeding is acknowledged as providing optimum nutrition for the young infant, the incidence and prevalence of breast-feeding after the first few months of life is low in many industrialized and developing countries. In the UK data from the 1995 Infant Feeding Survey (Foster et al., 1997) show a modest rise in the incidence of breast-feeding over the past decade, but the UK still lags behind other some European regions such as Scandinavia (Zetterstrom, 1999). The majority of mothers give up breast-feeding because they feel that they are producing insufficient milk to meet their infant's needs. Asian immigrants to the UK have a higher incidence of breast-feeding, but a much higher attrition rate (Thomas and Avery, 1997). Good support in the antenatal clinic, the hospital maternity unit and the community are likely to improve the incidence and duration of breast-feeding, but midwives in one study felt that their training

on practical aspects of breast-feeding was inadequate (Jaegar et al., 1997). WHO/UNICEF set up the Baby-Friendly Initiative during the 1980s to improve breast-feeding rates worldwide and have suggested 10 steps to successful breast-feeding, which include having a written breast-feeding policy (WHO, 1989; see Table 12.11).

The following points need to be considered when drawing up a policy for infant feeding for the first year. They have been largely derived from the most recent advice issued by the UK Department of Health (1988, 1991, 1994a).

Breast-feeding

Health-care professionals should be committed to the promotion, establishment and maintenance of full breast-feeding for all infants for 4–6 months or longer. Recently the World Health Assembly has changed its recommendations and has recommended that women exclusively breast-feed for a minimum of 6 months (see Chapter 9). It is unclear whether this recommendation will be adopted fully in the UK. There are few contraindications to breast-feeding. Infants with some inborn errors of metabolism, particularly galactosaemia,

Table 12.11   Ten steps to a baby-friendly environment

1. Have a written policy that is routinely communicated to all health-care staff
2. Train all health-care staff in skills necessary to implement this policy
3. Inform all pregnant women about the benefits and management of breast-feeding
4. Help mothers initiate breast-feeding within half an hour of birth
5. Show mothers how to breast-feed and how to maintain lactation even if they should be separated from their infants
6. Give newborn infants no food or drink other than breast-milk, unless medically indicated
7. Practice rooming-in so that mothers and infants can remain together 24 h a day
8. Encourage breast-feeding on demand
9. Give no artificial teats, pacifiers or soothers to breast-fed infants
10. Foster the establishment of breast-feeding support groups and refer mothers to them on discharge from hospital

Adapted from WHO/UNO (1989).

cannot receive breast milk. Maternal contra-indications include drug abuse, treatment with some prescription drugs and active tuberculosis. The position of women who are HIV-positive is less clear-cut. Where there is an alternative to breast milk in the form of safe water supplies and affordable suitable infant formula, women should consider whether the risks of vertical transmission outweigh the benefits of breast-feeding. In countries where these facilities are not universally available, breast-feeding is probably the safer option (Fowler *et al.*, 2000).

The necessary advice, reassurance and practical help to support breast-feeding should be available both immediately after delivery and in the mother's own home after discharge from hospital. The subject of infant feeding should be discussed with every parent early in pregnancy to enable ample time for decision-making before delivery. The benefits of exclusive breast-feeding for the infant and for the mother should be clearly pointed out.

Practical measures

Babies should be put to the breast as soon as possible (ideally within half an hour) after delivery. Mothers and babies should not be separated after birth and should be accommodated together in the same room.

Good positioning at the breast is important for successful breast-feeding; the baby should be supported so that he or she faces the breast without having to turn the head. The baby should have easy access to the nipple and should be brought to the breast so that both mother and baby are in a comfortable position during feeding. In order to empty the breast efficiently the baby must 'latch on' to the breast. This means that enough of the areola is drawn into the mouth to stimulate the mother's lactiferous sinuses and requires that the infant's mouth is opened sufficiently wide to accomplish this. Health-care professionals should be given the opportunity to watch successful breast-feeds before offering advice to mothers.

Babies should be demand fed and should not have a timetable imposed on them. Very young babies may need feeding very frequently, every 1–2 h, until a good milk supply is established. Feeding frequency decreases to an average of 8–9 times daily at 4 weeks and 6–7 times daily by age 4 months. Frequent feeding stimulates milk production and mothers who are exclusively breast-feeding should not feed less than six times daily during the first 3 months. Babies who are very sleepy may need waking for feeds.

Duration of feeding varies both between infants and in the same infant at different times during the day; the usual duration is 4–20 min per breast; younger infants are slower feeders than older ones. Infants signify that milk supply is exhausted or that they have fed sufficiently by changing their pattern of suckling or by sleeping.

Infants usually nurse from both breasts at each feeding session, although it is not essential to do so. Milk production is increased by frequent emptying of the breast; in addition the energy density of hind milk, produced towards the end of a feed, is higher than that produced at the beginning. For these reasons the first breast should be emptied before nursing from the second breast, and the first breast offered at each feed should be alternated.

Newborn infants should not be offered any fluids other than breast milk unless medically prescribed. The practice of giving infant formula, water or dextrose as a drink in between feeds should be strongly discouraged. The use of 'dummies' or pacifiers should likewise be discouraged at least until breast-feeding has become established.

Where breast-feeding is slow to become established it is important to take steps to maximize milk production by ensuring that the infant is latching on, that breasts are being emptied regularly and that feeding is sufficiently frequent. Undue emphasis should not be placed on the infant's weight and mothers should be reassured and supported so that they have confidence to persevere.

Where there is real concern over an infant's progress or there are perceived feeding difficulties the mother can express her milk and it can be given to the infant using a sterilized spoon or small cup. After lactation has become established (usually by about 2 weeks), then 'complementary' feeds, preferably of expressed breast milk, can be given from a bottle.

Formula-feeding

Whilst exclusive breast-feeding is acknowledged as being the optimum regimen for infants, the opinions and wishes of mothers who decide not to breast-feed should be respected; mothers should not be made to feel guilty once they have made a firm decision. Formula feeding should be discussed with all mothers during pregnancy. Mothers who decide to introduce formula feeds after discharge from hospital need to know the correct procedure for sterilization of equipment and

reconstitution of powdered formula. Alternatives to human milk for infant feeding are discussed in Chapter 8.

A variety of formulas suitable for newborn infants should be available in maternity units to avoid endorsement of a particular company's products.

Practical measures

There are a number of types of formula suitable for infant feeding. A whey-dominant feed is generally acknowledged as having a composition similar to human milk, and this type of formula is generally recommended for the first 3–4 months. Casein-dominant formulas, although having a slightly different composition, are also safe to use from birth, though they are more generally recommended after the age of 3–4 months. Table 12.12 gives details of compositional recommendations and nutrient content of these types of milk.

Many brands of milk are available as a powder, which is reconstituted with water, as a

Table 12.12 Compositional recommendations and nutrient composition of infant milk suitable from birth

Nutrient	Recommendation per 100 ml milk		Nutrient composition per 100 ml milk	
	Whey-dominant	Casein-dominant	Whey-dominant, e.g. SMA Gold[a]	Casein-dominant, e.g. Milumil[a]
Protein (g)	1.2–2.0	1.5–2.0	1.5	1.9
Energy (kcal)	60–75		67	69
(kJ)	250–315		280	290
Fat (g)	2.9–4.4		3.6	3.1
Carbohydrate (g)	4.2–10.5		7.2	8.4
Sodium (mg)	13.4–40.2		15.0	24.0
Calcium (mg)	Minimum 30		42.0	71.0
Iron (mg)	0.34–1.0		0.6	0.4
Vitamin C (mg)	Minimum 4.8		5.5	7.6
Vitamin D (µg)	0.6–1.87		1.0	1.0

EC Commision Directive 91/321/EC (OJ no. L175, 4.7.91). EC Commision Directive 96/4/EC (OJ no. L49, 28.2.96).
[a]Infant milk brands available in 2002 in the UK include: whey dominant – SMA gold (Wyeth), Premium (Nutricia), Aptamil (Milupa), Farley's First Milk; casein dominant – Milumil (Milupa), Plus (Nutricia), SMA White (Wyeth), Farley's Second Milk.

liquid concentrate that is diluted with water, or as a ready-to-feed preparation in a carton that can be decanted into a feeding bottle. Parents need to be informed about the relative merits and cost of each type of preparation.

All equipment for infant feeding must be sterilized for the first 6 months. After 6 months baby bottles and teats still need to be sterilized. Methods for sterilization comprise boiling in water for 10 min, soaking in suitable chemical sterilizing solution for a minimum of 30 min or steam sterilization following the manufacturer's instructions.

All babymilks in the UK are reconstituted using one level manufacturer's scoop of milk powder (approximately 3.6 g) for each 30 ml water. Outside the UK it is important to follow the manufacturer's instructions as there may be a different recipe. Water for reconstituting babymilk should be boiled at least until 6 months of age and longer if there is any doubt about the microbiological safety of the water supply. Water should be from a mains supply or bottled water with a sodium content of less than 10 mg/100 ml. Water softened with an ion-exchange system, natural mineral water, effervescent water and repeatedly boiled water should not be used as the sodium content is likely to be unacceptably high.

Follow-on formulas contain more protein and sodium than 'starter' formulas (see Table 12.13). In the UK they are not recommended for use before the age of 6 months; use is recommended to discontinue at the age of 1 year, when cow's milk is appropriate as the main drink. Follow-on formulas generally contain more iron than 'starter formulas' and may be advantageous where there is concern over iron deficiency (see section on iron nutrition in this chapter).

Bottle-fed infants should be fed on demand, and will move gradually from feeding 2–3 hourly to 4 hourly by about 8–10 weeks of age. The average fluid requirement for the first few months of life is approximately 150 ml/kg body weight.

Young infants require no food other than breast or modified formula milk for the first 4–6 months of life. Substances such as sugar, cereal or flavourings should never be added to baby bottles.

It is common for mothers to change the brand and/or the type of milk that they give their baby because they perceive that the baby is not satisfied. In theory casein-dominant milks empty from the stomach more slowly than whey-dominant milks. There are some disadvantages to continually changing milks: infants are sensitive to taste from a young age and introducing a variety of milks may confuse the infant. Other reasons for fractious behaviour such as colic, over- or underfeeding should be sought before recommending a change of formula.

Failure to gain adequate weight is not an indicator for changing the feed (see Failure to Thrive section), and a feed change may delay the diagnosis of an underlying condition. Where the mother feels that the baby is hungry, a feed change is preferable to the introduction of solid foods before the age of 4 months.

Table 12.13 Compositional recommendations and nutrient composition of follow-on formulas

	Recommendation per 100 ml milk	Content per 100 ml milk, e.g. Step Up[a]
Energy		
kJ	250–335	295
kcal	60–80	70
Protein (g)	1.6–3.15	1.8
Fat (g)	2.3–4.6	3.8
Carbohydrate (g)	4.9–9.8	7.2
Sodium (mg)	20–60	24
Vitamin D (μg)	0.7–2.1	2.1
Iron (mg)	0.7–1.4	1.3

EEC Commission Directive 91/321/EC (OJ no. L175/35, 4.7.91).
[a]Follow-on formulas available in 2002 in the UK, Europe and the USA include: Step Up (Nutricia), Progress (Wyeth), Milumil 3 (Milupa), Farley's Junior Milk.

Combined breast- and bottle-feeding

The introduction of 'complementary' milk feeds to breast-fed infants should be strongly discouraged whilst lactation is becoming established. However by the age of 3–4 months almost half of mothers in the UK who initially breast-fed their babies are giving some formula milk whilst continuing to breast-feed. Although exclusive breast-feeding is optimum for the infant, giving additional formula may enable mothers to continue to provide some breast-milk rather than abandon breast-feeding entirely, and health-care professionals should support mothers in their decision.

Other milks

Table 12.14 describes milks which may be used in some circumstances during infancy. Infants should receive an appropriately modified infant formula for at least the first year of life. Unmodified cow, goat and sheep milk is unsuitable as a main drink under the age of 1 year. All unmodified milks have a high renal solute load (due to a high protein and sodium content) and are low in iron and a number of important vitamins. After the age of 1 year goat and sheep milk can be used if parents wish, but all milk should be pasteurized and a suitable B vitamin supplement containing the RNI for folate should be used if there are any concerns over the adequacy of the rest of the diet.

Infant soya milks are suitable for use from birth onwards and are mainly used for infants with suspected or proven intolerance to cow's milk protein or lactose. Unmodified liquid soya milks are not suitable for use in children under the age of 1 year. Modified infant soya milks contain a similar level and range of nutrients to infant formula, and recommendations for micronutrient supplements are the same. Soya milks generally do not contain

foods originating from animals and are suitable for infants receiving a vegan diet – the Vegan Society (www.vegansociety.com) will supply the names of approved infant soya formulas. Soya formulas can be used to treat intolerances to milk protein or lactose, but have not been proved to be useful in preventing the development of allergy in high-risk infants (Zeiger, 2000).

Drinks other than milk

Infants need no fluid other than an adequate volume of breast milk or infant formula until the beginning of weaning with the introduction of solid foods after the age of 4 months. Rarely, if the infant is losing additional fluid because of sweating due to very high ambient temperatures or fever, diarrhoea or vomiting, then cooled boiled water can be given in between feeds. Fruit juice, baby juices and infant herbal teas are not a necessary part of the diet at any age. At the start of weaning the normal volume of breast milk or infant formula should be maintained. Once the infant is able to eat more than about 100 g purée foods per meal then one breast or bottle feed can be dropped and the fluid replaced by boiled water at the mealtime.

Weaning

Weaning is fully discussed in Chapter 9. The recommendations in this section are derived from the Department of Health (1994a). In Table 11.12 nutritional issues surrounding the developmental milestones from infancy to adulthood are described.

Foods other than milk should not be necessary before the age of 4 months. Nutritionally, milk supplies the whole of an infant's requirements until birth-weight has doubled. Young infants have poor head control and oro-motor development is not sufficient to permit

Table 12.14 Infant formulas adapted for special needs

Formula	Main ingredients	Characteristics	Recommended for	Prescribable*
SMA AR (Wyeth)	Whey + thickener	Pre-thickened milk	Gastro-oesophagal reflux	Yes
Emfamil AR (Mead Johnson)	Casein + whey + thickener	Pre-thickened milk	Gastro-oesophagal reflux	Yes
SMA LF (Wyeth)	Whey	Low lactose milk	Lactose intolerance	Yes
Enfamil Lactofree (Mead Johnson)	Casein + whey	Low lactose milk	Lactose intolerance	Yes
AL 110 (Nestlé)	Casein + whey	Low lactose milk	Lactose intolerance	Yes
Omneocomfort 1, Omneocomfort 2 (Cow + Gate)	Partially hydrolysed whey and thickener	Partially hydrolysed, pre-thickened, low lactose	Colic: Omneocomfort 1 for babies <6 months; Omneocomfort 2 for babies >6 months	No
Alfaré (Nestlé)	Extensively hydrolysed whey	Extensive hydrolysate, low lactose and medium chain triglycerides	Milk protein intolerance	Yes
Nutramigen (Mead Johnson)	Extensively hydrolysed casein	Extensive hydrolysate, low lactose	Milk protein intolerance	Yes
Peptijunor (Cow and Gate)	Extensively hydrolysed whey	Extensive hydrolysate, low lactose	Milk protein intolerance	Yes
Prejomin (Milupa)	Extensively hydrolysed soy and pork	Extensive hydrolysate, low lactose	Milk protein intolerance	Yes
Infatrini (Cow and Gate)	Whey and additional nutrients	High-energy infant formula (100 kcal/100 ml)	Malnutrition and failure to thrive	Yes
SMA High Energy (Wyeth)	Whey and additional nutrients	High-energy infant formula (91 kcal/100 ml)	Malnutrition and failure to thrive	Yes
Infasoy (Cow and Gate) Ostersoy (Farley's) Prosobee (Mead Johnson) Wysoy (Wyeth)	Soy protein isolate	Soy-based infant feed, lactose free	Malnutrition and failure to thrive	Yes

^aPrescribable for stated conditions (Advisory Committee on Borderline Substances), see British National Formulary and Monthly Index of Medical Specialties (MIMS). These products are available from retail pharmacies with a prescription from the family doctor on an FP10 form, free of charge for children.

coordinated movement of food through the mouth and coordinated swallowing. Early introduction of solids may cause choking and this is likely to cause rejection of foods from a spoon. Despite good reasons for not introducing solid foods before the age of 4 months, about half of infants in the UK are given solid foods before this age (Foster *et al.*, 1997). For nutritional reasons it is important that solid foods are introduced to supplement milk by the end of the sixth month (see Chaper 9).

Developmentally infants are ready to learn the more complex series of skills involved in weaning – taking food from a spoon, sealing the lips, moving a bolus of food to the back of the throat, achieving a safe swallow, chewing, biting and self-feeding. These skills develop over several months (see Table 11.2), but if an infant is not given the opportunity to develop these skills at the appropriate time, they may be slow to develop them later. Infants become increasingly inflexible about accepting different tastes and textures and are more likely to reject solid foods if they are introduced late.

For simplicity, weaning is often divided into three or four stages: stage 1, 4–6 months, learning to accept food from a spoon; stage 2, 5–7 months where a wider variety of tastes are introduced; stage 3, 6–10 months, learning to chew and accept different textures; and stage 4, > 10 months, learning to bite and to self-feed. In the UK recommendations stages 1 and 2 are combined. These divisions are in any case arbitrary and infants may progress at different rates. In practice, development should be continuous and once an infant has accepted food from one stage he or she should move on to the next. Suitable foods for the different stages of weaning are shown in Tables 12.15–12.17.

Whilst the use of hygienically prepared home-cooked foods probably represents the ideal, there is a wide variety of commercially produced infant weaning foods available. Products are available as a dried powder, which is reconstituted with water, and ready prepared in cans, jars or frozen. Stage 1 foods are a smooth purée intended for the start of weaning; stage 2 foods contain soft lumps; and stage 3 toddler meals contain food of a firmer texture. Exclusive use of ready-prepared weaning foods should be discouraged, as it is difficult to wean infants on to family meals later. However, they do have some advantages – they are prepared under strict hygienic conditions, do not contain salt or food additives and may enable the infant to enjoy a greater variety of foods. Nutritionally they may be more nutrient dense than some home prepared foods (Stordy et al., 1995), particularly for iron, as many savoury foods are fortified with iron.

Practical measures

Foods other than milk should not normally be given until the age of 4 months, but should be introduced by the end of the sixth month. If parents wish to wean their infant before the age of 4 months they should be encouraged to try other measures first, such as increasing the volume or frequency of milk feeds.

Where infants are weaned before 4 months it is particularly important that foods have a low renal solute load (i.e. are low in protein and sodium) and are of low allergenicity. Baby cereals, potatoes and vegetables are the most suitable items in this situation.

Foods should not be added to baby bottles, but should be offered from a suitable soft spoon.

Care should be taken to ensure that all equipment used in the preparation and serving of food is very clean. Sterilization should not be necessary in the infant's own home, but may be advisable in a nursery or day-care setting.

Food for infants should ideally be cooked without salt. Strong spices such as garlic and chilli should also be avoided. Foods should be prepared with a minimum of sugar – small amounts may be added to fruit to improve palatability. Wheat-containing foods should not be introduced before the age of 6 months. Up until 1 year of age eggs should be well cooked so that the yolk and white are solid. Fibre-enriched and very high fibre foods should be avoided until the age of about 1 year, although wholegrain cereals and bread can be used after the initial stage of weaning.

Although cow's milk should not be used to replace breast milk or formula as the main drink before the age of 1 year, it can be used as part of the weaning diet in the form of cheese, yoghurt, custard, etc. once weaning has become established.

Initially only tastes of bland smooth purée food should be offered at one feed during the day. The quantity and variety of foods can be increased once the infant accepts food from a

Table 12.15 Foods suitable for stage 1 and 2 weaning at 4–7 months

Food	Normal diet	Vegeterian diet	Vegan diet
Milk	Minimum 600–800 ml breast or infant formula daily	As for normal diet	Minimum 600–800 ml breast or infant soya formula daily
Milk products	Cow's milk and products can be used in weaning after 4 months, e.g. yoghurt, custard, cheese, cheese sauce	As for normal diet	Soya milk can be used to make custard and sauces and can be added to cereal
Starchy foods	Mix smooth cereal (e.g. rice cereal) with breast, formula or cow's milk. Use an iron-fortified cereal where possible. Do not use wheat-based cereals or pasta. Boiled rice can be puréed. Potatoes, swede, turnip etc. can be puréed using milk and butter or margarine	As for normal diet	Mix smooth cereal (e.g. rice cereal) with breast milk or infant soya formula. Use an iron-fortified cereal where possible. Do not use wheat-based cereals or pasta. Boiled rice can be puréed. Potatoes, swede, turnip can be puréed using soya milk and/or vegetable oil or margarine
Vegetables and fruits	Use soft-cooked vegetables and fruits as a smooth purée. Soft raw fruits such as banana can be mashed. All fruit and vegetables are suitable for stage 1	As for normal diet	As for normal diet
Meat	Use soft cooked meat or poultry as a purée once a day. Add only a minimal amount of salt during cooking	Give well-cooked pulses or eggs as a purée once a day to increase iron uptake	As for vegetarian diet
Pulses	Small quantities of well-cooked peas, beans and lentils can be included	As for normal diet	As for normal diet
Eggs	Use hard-boiled egg mashed or as a purée	As for normal diet	See advice for meat
Fish	Ensure fish has no bones – purée with potatoes or a sauce. Do not give canned fish as it is too salty	See advice for meat	See advice for meat
Nuts	Avoid nuts under 6 months	As for normal diet	As for normal diet
Flavourings	Avoid very spicy and salty foods including yeast extracts. Try not to add salt when cooking. Herbs can be used for flavourings. Use only a minimum amount of sugar in cooking and avoid very sugary foods	As for normal diet	As for normal diet
Other drinks	Breast or formula milk is sufficient up to 4–6 months. Boiled water can be given with meals. Avoid baby juices and fruit juice or give diluted with water. Do not give tea, coffee, squash or fizzy drinks	As for normal diet	As for normal diet

spoon. It is not necessary to introduce foods one at a time except where there is risk of allergy (see section on allergy in this chapter), once infants have learnt to eat from a spoon. Savoury foods and unsweetened cereals and fruit should be accepted before sweetened foods, such as desserts, are offered.

The addition of a fat source (butter, margarine, olive and other vegetable oils) to purée foods such as potatoes and vegetables, which have a low fat content, may be desirable to increase the energy density. The texture should progress from smooth purée to food of a mashed texture containing small lumps. Chewing of lumpy foods can be expected by about 3 months after the commencement of weaning. Infants should be given food to hold and begin to self-feed after about 7 months of age.

The usual volume of milk should be continued during the initial stages of weaning, but should be decreased as weaning progresses. The fluid can be replaced by water or by very dilute fruit juice in limited quantities.

The use of a baby bottle should be gradually reduced after the age of 6 months. A feeding beaker can be used and by the age of 1 year children should only receive an occasional bottle.

By the end of the first year infants should be consuming four portions of cereal, four portions of fruit and vegetables, two portions from the milk group (approximately 350 ml whole milk or equivalent; Figure 9.9) and two portions of meat or alternatives daily. They should consume a meal pattern of three meals and two to three snacks (which may consist of a milk drink) and should be drinking mainly from a cup.

Vitamins

A supplement of vitamins A (200 µg per dose), D (7 µg per dose) and C (20 mg per dose) is currently available under Welfare Food Scheme. The Department of Health (1994a)

recommendations for these are set out below. There are few dietary sources of vitamin D (see Table 12.4), and most individuals rely upon synthesis of cholecalciferol in skin that is exposed to ultra-violet light. Children with dark skins and those who are not regularly exposed to sunlight are at risk of vitamin D deficiency. There is a particular problem with vitamin D deficiency in young Asian children (Lawson and Thomas, 1999).

The subject of micronutrient intakes and deficiency in childhood is discussed in Chapter 11. The most recent National Diet and Nutrition Surveys of Children (Gregory et al., 1995, 2000) showed that intake of a number of vitamins and minerals was below dietary recommendations and some children had low blood levels of micronutrients. Although a varied and balanced diet will provide adequate micronutrients for all ages, many children do not receive such a diet. Children at risk of deficiency because of a poor dietary intake or increased requirements may benefit from a general multinutrient supplement. In general these supplements are not prescribable and can be bought over the counter. Supplements should be specifically designed for young children and should not contain more than the daily RNI for age. The fat-soluble vitamins A and D are toxic and children should not receive excess quantities, for instance from a fortified infant formula plus a supplement.

Practical measures

A vitamin supplement is not necessary for infants aged under 6 months who are breast-fed by a healthy mother. Between the ages of 6 and 12 months breast-fed infants should receive the recommended doses of vitamins A, D and C. Where there is concern over the mother's nutritional status, breast-fed infants should receive the recommended doses of vitamins A, D and C from 2 months of age.

Table 12.16 Foods suitable for stage 3 weaning 6–10 months

Food	Normal diet	Vegetarian diet	Vegan diet
Milk	500–900 ml breast milk, infant formula or follow-on formula. Do not give unmodified cow's milk as a main drink	As for normal diet	500–900 ml breast milk or modified infant soya formula. Do not give adult-type soya milk as a main drink. Breast-fed infants may need a supplementary drink of infant soya milk if there are concerns about weight gain
Milk products	Hard cheese can be grated or cut into small cubes and used as a 'finger food'	As for normal diet	Infant soya formula (or adult soya milk in small quantities) should be used to mix with cereal and to make sauces. Tofu can be introduced and soya yoghurts and desserts can be used
Starchy foods	Wheat-based breakfast cereals can be used, but avoid ones that are very high in fibre. Bread, rusks or pasta can be introduced. Use a variety of whole grain and white cereal products. Potatoes and other starchy vegetables can be mashed or cubed to use as 'finger food'. Aim for 2–3 portions of starchy foods each day	As for normal diet	As for normal diet
Vegetables and fruit	Cooked vegetables and fruit (with minimum added salt/sugar) can be mashed or cubed to use as 'finger food'. Soft raw vegetables and fruit (banana/melon/tomato) can be used as 'finger food'. Aim for a minimum of 2 portions of fruit and vegetables each day	As for normal diet	As for normal diet
Meat, fish and pulses	Meat and poultry can be minced, fish (no bones) can be mashed. Encourage oily fish (sardine, mackerel). Small amounts of canned fish can be used. Aim for 1 portion of meat or fish or egg each day	Give pulses, baked beans, peas, lentils, nuts, tofu, meat substitute or egg once a day to increase iron and protein intake. Mix these foods with cereal to improve protein quality, e.g. macaroni cheese. Aim for 1–2 portions each day. Egg or nut butter can be used for one portion	Give pulses, baked beans, peas, lentils, nuts, tofu, meat substitute once a day to increase iron and protein uptake. Mix these foods with cereal to improve protein quality, e.g. dhal and rice. Aim for 1–2 portions each day. Nut butter can replace one portion

(continued)

Table 12.16 (*continued*)

Food	Normal diet	Vegetarian diet	Vegan diet
Egg	Hard-boiled egg can be chopped and used as finger food. Do not give soft-cooked egg yet	As for normal diet	See advice for meat
Nuts	Nut butters can be introduced. Do not give whole nuts to children under the age of 5 years	As for normal diet	As for normal diet
Flavourings	Avoid salty and sugary foods. Small amounts of yeast extract can be introduced	As for normal diet	As for normal diet
Drinks and other foods	Water or very dilute fruit juice can be given with meals. Do not give tea, coffee, squash or fizzy drinks. Do not give too many fried foods. Encourage savoury rather than sweet foods. Avoid giving cakes, very sweet biscuits, and crisp-type products as in-between-meal snacks	As for normal diet	A vegan diet can be low in energy, and it is important to include sufficient fat in the diet. It may be necessary to add vegetable oil or margarine to meals to increase energy uptake. Give a starchy snack (e.g. plain biscuit) in between meals
Supplements	A supplement of vitamin A, D, and C is recommended for infants who are breast-fed after 6 months. A supplement is not necessary for infants taking at least 500 ml infant formula	As for normal diet	A supplement of vitamins A, D and C is recommended for infants who are breast-fed after 6 months. A supplement of vitamin B_{12} may also be necessary. A supplement is not necessary for infants taking at least 500 ml of a fortified infant soya formula

A formula-fed infant under the age of 1 year does not require a supplement unless the intake of standard or follow-on formula falls below 500 ml per day. For children aged 1–5 years where infant formula is not the main drink, a supplement of vitamins A, D and C should be considered unless the health-care professional is confident that the child is receiving sufficient intake from the diet (see Table 12.4) or, in the case of vitamin D, the skin is regularly exposed to sunlight. Special consideration should be given to encouraging Asian families to supplement children with 7–10 µg vitamin D daily up to the age of 5 years.

The health-care team should agree on suitable over-the-counter multivitamin prepara-

tions available in their area, which can be recommended to children at risk. Where there is concern over a child's dietary intake, change to a varied and balanced diet must be encouraged. Where changes are not accepted a suitable multivitamin supplement can be recommended.

Iron

Iron deficiency is the commonest nutritional deficiency in the UK and is seen in about 12 per cent of children aged 18–29 months (Gregory *et al.*, 1997). It is particularly high in areas of deprivation and in children from minority ethnic groups (James *et al.*, 1988; Lawson *et al.*, 1998). Iron deficiency is discussed in Chapter 11. The iron found in meat has a high bioavailability and is easily absorbed. Non-haem iron found in foods of plant origin is less readily absorbed and needs vitamin C to be consumed at the same meal to optimize absorption. Breast milk is fairly low in iron but the iron is in a readily available form. After the age of about 6 months additional iron from the diet is necessary to prevent iron deficiency in breast-fed infants. Infant formulas sold in the UK are fortified with iron (0.6 mg/100 ml); follow-on formulas have a higher level of fortification (1.2 mg/100 ml) and usually provide sufficient iron, although it is not well absorbed. Cow's milk is low in iron and the iron present is poorly available.

Practical measures

Unmodified milks (cow, sheep, goat) should not be used as a drink until at least 12 months of age. The use of breast milk or a fortified infant formula should be continued until 1 year. Small amounts of milk can be used as part of the diet, as sauces, yoghurt, desserts and cheese, before the age of 12 months (see Weaning section in this chapter).

After the age of 1 year, continued use of a fortified infant milk or a follow-on formula can be considered for children who eat poorly or who have a low iron intake. After the age of 1 year a maximum of 500 ml (1 pint) of unmodified milk should be given. An iron-fortified infant cereal or adult breakfast cereal can be used for infants and children.

One serving of meat, poultry or fish should be included in the diet each day. For children who do not eat meat iron-rich foods should be included (see Tables 12.7 and 12.9) accompanied by vitamin C-rich food or drink at two meals each day. Iron-rich snacks (see Table 12.8) should be used in place of crisps and soft drinks.

Where there is concern about a child's iron intake, a finger prick blood sample should be tested for haemoglobin and ideally ferritin levels. If iron-deficiency anaemia is diagnosed an iron supplement should be prescribed for 6 months.

Minerals and trace elements

The major minerals and trace elements likely to be deficient in the diets are calcium, magnesium and zinc (see Chapter 11). For food sources of these, see Table 12.2. Mineral supplements are rarely required for young children, although some trace elements may be included in over-the-counter multinutrient supplements for young children. For children receiving a milk-free diet a calcium supplement will be required if a milk substitute is not taken, but intake and requirements for all such children should be formally assessed.

Problems Associated with Feeding Infants and Young Children

Rationale for nutrition policy

Parents' perceptions of feeding difficulties during infancy and early childhood may differ from those of the health-care professional. Feeding of infants is seen as probably the most important function of a parent and is the cause of a great deal of anxiety. It is important that a policy is adopted for dealing with problems so that consistent advice is given to prevent confusion and further anxiety for parents. Many feeding difficulties cause no ill-effects and the infant or child will grow out of them in the course of time. It is important that a local infant and child nutrition policy includes within it a policy for the regular weighing and recording of weights for children. Most

Table 12.17   Foods suitable for stage 4 weaning at > 10 months

Food	Normal diet	Vegetarian diet	Vegan diet
Milk	About 500–600 ml breast milk or infant formula each day	As for normal diet	About 500–600 ml breast milk or modified infant soya formula each day
Milk products	Milk products such as yoghurt and cheese can partly replace breast milk or infant formula, but see supplements section below	As for normal diet	Soya products such as tofu can partly replace breast milk or infant soya formula, but see supplement section below
Starchy foods	Starchy foods can be normal adult texture. Encourage wholegrain breakfast cereal, bread, pasta and rice. Discourage foods with added sugar such as sweet biscuits and cakes, and very fatty foods such as crisps and chips. Aim for 3–4 portions per day	As for normal diet. Breakfast cereals fortified with iron are particularly important in meat-free diets	As for vegetarian diet
Vegetables and fruit	Encourage lightly cooked or raw fruit and vegetables as well as cooked. Aim for 3–4 portions daily	As for normal diet	As for normal diet
Meat, fish, egg, pulses and nuts	Continue to mince meat. Poultry may be very finely chopped. Avoid salty and fatty processed meat products such as burgers and pies. Minimum 1 portion daily	Use egg, milk products, peas, beans, lentils, soya products, nut butters and meat substitutes in place of meat and fish. Mix pulses with cereals to improve protein quality. Minimum 2 portions daily or 1 egg	Use soya dairy-type products, peas, beans, lentils, nut butters, and meat substitutes in place of meat, fish and egg. Mix pulses with cereals to improve protein quality. Minimum 2 portions daily
Flavourings	Limit fried, fatty, salty and sugary foods	As for normal diet	As for normal diet
Drinks and other foods	As for stage 2	As for stage 2	As for stage 2
Supplements	A supplement of vitamins A, D and C is recommended if consumption of infant formula falls below 500 ml daily	As for normal diet	A supplement of vitamins A, D and C (and possibly vitamin B_{12}) is recommended if consumption of a fortified infant soya milk falls below 500 ml daily

feeding difficulties which lead to adverse consequences are characterized by a failure to gain weight or weight faltering. Adequate equipment such as a self-calibrating stadiometer and accurate scales with 10 g increments for infants and 50 g increments for children should be available to all health-care professionals so that an accurate weight and length or height can be easily obtained. Centile charts should be appropriate for the country and follow current recommendations. The Child Growth Foundation (www.cgf.org.uk) will advise on appropriate equipment and charts. Recommendations for frequency of weighing and measuring have been agreed in the UK (Wright, 2000; Hall, 2000). Infants who are growing normally should not be weighed more frequently than every 2 weeks under the age of 6 months and every month thereafter. Where there is clinical concern about an infant or child both weight and height should be measured. Slow growth is discussed in the section on failure to thrive.

Feeding infants and children with special needs or those who require a therapeutic diet is outside the remit of this chapter and the reader is directed to a text book on this specialist subject, such as *Clinical Paediatric Dietetics* (Shaw and Lawson, 2001).

Colic

Colic occurs with equal frequency in breast- and bottle-fed infants, usually between the ages of 6 weeks and 3 months. Characteristically infants with colic cry vigorously and draw their legs up towards the chest. This behaviour occurs most frequently during the evening and is typically repeated at the same time each day. The infant may be inconsolable, causing distress and anxiety for the parents. The pain is thought to be due to spasm of the gut wall in the colon, which may be due to distension by gas, although the exact aetiology is poorly understood (Lucassen and Assendelft, 2001). A direct connection with the diet has not been shown, and first-line advice should not be to change either the mother's diet (if breast-feeding) or the type of feed in formula-fed infants. If the infant is gaining weight adequately and is happy during the rest of the day then it is unlikely that the cause is a medical problem, but reflux, food allergy or malab-

sorption (often coeliac disease) should be considered.

Practical measures

Check that the formula fed baby is not being over- or underfed – at age 0–6 months the infant should receive approximately 150 ml/kg, 7–12 months 120 ml/kg body weight. The use of a proprietary colic medication may help. These may be purchased over the counter or prescribed by the family doctor. These mainly act to reduce flatulence. The infant should be positioned at the breast or bottle in a way to reduce excessive air swallowing. Common causes for air swallowing are too rapid or too slow a delivery of feed (breast or bottle), or the baby bottle being vigorously shaken prior to or during the feed.

Infant herbal drinks, such as fennel, are not indicated for colic, but if the carers feel that a warm drink of a sugar-free preparation alleviates symptoms there is no harm in the practice. It is important that the feeding bottle is held tilted towards the baby to avoid air entering the teat. The teat should be removed from the mouth at intervals to prevent it collapsing. Feeds should be interrupted at least once in order to hold the baby in an upright position to allow any swallowed air to be voided. Breast-fed babies should have a good seal around the nipple with their lips to avoid air ingestion.

Various devices are marketed for bottle-fed infants and these can be tried, although none are universally efficacious. Bottles with disposable inner bags and those with a tilted head may reduce air swallowing. Anti-colic teats are also available.

Reassurance that colic is a normal phenomenon and that the cause is unlikely to be due to a medical problem is important for parents. If the simple measures outlined above are not successful, then food intolerance may be suspected.

A few breast-feeding mothers find that removal of one or more items regularly consumed from the diet alleviates symptoms. If cow's milk and dairy products (including cheese) are removed, care should be taken that the mother has an adequate calcium intake (see Tables 12.2 and 12.10).

Colic is not an indication to stop breast-feeding and the switching from one brand of milk to another or from a whey- to a casein-based feed has not been shown to be helpful. If food intolerance is suspected the culprit may be lactose or milk protein. Formulas that are low in lactose may be used. One milk (Omneocomfort) is marketed in the UK specifically for the management of colic. It contains hydrolysed milk protein, which may in theory be less antigenic than whole protein, and is also low in lactose. Milks of this kind still contain substantial quantities of whole milk protein and should not be used for the management of proven food allergy. Table 12.14 lists specialised milks that may be useful for the management of colic.

If none of the above solutions work then complete removal of milk from the diet should be considered. Substitution of infant formula for infant soya milk is usually not helpful, as many food allergic infants become intolerant to soya. A fully hydrolysed feed should be prescribed by the family doctor and all traces of milk protein removed from the weaning diet. An outline of a milk-free regimen is given in Table 12.6. Removal of one or more items from the diet of an infant may give rise to nutritional deficiencies and it is important that restricted diets are supervised by a paediatric dietician.

Acute diarrhoea

Acute diarrhoea accounts for a substantial proportion of paediatric consultations and morbidity in children under 5 years of age in Western countries and is a major cause of infant mortality in developing countries. Management of acute gastroenteritis in developing countries has been reviewed extensively (WHO, 1990) and will not be considered further in this chapter. Guidelines for management of acute diarrhoea for well-nourished children in industrialized countries have been published by the Royal College of Paediatrics and Child Health (Armon et al., 2001) and the American Academy of Pediatrics (1996). Dehydration and hypernatraemia are potentially fatal to infants and most cases of acute diarrhoea, particularly if accompanied by vomiting, should be referred to a paediatrician as an emergency.

Practical measures

Infants and children who present acutely unwell with diarrhoea must be assessed by a paediatrician to exclude conditions other than an acute infection and to estimate the degree of dehydration. If the diarrhoea is of recent origin, is not severe (i.e. stools not watery, < 8 per 24 hours) and the infant is not dehydrated, then normal fluids (breast or formula milk) should be given in small aliquots at about 150 ml/kg and the situation reviewed in 2–4 h.

Most cases with mild to moderate dehydration will require oral rehydration fluids (Table 12.18) and should be observed in a paediatric unit for a period of up to 6 h to ensure successful rehydration. In mild to moderate dehydration oral rehydration fluids are given to replace fluid lost, in small aliquots over a period of 4 h. After 4 h normal feeds can be resumed. More severe diarrhoea with or without vomiting may need oral rehydration via a naso-gastric tube or by intravenous infusion.

Vomiting, posseting and gastro-oesophageal reflux

Clear definition of these terms should be agreed by health-care professionals as management

Table 12.18 Oral rehydration solutions

	Glucose (g/l)	Sodium (mmol/l)	Potassium (mmol/l)	Chloride (mmol/l)	Base (mmol/l)
Dioralyte (SmithKline Beecham Healthcare)	16	60	20	60	Citrate 10
Dioralyte Relief (SmithKline Beecham Healthcare)	30 g rice starch	60	50	20	Citrate 10
Diocalm Junior (Rhone-Poulenc Rorer)	20	60	20	50	Citrate 10
Rehidrat (Searle)	50	50	20	50	Bicarbonate 20 Citrate 10
Electrolade (Eastern)	20	50	20	40	Bicarbonate 30

depends upon the nature and the cause of symptoms. True vomiting is preceded by a pro-dromal phase where the infant shows some distress. Vomitus is forcibly ejected and persistent vomiting is usually associated with gastro-intestinal infection or with fever. If vomiting continues for more than a few hours there is a danger of dehydration and the infant should be seen by a paediatrician as an emergency.

Posseting, 'spitting up' or regurgitation without other symptoms is common during infancy and is usually due to an immature oesophageal sphincter. The condition is normally benign and improves with age as the infant matures and progresses onto a less bulky diet. Posseting that is accompanied by other symptoms such as failure to thrive, colic, distress on feeding, chest infections or wheeze may be due to conditions such as oro-motor dysfunction, hiatus hernia or milk protein intolerance. The European Society for Pediatric Gastroenterology, Hepatology and Nutrition has issued guidelines for the management of gastro-oesophageal reflux (Vandenplas *et al.*, 1996).

Practical measures

Projectile vomiting that develops within the first 2 weeks of life may be due to pyloric stenosis and requires an urgent referral to a paediatrician. Where vomiting is accompanied by diarrhoea an oral rehydration regimen should be started without delay.

Check that fluid volume is not excessive. Give smaller more frequent feeds if appropriate. Infants should be maintained in an upright position after feeding and watched to see if they put their hand into their mouth, which may induce vomiting. For infants over 13 weeks of age a small amount of solid food can replace some milk e.g. babyrice mixed with breast or formula milk. Formula feeds can be thickened, either by the addition of a proprietary feed thickener or by the use of a pre-thickened feed (see Table 12.14). A feed thickener can be mixed with expressed breast milk or boiled water and given on a teaspoon before a breast-feed. Anti-reflux medication may be prescribed by the GP if simple behavioural and dietary measures are not effective.

Constipation

Constipation is defined as the infrequent passing of hard stools. The bowel habits of normal infants and children vary considerably (Tham *et al.*, 1996). Breast-fed infants are less likely to be constipated because fat is more completely absorbed, leaving less insoluble calcium soaps in the large intestine. However stool frequency may be only every 3–4 days. Bottle-fed babies may pass stools every second day and stools will be harder than in breast-fed infants. If the infant seems to experience no difficulty or pain it is unlikely that constipation is serious. Severe constipation can be due to conditions such as Hirschsprung's disease, and cow's milk protein intolerance can lead to constipation. The presence of organic conditions causing constipation is often associated with poor appetite and failure to thrive.

Practical measures

Check that the infant is clinically constipated – obtain a record of stool frequency, consistency and difficulty or pain on passing stools. Check that the fluid volume is adequate, that formula feeds are not being overconcentrated, and that additions are not being put into baby bottles. Offer additional drinks of pure orange juice diluted 1 part juice plus 2 parts boiled water.

For infants over the age of 13 weeks, offer puréed fruit and vegetables. For infants over the age of 17 weeks offer puréed beans or lentils. For infants over the age of 6 months wholegrain cereals can be used, e.g. wholewheat breakfast cereal, wholegrain rice and pasta. Unprocessed bran or fibre-enriched cereals should not be given to infants and young children.

If these measures are unsuccessful the infant should be referred to a paediatrician for further investigation.

Food intolerance and allergy

It is common for many parents to think that their child suffers from a food allergy, and many go on to restrict some dietary components. The prevalence of food allergy is increasing and is most common in early life – up to 5 per cent of infants under the age of 1 year, and 1–2 per cent in pre-school-aged children. Not all adverse reactions to food are caused by allergy (see Figure 12.2). It is important that if food allergy is suspected children are referred for a paediatric opinion so that a diagnosis is made and dietary advice is obtained.

The commonest allergens are cow's milk, egg, wheat, peanuts, tree nuts and soya. Allergy to food additives, often suspected by parents, is rare, affecting only 0.03 per cent of the population. Symptoms of true food allergy may include skin reactions such as dermatitis, gastro-intestinal symptoms such as reflux, vomiting and diarrhoea and respiratory symptoms such as asthma and wheezing. Hyperactivity, which affects 1–5 per cent of children, may be caused by an adverse reaction to food in a small proportion of children.

Most children grow out of allergies, particularly if they have developed during infancy. Some 45–50 per cent of infants with cow's milk protein intolerance recover by the age of 1 year, and 85–90 per cent by the age of 3 years (Ahmed and Fuchs, 1997). Peanut allergy is an exception and is likely to be lifelong. Coeliac disease, which is a permanent intolerance to wheat gluten, is also a lifelong condition affecting 1 in 1500 people in the UK. It is important that a proper diagnosis (such as small intestinal biopsy or anti-endomysial antibodies in blood) is made to distinguish coeliac disease from temporary wheat intolerance.

The subject of food allergy has been extensively reviewed in the publications *Adverse Reactions to Food and Food Ingredients* and *Peanut Allergy* (Committee on Toxicology of Chemicals in Food, Consumer Products and the Environment 1998, 2000) and *Adverse Reactions to Food* (British Nutrition Foundation, 2002).

Practical measures

Weight gain is often slow in an infant with food allergy and poor weight gain may be the presenting symptom in food intolerance. An adverse reaction to a food on one occasion may not be significant. If the reaction is not severe the infant should be tried with the food on two or three occasions several days apart. Infants are considered to be at high risk of allergy if there is a parental family history of allergy.

Mothers of high-risk infants should be encouraged to exclusively breast-feed for the first 6 months. Although there is no conclusive evidence of efficacy, some mothers may wish to exclude milk and dairy products and peanuts whilst they are breast-feeding (see Table 12.6).

Solids should not be introduced before the age of 6 months in high-risk infants. First foods introduced should be of low allergenicity, e.g. rice, potato, vegetables and fruit (excluding tomato and citrus fruits).

Foods with a higher allergenicity, such as milk and milk products, egg and wheat, should be introduced singly with a period of 24–48 h between each new food. Potentially allergenic foods should be delayed until the age of 6–9 months. High-risk infants (i.e. those with an atopic family history) should avoid peanuts and peanut products until the age of 3 years. Nut oils are usually tolerated. Soya milk is not useful for the prevention of allergy in high-risk infants, because allergy to soya can develop.

If breast-feeding is not possible in high-risk infants the use of an extensively hydrolysed formula (see Table 12.14) should be considered. Formulas based on partially hydrolysed milks are marketed in Europe, the UK and the USA for the prevention of allergy. Their usefulness in preventing food allergy in high-risk infants has not been fully evaluated.

If a breast-fed infant appears to react to cow's milk or infant formula the mother should be encouraged to continue breast-feeding for at least 6 months. For breast-fed infants who appear to react to cow's milk, solids should be delayed until after 6 months and the infant treated as high risk when introducing foods.

For formula-fed infants who are suspected of reacting to cow's milk with skin or respiratory symptoms a modified infant soya formula (Table 12.14) can be tried. For longer term use these formulas are prescribable by the family doctor. Formula-fed infants with gastrointestinal symptoms should not be given a soya formula. An extensively hydrolysed formula (Table 12.14) is recommended; these milks are only available on prescription from the family doctor.

It is important that all sources of the potential allergen are removed from the diet. For a milk protein-free diet see Table 12.6. Milk is very often added to commercially prepared baby foods and parents should read the label attached to all prepared foods. If the infant appears to respond to removal of an allergen such as milk, he or she should be referred to a paediatrician and paediatric dietitian for diagnosis and dietary advice because nutritional deficiencies are likely in infants receiving a restricted diet.

If more than one allergen is suspected (e.g. milk and wheat or milk and soya) it is essential that advice from a paediatric dietitian is sought, as there is a high risk of nutritional deficiencies resulting from such a restricted diet. Foods removed from the diet because of allergy can be slowly reintroduced in very small amounts between the ages of 1 and 2 years. It is essential that this is done under expert medical supervision, as there is a risk of an anaphylactic reaction.

Failure-to-thrive

Failure-to-thrive is a relatively common condition and may affect up to 5 per cent of children overall and 10 per cent of children from families with medical or socio-economic

Table 12.19 Definitions of failure-to-thrive

Infants – take as baseline maximum weight centile at 4–6 weeks
Unexplained weight of <0.4 centile
Downward weight track crossing >2 centiles
Persistent weight gain less than minimal thrive lines (see text)

Children
Unexplained weight of <0.4 centile
Downward weight track crossing >2 centiles
Weight >2 centiles below height centile
Body mass index <10th centile

---

problems (Underdown and Birks, 1999). The majority of cases occur before the age of 18 months, most commonly during the second 6 months of life when growth is rapid and nutrient requirements are high. The term 'failure to thrive' is generally understood to describe growth velocity that is less than expected for a child's age and size. Because failure to thrive is described in terms of velocity it cannot be diagnosed on the basis of a single measurement – a minimum of two (and preferably more) measurements are required over a period of several weeks. There is no commonly agreed definition for failure to thrive, although a number have been suggested (Wright, 2000) and these are summarized in Table 12.19. Two charts are produced which define the lower limit of normal weight velocity in infants (Cole, 1995; Wright *et al.*, 1998) and from birth to 5 years. In addition a set of 'thrive line' acetates have been produced by the Child Growth Foundation to overlay the Child Health Record and (from 2002) the standard British four in one growth charts.

No single or group of tests adequately identifies infants and children with faltering growth and it is important to use any growth monitoring tool carefully. Parental height must be taken into account when considering the height of a child. Babies who are born large

and those who are small at birth have a tendency to revert to the mean, so that large babies may not gain as much weight as small babies and may fall through two weight centiles as part of their normal growth pattern. Small babies are less likely to decrease their weight centile. Breast-fed infants gain weight more slowly than formula-fed ones and normal growth charts for breast-fed infants are available from the Child Growth Foundation.

The basic cause of failure-to-thrive (except in some genetic conditions) is a nutrient intake that is inadequate to support normal growth. There are a variety of reasons for an inadequate intake, and these are summarized in Table 11.3. In many cases the aetiology is multifactorial, with behavioural, socio-economic and organic diseases playing a part. The cause of the poor intake should be sought, as this provides the rationale and basis for treatment; management should be via a multidisciplinary team based in the community.

Slow growth during the first year of life is particularly worrying to parents and there is some evidence that low weight gain during this period affects health outcomes in later life (Lucas *et al.*, 1999). Most children referred for faltering growth do not entirely catch up to their projected height or weight centile. Poor appetite and difficulties with food often remain a problem in the long term. There appears to be no major long-term adverse effect on cognition, although short-term deficits have been described (Drewett *et al.*, 1999). A range of therapeutic interventions have been reviewed by The Children's Society (Batchelor, 1999; Underdown and Birks, 1999) and serve as a good basis for a local policy.

Practical measures

Infants and children suspected of failure to thrive should be weighed regularly – infants fortnightly and children over the age of 1 year monthly. Local facilities should agree on criteria for the diagnosis of failure to thrive and criteria for referral for investigation (see Table 12.19). Poor growth due to organic conditions must always be excluded before behavioural or environmental issues are blamed.

A qualitative diet history should be taken in order to assess usual feeding pattern and type and quantity of foods eaten. There is no need to estimate the nutrient content of the diet. Where possible, a mealtime should be observed with the child's usual carer to assess the environment and carer–child interaction.

Signs of distress, choking, coughing and wheezing associated with feeding may indicate oro-motor dysfunction or dysphagia and the child should be referred to a paediatrician for further investigation. The initial intervention should seek to increase food intake by addressing parenting skills, the feeding environment and the child's behaviour (see Table 12.20). The energy content of the diet should be

Table 12.20 Strategies for feeding problems in children aged over 1 year

---

Foods
Not more than 500 ml of milk daily
Restrict fruit juice
Restrict fluids at mealtimes
Restrict in-between meal snacks – discourage 'grazing'
Restrict alternative foods offered

Presentation
Discourage baby bottles
Small attractive meals
Easy to eat – chopped or finger foods
Appropriate seating and utensils
Allow child to self-feed part of meal
Set time limit on meals
No bribery with sweet foods
Three meals and three snacks daily

Feeding environment
No force-feeding
Individual attention and help from carer
Eat with family, not alone
Not too many distractions (e.g. loud TV or music)
No anger shown at food rejected

Table 12.21 Increasing energy density of the diet – children over 1 year

---

Limit the amount of plain water and low-energy drinks
Use whole milk (3.8 per cent fat) or 'Breakfast' milk (4.8 per cent fat)
Avoid an adult-type low-fat high-fibre 'healthy' diet
Add butter, margarine or vegetable oil to mashed potato and vegetables
Add cream or cheese to soups, vegetables, desserts, cereals
Fry foods in vegetable oil – chips, fried bread, vegetables

---

increased using normal foods (see Table 12.21). An age-appropriate multivitamin and mineral supplement may be useful to alleviate parental concerns whilst the reasons for poor food intake are being addressed.

Where failure to thrive is due to organic illness or where measures to improve growth using normal foods and behavioural techniques have failed, it may be necessary to use an energy supplement. A glucose polymer or a powder or liquid containing fat and carbohydrate can be prescribed by the family doctor for failure to thrive and can be added to the food of children over the age of 1 year.

For infants under the age of a year who are largely dependent on milk it is important that there is sufficient protein to ensure growth of lean tissue. If a protein:energy ratio of less than 9 per cent is given then weight gain will comprise largely adipose tissue and water. Energy supplements alone should not be added to infant formula. The use of a nutrient-dense high-energy formula formulated to encourage optimum catch-up growth should be considered. These products are prescribable by the family doctor and are described in Table 12.14.

Recovery from failure to thrive is considered to be adequate when weight returns to within one centile band of the original centile and weight velocity is progressing normally.

Feeding Children Aged 1–5 Years

Rationale for nutrition policy

Growth velocity decreases with increasing age and nutrient requirements expressed per unit of body weight decline. By the age of 1 year most children should be consuming a diet that, although modified in texture, is similar to that of an adult (see Table 11.12). Nutrient deficiencies are still likely in this age group and the UK National Diet and Nutrition Survey of children aged $1\frac{1}{2}$–$4\frac{1}{2}$ years (Gregory *et al.*, 1995) highlighted the fact that, although iron is the most common dietary deficiency, intake of other nutrients may be marginal for some children. Many children in this age group are looked after by carers or attend nursery school for some of their meals. The Department for Education and Employment (2000a) has published guidelines towards achieving the standards for healthy school lunches in nursery schools/units. Table 12.17 suggests foods that are suitable for this age group. Health professionals have an important role in providing education for those caring for the under 5 age group both at home and in private and public sector childcare facilities.

Practical measures

Young children should be encouraged to eat as wide a variety of foods as possible as this period lays the foundations for the child to choose a healthy diet in the future. Three main meals and two to three snacks should be the eating pattern. A bedtime snack or milk drink may be beneficial. Frequent eating between meals or 'grazing' should be discouraged. If children complain of hunger outside their normal meal or snack time then fruit or water can be offered rather than crisps, sweets or biscuits and soft drinks.

An adult pattern of eating based on the Balance of Good Health (Figure 9.9) should be aimed for, although fat may still provide a greater proportion of dietary energy than is recommended for adults. The diet from now on should include five portions of fruit and vegetables, one portion of meat or one to two portions of meat alternatives (pulses or nut butters) and four to five portions of starchy foods each day. Whole nuts should not be given to children under the age of 5 years because there is a danger of choking.

After the age of 1 year about 350 ml milk or two foods from the milk group (Figure 9.9) will satisfy calcium requirements. Whole milk should be used until 2 years. After the age of 2 years semi-skimmed milk can be introduced if the child is gaining weight adequately. Skimmed milk can be used from the age of 5 years.

Cultural Influences on diet

Religious and ethical beliefs cause parents to choose particular foods and eating patterns that deviate from a traditional diet. In most cases these diets are perfectly adequate for infants and young children. Food rules pertaining to the main world religions are shown in Table 12.22. Vegetarian diets are defined as excluding meat and fish but including milk and egg and should be adequate for the needs of the growing child, although iron deficiency may be a problem. Vegan diets, which exclude all animal products (including milk) present more difficulty for the young child, since such diets are less energy dense and require a greater bulk of food to be eaten to achieve an adequate nutrient intake. Nutrients which may be deficient include protein, calcium, iron, iodine and vitamin B_{12}. More restricted diets such as fruitarian, raw vegan and macrobiotic diets are very bulky and in general do not provide adequate nutrients for children under the age of 5 years unless a supplement such as a fortified soya formula is given (Table 12.14).

Table 12.22 Cultural and religious influences on diet

Food	Lacto-ovo vegetarian	Vegan	Jewish	Moslem	Sikh	Hindu	Buddhist
Milk + milk products	✓	✗	Not with meat	✓	✓	✓	✓
Eggs	✓	✗	✓	✓	✓	*	*
Chicken	✗	✗	Kosher	Halal	*	*	*
Lamb/mutton	✗	✗	Kosher	Halal	✓	*	*
Beef	✗	✗	Kosher	Halal	✗	✗	*
Pork	✗	✗	✗	✗	*	*	*
Fish	✗	✗	No shellfish	Halal	*	*	*
Alcohol	✓	✓	✓	✗	✓	✓	*
Fasting	✗	✗	Yom Kippur	Ramadam	✗	Individual	Individual
Fruit and vegetables	✓	✓	✓	✓	✓	✓	✓
Pulses	✓	✓	✓	✓	✓	*	✓

*Not taken by very orthodox adherents.
Kosher – prepared according to Jewish food laws. Yom Kippur – Jewish religious festival.
Halal – prepared according to Moslem food laws. Ramadam – Moslem month of fasting during daylight hours

Practical measures

Practical suggestion for weaning foods for vegetarian and vegan diets are given in Tables 12.15–12.17. Vegetarian and vegan diets should contain foods from the four main food groups (Figure 9.9). At least four portions of processed cereal (bread, breakfast cereal, pasta etc.) and two portions of meat substitute (pulses and nuts) should be taken each day to ensure an adequate protein intake.

Vegetable proteins should be combined at the same time as proteins with a higher biological value such as milk, egg, pulses and cereal (e.g. baked beans on toast) to ensure a beneficial balance of amino acids. Three portions of vegetarian iron-containing foods (see Table 12.9) should be taken each day along with a source of vitamin C at the same meal.

If milk and milk products are excluded from the diet at least 500 ml of a fortified infant soya formula (Table 12.14) should be taken until the age of 2 years. After this a calcium-enriched adult soya milk can be used. Milk substitutes prepared from other ingredients such as rice, oats or nuts are nutritionally inadequate for young children if used as a main drink.

A supplement of vitamin D is recommended for vegan children under the age of 5, as a vegan diet contains none. A supplement containing iodine and riboflavin should be considered if there are no dietary sources (Table 12.4).

Fussy eaters

Food refusal often becomes an issue at about 2 years of age as the toddler begins to assert his or her independence. It is important that children are able to exercise some control over their feeding and they should be encouraged to participate in self-feeding and to choose some food. However nutritional problems are likely if a young child is allowed to have complete control over food choice. Many children dislike vegetables, but will perhaps eat a limited range (peas are often popular) or fruit. Selective and faddy eating is a phase through which most children pass fairly quickly if parents show some tolerance. Short periods of a less than adequate diet will do no harm to a well-nourished child with a normal weight.

Practical measures

A multivitamin supplement designed for young children which contains no more than the RNI for micronutrients may allay parental anxiety during times of poor feeding. Weight should be monitored as suggested in the failure to thrive section, and appropriate action taken.

Excessive fluid consumption should be restricted and mainly water or milk given in between meals. Restrict milk intake to not more than 500 ml per day. Continual 'grazing' on high-energy low-nutrient foods such as confectionery should be discouraged and three meals and two to three snacks aimed for each day.

Carers should not offer too many alternatives if a food is disliked. Plain starchy foods (e.g. sandwiches) or fruit or milk should be offered as a replacement rather than preferred foods such as confectionery or crisps. Continued exposure to disliked foods such as vegetables encourages eventual acceptance, so parents should continue to place small quantities of food onto the child's plate, although they do not have to eat it.

Alternative ways of serving disliked foods can be tried – minced meat made into burgers or puréed meat as a home made soup may be preferred to slices of meat. Grated raw carrot can replace cooked vegetables and raw or cooked baby sweetcorn is a popular 'finger food'. It may be useful to allow only a maximum number of 'disliked' foods (e.g. six items) that need not be eaten in the diet. If feeding difficulties become prolonged or cause a lot of anxiety and tension some of the strategies suggested in Tables 12.21 and 12.22 can be tried.

Healthy eating recommendations for pre-school children

A number of recommendations for healthy eating and the prevention of cardiovascular disease in later life have been published (American Academy of Pediatrics, 1995; Department of Health, 1994b; Aggett et al., 1994) and these are summarized in Table 12.23. In all reports, dietary modification to reduce fat and increase fibre are not recommended before the age of 2 years. By the time the child is 5 years old the percentage energy derived from total fat should not exceed 35 per cent. It is important that the pre-school child obtains sufficient energy and other nutrients from the diet and that nutrient intake is not compromised by a diet that is inappropriately low in fat or high in fibre. The timing of the change from an infant high-fat low-fibre diet to an adult diet where fat is replaced by complex carbohydrates should be

Table 12.23 Healthy eating recommendations, USA, UK and Europe

	UK	USA	Europe
Age at which recommendations apply	>2–5 years	>2 years	>2–3 years
Total fat as percentage of energy	35	30	30–35
Saturated fat as percentage of energy	10	8–10	8–12
Carbohydrate as percentage of energy	–	55	–
Protein as percentage of energy	–	15	–
Fibre (g/day)	–	5–10 g	–

– No recommendation given. UK, Department of Health (1994b). USA, American Academy of Pediatrics (1995). Europe, Aggett et al. (1994).

flexible. The recommendations outlined below can be used from the age of 2 years in children with normal growth and weight gain. For children who are slow to gain weight some of the modifications (such as changing to low-fat milk products) should not be started until nearer the age of 5 years.

Practical measures

Encourage the consumption of cereals and starchy foods (including potato). Four portions should be included daily at age two to three and five portions daily by the age of 5 years. Cereals should preferably be wholegrain. Encourage consumption of vegetables and fruit – four portions daily at 2–3 years, five portions daily at 5 years.

Two portions (cups) of milk or dairy products such as yoghurt, fromage frais and cheese should be included each day. Semi-skimmed milk and low-fat dairy products should be used. Lean meats can be used in moderation – one to two portions daily. Oily fish – mackerel, herring, sardine and tuna should be included once to twice weekly. Encourage the use of non-meat non-dairy protein foods such as peas, beans, baked beans, lentils and nut butters (e.g. peanut butter).

Sugar, salt and fatty foods should be kept to a minimum (savoury snacks, sweets, cakes, biscuits and chocolate). They need not be entirely excluded from the diet but should not be used every day.

The amount of animal fats should be reduced by cutting visible fat off meat, buying lower fat minced meat, avoiding fatty meats such as duck, sausages and convenience meat foods. The amount of lard, butter and cream consumed should be limited.

Fried foods should not be given every day; when frying foods a minimum amount of oils should be used, such as seed oil (sunflower, corn, soya) or other unsaturated oils (e.g. olive, rapeseed). Foods should not be fried in hard margarine, butter, coconut oil or lard. Polyunsaturated margarines should be used in place of hard margarine and butter.

School-age Children

Rationale for nutrition policy

Today's children appear to have fewer health problems than any previous generations. However there is concern that unhealthy lifestyles, including diet, may be storing up problems for the future: coronary heart disease, stroke, osteoporosis and some cancers are all nutrition-linked and are potentially preventable. The National Diet and Nutrition Survey of children aged 4–18 years in the UK (Gregory *et al.*, 2000) showed that the majority of children under the age of 10 years had an adequate intake of most nutrients. Fat and sugar intake was higher than recommendations and many children consumed low quantities of fruit and green vegetables. Dietary fibre intakes were generally lower than recommendations and this has implications for a number of nutrition-related diseases.

Obesity is becoming increasingly common in this age group, and children surveyed appeared to be far less active than recommendations made by the Health Education Authority (see Practical Measures below; Biddle, 1998). It is important to ensure a varied and nutrient-dense diet as eating habits are becoming established during this period. The school and school meals as well as parents are important sources of experience and education about food and nutrition for school-age children. Local Health Educators have the opportunity to become involved in the Healthy Schools project (Department for Education and Employment, 1999) and similar local initiatives. Standards for catering for primary schools have been published (Department for

Table 12.24 Recommendations for school meals[a]

Nursery schools/units
Foods from the following food groups should be available as part of the lunch:
1. Starchy foods
2. Fruit and vegetables
3. Milk/dairy foods
4. Meat/fish or non-dairy sources of protein

Primary schools
Foods from above food groups should be available each day
Oil-cooked starchy foods (e.g. chips) should not be available more than three times a week
Red meat should be offered at least twice a week and fish once a week
Fresh fruit, fruit canned in juice or fruit salad should be offered at least twice a week

Secondary schools
A choice of two foods from the above food groups should be offered each day
At least one of the starchy foods should not be fried or cooked in oil
Red meat should be available at least three days a week and fish at least twice a week
Both a fruit and a vegetable should be offered each day

---

[a]Department for Education and Employment (2000a–c).

Education and Employment, 2000b) and are summarized in Table 12.24.

Practical measures

The daily meal pattern should remain as three meals and two to three snacks (or milk drinks). Semi-skimmed should be encouraged for this age group or skimmed milk is suitable from the age of 5 years. Approximately 350–500 ml milk daily will meet the calcium requirements of this age group.

Snacks should be based on starchy foods and fruit rather than those that are high in sugar, fat and salt (Figure 9.9).

Activity – walking, swimming, cycling and games – should be encouraged. Children should undertake activity of moderate intensity (sufficient to make participant slightly breathless) for at least 1 h each day. At least twice a week activities should be those that promote bone health and maintain muscular strength (e.g. running, brisk walking, gym training).

Adolescents

Rationale for nutrition policy

Adolescents tend to move away from traditional influences such as parents and school and are far more influenced by peer pressure and media. Health messages from statutory bodies and school are perceived as less relevant to adolescent lifestyle. Messages should be holistic, not just aimed at food and nutrient intake. Information on drugs, smoking and safe sex need to be given as a package about healthy behaviour. Schools that adopt an integrated approach to promoting healthy eating through the curriculum (teaching, catering, vending machines, physical activity) are more likely to be successful than those who teach health subjects in isolation. School meals standards exist for pupils in secondary schools (Department for Education and Employment, 2000c) and see Table 12.24.

The National Diet and Nutrition Survey of children aged 4–18 years (Gregory *et al.*, 2000) showed that intakes and blood levels of certain nutrients were low in the older age goups (11–18 years), particularly in girls. The major nutrients of concern were riboflavin, vitamin D, iron (9 per cent of girls aged 11–14 had haemoglobin levels $<110\,g/l$), zinc and calcium. The demands of puberty and the associated growth spurt make the requirements high for iron and calcium. Puberty is an important time for the deposition of calcium in bone and 60 per cent of adult peak bone mass is accrued at this time. Adolescents have a high intake of saturated fats, salt and sugar associated with snacking and fast foods and a low consumption of fruit and vegetables. Ten per cent of girls aged 15–18 reported that they ate a vegetarian diet and 16 per cent of girls of this age were 'dieting' to lose weight. Both obesity and eating disorders may develop in adolescence, and it is important that health-care professionals are aware of changes in body size and can offer appropriate advice in a sensitive way.

Practical measures

Dietary patterns and recommendations on exercise are similar to those described above for school-age children. Table 11.13 provides an outline of the principles for good nutrition in childhood and adolescence and this complements the advice given here.

The consumption of about 500 ml (or two large portions) of low-fat milks and cheeses should be encouraged. Low-fat milk, yoghurt and cheese should be available as snacks and at mealtimes at school. Iron-rich foods should be consumed at the three main meals of the day (see section on iron). Iron-fortified breakfast cereals can make a significant contribution to iron intake in this age group.

Encourage the consumption of cereal (preferably wholegrain) and fruit and vegetables in place of snacks that are high in fat, sugar and salt. Parents and health-care workers should exert pressure on schools to ensure that vending machines and school shops sell a variety of 'healthy' snacks and not just soft drinks and confectionery. Advice should be made available on alternatives for snack foods which are lower in fat (see Table 12.25).

Emphasis should be placed on the desirability of fitness and health rather than on slimness. Adolescent boys and girls benefit from learning to cook simple healthy meals and snacks. This should be included as part of the curriculum, but could also be taught in the context of an after-school optional activity.

Obesity

Rationale for nutrition policy

The growing trend of childhood obesity is discussed in Chapter 11 along with suggestions for management and prevention. Recommendations for treatment of childhood obesity have been published (Barlow and Dietz, 1998) and could form the basis for a nutrition policy for prevention and management of childhood obesity in a population. There is some controversy over the most appropriate age to begin counselling for weight management, and health-care staff have been reluctant to offer advice because there is a belief that plump babies or young children will 'grow out of it'. The childhood risk factors for developing obesity have been analysed (Parsons *et al.*, 1999) and high-risk families with a large baby who is growing rapidly should be counselled during the first year of life. Growth charts which show the 95th centile for weight velocity will be available by 2003 (Child Growth Foundation) and this will give staff the opportunity for early intervention. Advice for young children should focus on avoiding very energy-dense foods, not interpreting crying or

Table 12.25   Alternatives to high energy foods

Foods with high energy density	Alternative (not necessarily low in energy, but an alternative to higher-energy foods)
Butter, margarine	Low-fat spreads
Whole milk and products made from it	Low-fat (skimmed) milk and low-fat desserts (e.g. yoghurt)
Ice cream	Sorbet, ice lollies
Fats, oils and fried foods	Grilled or baked foods 'fried' using low-fat oil spray
Chips	Oven chips
Crisps	Low-fat crisps
	Popcorn
	Twiglets
	Extruded starch products (e.g 'Monster Munch')
Cakes and biscuits	Rice cakes with jam (no butter)
	Crispbread with yeast extract
	Cereal bars
	Fruit
	Breakfast cereal and skimmed milk
	Wholemeal sandwiches with low-fat spread and banana, Marmite etc.
Chocolate	'Low-calorie' chocolate bars
	Fruit gums and hard fruit confectionery
	Chewing gum
Soft drinks	Mineral water
	Low-calorie squash and fizzy drinks

fussiness as hunger and increasing activity rather than on traditional weight management advice. For toddlers and older children the emphasis should be on healthy eating and an active healthy lifestyle rather than on weight reduction or dieting.

Practical measures

Assess current food intake (a detailed calculation of energy intake is not helpful). Advice for weight control should be based on about two-thirds of current intake. Very-low-calorie diets – below 600 kcal are not suitable for children or adolescents; they provide an inappropriate balance of nutrients and may compromise longitudinal growth. Commercially available meal replacements in the form of bars or drinks may be useful for older children, provided they form part of an otherwise balanced diet and are not used for more than one meal per day.

Ensure that balance of foods from four main food groups are included – five portions of cereal (preferably wholemeal), five portions of fruit and vegetables, two portions of low fat milk and one to two portions of meat or meat alternatives. Skimmed milk can be used in place of whole or semi-skimmed milk from the age of 2 years if obesity is a problem. If skimmed milk is used for children under 5 a supplement of vitamins A and D should always be given.

If the energy intake is judged to be less than 1000 kcal/day, or if the meal pattern omits some major nutrient-rich foods, a micronutrient supplement should be considered. The eating pattern should be based on three meals per day and meals should not be omitted. Low-calorie snacks or drinks in between meals may also be included. Food consumption should be restricted to designated meal and snack times rather than constant 'grazing' throughout the day. Alternatives to high energy-density foods should be suggested (see Table 2.25).

The importance of activity must be emphasized. Pre-school-aged children need to be able to run and play games every day. Avoid using a baby buggy or push chair and encourage toddlers to walk. For older children see guidelines for physical activity in section on school children. Pursuits that encourage low activity and snack consumption – particularly television viewing and personal computer use – should be restricted; encourage activities that will reduce time watching television as this is often a prompt for snacking.

The aim should be to maintain weight in all but the most obese children, or a maximum loss of 500 g/month. As children increase in height the BMI decreases if body weight remains static. Children should not be weighed more than once per week – less often may be preferable. Older children may benefit from attending an adult slimming club, provided that the regimen suggested is suitable for a child.

Advice on healthy eating and lifestyle, including increased activity, should be directed towards the whole family and all members need to change their eating habits and behaviour. Undesirable foods (crisps, chocolate etc.) should not be kept in the house and all members of the family should agree not to consume these when the child is present. Convenience foods that require minimal preparation and cooking in the home tend to be high in fat and therefore energy-dense. Families of obese children need to consider using more basic ingredients and home-based cooking. Eating as a family group rather than individually encourages restraint in eating and emphasizes the social aspects of eating.

Conclusion

A coherent nutrition policy, as part of a more general health policy, is essential if meaningful health education messages are to be presented to populations in a practical and understandable way. All areas of developmental nutrition, including maternal health prior to conception, during pregnancy and lactation, infancy, childhood and adolescence are important. Nutrition during fetal life, infancy and childhood affects the subsequent health and well-being of the child and is likely to affect lifelong health and disease susceptibility. Eating habits and lifestyle factors learned in childhood are likely to persist into adult life. Both policy-makers and practitioners in health-care need to use the opportunities offered at (for example) prenatal and pregnancy counselling, consultation with individual carers, parent groups, nurseries, schools and youth groups to provide information and advice to parents, other carers and children themselves.

References

Aggett PJ, Haschke F, Heine W, Hernell O, Koletzko B, Lafeber H, Ormission A, Rey J and Tormo R (1994) Committee report: childhood diet and prevention of coronary heart disease. ESPGAN Committee on Nutrition. European Society of Pediatric Gastroenterology and Nutrition. *J. Pediatr. Gastroenterol. Nutr.* **19**, 261–269.

Ahmed T and Fuchs GJ (1997) Gastrointestinal allergy to food: a review. *J. Diarrh. Dis. Res.* **15**, 211–223.

American Academy of Pediatrics (1995) National Cholesterol Education Program: Report of the Expert Panel on Blood Cholesterol Levels in Children and Adolescents 1992. *Pediatrics* **89**, 525–584.

American Academy of Pediatrics (1996) Practice parameter: the management of acute gastroenteritis in young children. Provisional Committee on Quality Improvement, Subcommittee on Acute Gastroenteritis. *Pediatrics* **97**, 424–435.

Armon K, Stephenson T, MacFaul R, Eccleston P and Werneke U (2001) An evidence and consensus based guideline for acute diarrhoea management. *Arch. Dis. Child.* **85**, 132–142.

Barlow SE and Dietz WH (1998) Obesity evaluation and treatment: Expert Committee recommendations. The Maternal and Child Health Bureau, Health Resources and Services Administration and the Department of Health and Human Services. *Pediatrics* **102**, E29.

Batchelor J (1999) *Failure to Thrive in Young Children: Research and Practice Evaluated.* The Children's Society, London.

Biddle P (1998) *Young and Active? Young People and Health-enhancing Physical Activity: Evidence and Implications.* Health Education Authority, London.

British Nutrition Foundation (2002) *Adverse Reactions to Food.* Blackwell Science, London.

Cole TJ (1995) Conditional reference charts to assess weight gain in British infants. *Arch. Dis. Child.* **73**, 8–16.

Committee on Toxicity of Chemicals in Food, Consumer Products and the Environment (1997) *Peanut Allergy.* HMSO, London.

Committee on Toxicity of Chemicals in Food, Consumer Products and the Environment (2000) *Adverse Reactions to Food and Food Ingredients.* Food Standards Agency, London.

Department for Education and Employment (1999) *National Healthy School Standards Guidance.* Department of Education and Employment Publications, Nottingham.

Department for Education and Employment (2000a) *Healthy School Lunches for Pupils in Nursery Schools/Units.* Department of Education and Employment Publications, Nottingham.

Department for Education and Employment (2000b) *Healthy School Lunches for Pupils in Primary Schools.* Department of Education and Employment Publications, Nottingham.

Department for Education and Employment (2000c) *Healthy School Lunches for Students in Secondary Schools.* Department of Education and Employment Publications, Nottingham.

Department of Health (1988) *Present Day Practice in Infant Feeding: Third Report.* Report on Health and Social Subjects no. 32. HMSO, London.

Department of Health (1991) *Dietary Reference Values for Food Energy and Nutrients for the United Kingdom.* Report on Health and Social Subjects no. 41. HMSO, London.

Department of Health (1994a) *Weaning and the Weaning Diet.* Report on Health and Social Subjects no. 45. HMSO, London.

Department of Health (1994b) *Nutritional Aspects of Cardiovascular Disease.* Report on Health and Social Subjects no. 46. HMSO, London.

Department of Health (1995) *Sensible Drinking.* The report of an inter-departmental working group. Department of Health, London.

Department of Health (1996) *While you are Pregnant: Safe Eating and How to Avoid Infection from Food and Animals.* Department of Health, London.

Department of Health (2000) *Folic Acid and the Prevention of Disease.* Report on Health and Social Subjects no. 50. The Stationery Office, London.

Drewett RF, Corbett SS and Wright CM (1999) Cognitive and educational attainments at school age of children who failed to thrive in infancy: a population-based study. *J. Child Psychol. Psychiat.* **40**, 551–561.

Feig DS and Naylor CD (1998) Eating for two: are guidelines for weight gain during pregnancy too liberal? *Lancet* **351**, 1054–1055.

Foster K, Lader D and Cheesbrough S (1997) *Infant Feeding 1995.* HMSO, London.

Fowler MG, Simonds RJ and Roongpisuthipong A (2000) Update on perinatal HIV transmission. *Pediatr. Clin. N. Am.* **47**, 21–38.

Gregory JR, Collins DL, Davies PSW, Hughes JM and Clarke PC (1995) *National Diet and Nutrition Survey: Children Aged $1\frac{1}{2}$ to $4\frac{1}{2}$ years; Vol. 1: Report of the Diet and Nutrition Survey.* HMSO, London.

Gregory J, Lowe S, Bates CJ, Prentice A, Jackson LV, Smithers G, Wenlcok R and Farron M (2000) *National Diet and Nutrition Survey: Young People Aged 4 to 18 years; Vol. 1: Report of the Diet and Nutrition Survey.* The Stationery Office, London.

Grossman J and Webb K (1991) Local food and nutrition policy. *Aust. J. Public Health* **15**, 271–276.

Hall DMB (2000) Growth monitoring. *Arch. Dis. Child.* **82**, 10–15.

Helsing E (1997) The history of nutrition policy. *Nutr. Rev.* **55**, S1–S3.

Jaegar MC, Lawson MS and Filteau S (1997) The impact of prematurity and neonatal illness on the decision to breastfeed. *J. Adv. Nurs.* **25**, 729–737.

James J, Evans J, Male P, Pallister C, Hendrikz JK and Oakhill A (1988) Iron deficiency in inner city pre-school children: development of a general practice screening programme. *J. R. Coll. Gen. Pract.* **38**, 250–252.

James WP, Ralph A and Bellizzi M (1997) Nutrition policies in western Europe: national policies in Belgium, The Netherlands, France, Ireland, and the United Kingdom. *Nutr. Rev.* **55**, S4–20.

Kennedy E and Cooney E (2001) Development of the child nutrition programs in the United States. *J. Nutr.* **131**, 431S–436S.

Lawson MS and Thomas M (1999) Low vitamin D status of Asian two year olds living in England. *Br. Med. J.* **1**, 218.

Lawson MS, Thomas M and Hardiman A (1998) Iron status of Asian children aged 2 years living in England. *Arch. Dis. Child.* **78**, 420–426.

Lucas A, Fewtrell MS and Cole TJ (1999) Fetal origins of adult disease – the hypothesis revisited. *Br. Med. J.* **319**, 245.

Lucassen PL and Assendelft WJ (2001) Systematic review of treatments for infant colic. *Pediatrics* **108**, 1047–1048.

Parsons TJ, Power C, Logan S and Summerbell CD (1999) Childhood predictors of adult obesity: a systematic review. *Int. J. Obes. Relat. Metab. Disord.* **23**, S1–S107.

Shaw V and Lawson M (eds) (2001) *Clinical Paediatric Dietetics*. Blackwell, Oxford.

Stordy BJ, Redfern AM and Morgan JB (1995) Healthy eating for infants – mothers' actions. *Acta Paediatr.* **84**, 753–741.

Tham EB, Nathan R, Davidson GP and Moore DJ (1996) Bowel habits of healthy Australian children aged 0–2 years. *J. Paediatr. Child Health* **32**, 504–507.

Thomas M and Avery V (1977) *Infant Feeding in Asian Families*. Office for National Statistics. HMSO, London.

Underdown A and Birks E (1999) *Faltering Growth – Taking the Failure out of Failure to Thrive*. The Children's Society, London.

Vandenplas Y, Belli D, Benhamou P, Cadranel S, Cezard JP, Cucchiara S, Dupont C, Faure C, Gottrand F, Hassall E, Heymans H, Kneepkens CM and Sandhu B (1997) A critical appraisal of current management practices for infant regurgitation – recommendations of a working party. *Eur. J. Pediatr.* **156**, 343–357.

WHO (1989) *Protecting, Promoting and Supporting Breastfeeding: the Special Role of Maternity Services – a Joint WHO/UNICEF Statement*. WHO, Geneva.

WHO (1990) *A Manual for the Treatment of Diarrhoea*. Programme for the control of diarrhoeal diseases. WHO/CDD, Geneva.

Wright CM (2000) Identification and management of failure to thrive: a community perspective. *Arch. Dis. Child.* **85**, 132–142.

Wright C, Avery A, Epstein M, Birks E and Croft D (1998) New chart to evaluate weight faltering. *Arch. Dis. Child.* **78**, 40–43.

Yip R, Binkin NJ, Fleshood, L and Trowbridge FL (1987) Declining prevalence of anemia among low-income children in the United States. *JAMA* **258**, 1619–1623.

Zeiger RS (2000) Dietary aspects of food allergy prevention in infants and children. *J. Pediatr. Gastroenterol. Nutr.* **30**(Suppl.), S77–S86.

Zetterstrom R (1999) Breastfeeding and infant-mother interaction. *Acta Paediatr.* **88**(Suppl.), 1–6.

INDEX

Page numbers in bold refer to figures, while page numbers in italic signify tables